Carbohydrates 2018

Carbohydrates 2018

Special Issue Editors

Amélia Pilar Rauter
Nuno Manuel Xavier

MDPI • Basel • Beijing • Wuhan • Barcelona • Belgrade • Manchester • Tokyo • Cluj • Tianjin

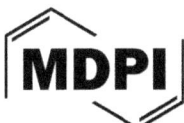

Special Issue Editors
Amélia Pilar Rauter
Universidade de Lisboa
Portugal

Nuno Manuel Xavier
Universidade de Lisboa
Portugal

Editorial Office
MDPI
St. Alban-Anlage 66
4052 Basel, Switzerland

This is a reprint of articles from the Special Issue published online in the open access journal *Pharmaceuticals* (ISSN 1424-8247) (available at: https://www.mdpi.com/journal/pharmaceuticals/special_issues/carbohydrates2018).

For citation purposes, cite each article independently as indicated on the article page online and as indicated below:

LastName, A.A.; LastName, B.B.; LastName, C.C. Article Title. *Journal Name* **Year**, *Article Number*, Page Range.

ISBN 978-3-03928-316-3 (Pbk)
ISBN 978-3-03928-317-0 (PDF)

© 2020 by the authors. Articles in this book are Open Access and distributed under the Creative Commons Attribution (CC BY) license, which allows users to download, copy and build upon published articles, as long as the author and publisher are properly credited, which ensures maximum dissemination and a wider impact of our publications.

The book as a whole is distributed by MDPI under the terms and conditions of the Creative Commons license CC BY-NC-ND.

Contents

About the Special Issue Editors vii

Amélia Pilar Rauter and Nuno Manuel Xavier
Special Issue "Carbohydrates 2018"
Reprinted from: *Pharmaceuticals* **2020**, *13*, 5, doi:10.3390/ph13010005 1

Luís O. B. Zamoner, Valquiria Aragão-Leoneti and Ivone Carvalho
Iminosugars: Effects of Stereochemistry, Ring Size, and *N*-Substituents on Glucosidase Activities
Reprinted from: *Pharmaceuticals* **2019**, *12*, 108, doi:10.3390/ph12030108 3

Nuno M. Xavier, Eduardo C. de Sousa, Margarida P. Pereira, Anne Loesche, Immo Serbian, René Csuk and M. Conceição Oliveira
Synthesis and Biological Evaluation of Structurally Varied 5′-/6′-Isonucleosides and Theobromine-Containing *N*-Isonucleosidyl Derivatives
Reprinted from: *Pharmaceuticals* **2019**, *12*, 103, doi:10.3390/ph12030103 17

Ana M. de Matos, Alice Martins, Teresa Man, David Evans, Magnus Walter, Maria Conceição Oliveira, Óscar López, José G. Fernandez-Bolaños, Philipp Dätwyler, Beat Ernst, M. Paula Macedo, Marialessandra Contino, Nicola A. Colabufo and Amélia P. Rauter
Design and Synthesis of CNS-targeted Flavones and Analogues with Neuroprotective Potential Against H_2O_2- and $A\beta_{1-42}$-Induced Toxicity in SH-SY5Y Human Neuroblastoma Cells
Reprinted from: *Pharmaceuticals* **2019**, *12*, 98, doi:10.3390/ph12020098 39

Juan C. Estévez, Marcos A. González, M. Carmen Villaverde, Yuki Hirokami, Atsushi Kato, Fredy Sussman, David Reza and Ramón J. Estévez
Chain-Branched Polyhydroxylated Octahydro-*1H*-Indoles as Potential Leads against Lysosomal Storage Diseases
Reprinted from: *Pharmaceuticals* **2019**, *12*, 47, doi:10.3390/ph12020047 57

Katherine McReynolds, Dustin Dimas, Grace Floyd and Kara Zeman
Development of a Microwave-assisted Chemoselective Synthesis of Oxime-linked Sugar Linkers and Trivalent Glycoclusters
Reprinted from: *Pharmaceuticals* **2019**, *12*, 39, doi:10.3390/ph12010039 71

Patrícia Batista, Pedro Castro, Ana Raquel Madureira, Bruno Sarmento and Manuela Pintado
Development and Characterization of Chitosan Microparticles-in-Films for Buccal Delivery of Bioactive Peptides
Reprinted from: *Pharmaceuticals* **2019**, *12*, 32, doi:10.3390/ph12010032 85

Michelle M. Kuttel and Neil Ravenscroft
Conformation and Cross-Protection in Group B Streptococcus Serotype III and *Streptococcus pneumoniae* Serotype 14: A Molecular Modeling Study
Reprinted from: *Pharmaceuticals* **2019**, *12*, 28, doi:10.3390/ph12010028 101

Farzana Hossain and Peter R. Andreana
Developments in Carbohydrate-Based Cancer Therapeutics
Reprinted from: *Pharmaceuticals* **2019**, *12*, 84, doi:10.3390/ph12020084 119

Rachel Hevey
Strategies for the Development of Glycomimetic Drug Candidates
Reprinted from: *Pharmaceuticals* **2019**, *12*, 55, doi:10.3390/ph12020055 137

About the Special Issue Editors

Amélia Pilar Rauter is Full Professor of Organic Chemistry and the President of the Department of Chemistry and Biochemistry of Faculdade de Ciências, Universidade de Lisboa (Ciências ULisboa), and the Coordinator of the Carbohydrate Chemistry Group (Group 11) of the Centro de Química Estrutural (CQE). She is the President of the International Carbohydrate Organisation and the Secretary of the European Carbohydrate Organisation, and serves IUPAC as Vice-President of the IUPAC Division of Organic and Biomolecular Chemistry, as Titular Member of IUPAC Division of Chemical Nomenclature and Structure Representation and as Associate Member of its Interdivisional Committee on Terminology, Nomenclature and Symbols. She is the founder of the Portuguese Chemical Society Carbohydrate Group. Her research covers the development of new carbohydrate-based molecular entities for the treatment/prevention of metabolic (diabetes), degenerative diseases (Alzheimer's and Prion diseases, cancer), and infection, either inspired in nature or accessed through rational design and synthesis. She is Editor of the Royal Society of Chemistry Carbohydrate Chemistry book series, Associated Editor of the Mediterranean Journal of Chemistry, and member of journals advisory/editorial boards in Medicinal/Organic/Carbohydrate Chemistry, namely the European Journal of Organic Chemistry (Wiley), Medicinal Chemistry (Bentham Science), Pharmaceuticals (MDPI), Journal of Carbohydrate Chemistry (Taylor & Francis), among others. She has published more than 150 papers and book chapters, authored 8 granted patents and has been invited as speaker of national and international meetings e.g., Gordon Conference, ECO and ICS meetings. Among her honors, she was awarded with the Mention of Excellency by Faculdade de Ciências, Universidade de Lisboa since 2007, she is Fellow of the Royal Society of Chemistry and received the Madinaveitia-Lourenço Prize given by the Spanish Royal Chemical Society in 2017.

Nuno Manuel Xavier (Dr.) is a Researcher at Centro de Química Estrutural (CQE), Faculdade de Ciências, Universidade de Lisboa (Ciências Ulisboa). He received a double PhD degree in Chemistry (Organic Chemistry) from the University of Lisbon and from the National Institute of Applied Sciences of Lyon in 2011. He was then a Postdoctoral Research Fellow at the University of Natural Resources and Life Sciences of Vienna and afterwards a post-Doc at Prof. Rauter Carbohydrate Chemistry Group at Ciências ULisboa. In 2014 he was awarded an Investigator Starting Grant at Ciências ULisboa and recently he has been selected as Assistant Researcher at CQE, both of which under highly competitive calls from the Portuguese Foundation for Science and Technology (FCT). His research has been devoted to the development of efficient synthetic methodologies for novel bioactive carbohydrate-based molecules, for which he has been internationally recognized with various Young Scientist Awards (e.g., IUPAC, Alberta Ingenuity Centre for Carbohydrate Science - Canada, Groupe Lyonnais des Glyco-Sciences - France) and an Innovation Award at the International Carbohydrate Symposium 2018. He has been particularly focused on medicinal chemistry of nucleos(t)ides towards new therapeutic lead compounds. He was the PI of an FCT-funded R&D exploratory project and Team Member of 8 projects funded by national or international entities. His research activities have been reported in ca. 40 publications and he has been Speaker of more than 30 lectures in international and national Symposia.

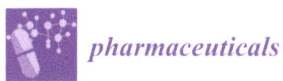

Editorial

Special Issue "Carbohydrates 2018"

Amélia Pilar Rauter [1,2,*] and Nuno Manuel Xavier [1,2]

1. Centro de Química e Bioquímica, Faculdade de Ciências, Universidade de Lisboa, Ed. C8, 5° Piso, Campo Grande, 1749-016 Lisboa, Portugal; nmxavier@fc.ul.pt
2. Centro de Química Estrutural, Faculdade de Ciências, Universidade de Lisboa, Ed. C8, 5° Piso, Campo Grande, 1749-016 Lisboa, Portugal
* Correspondence: aprauter@fc.ul.pt

Received: 20 December 2019; Accepted: 20 December 2019; Published: 29 December 2019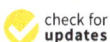

This special issue of Pharmaceuticals has been dedicated to Carbohydrates on the occasion of the 29th International Carbohydrate Symposium, held at the Universidade de Lisboa from 15–19 July 2018. Recent findings and trends in carbohydrate science are presented and discussed in its nine articles. They are demonstrative of the relevance of carbohydrate research in medicinal chemistry and pharmaceutical sciences, and of the exciting opportunities that carbohydrate-based structures offer for the discovery of new solutions for therapy and diagnosis.

Carbohydrates are natural, multifunctional, and stereochemically rich molecules, playing important roles in biological processes relevant for health and disease. Embodying such structural features, these unique molecular entities can be transformed in a diversity of compounds applied as drugs, food supplements, as biologically active materials, in cosmetics, just to name a few of the wide uses of carbohydrates and their mimetics. Research in carbohydrates also covers a diversity of domains as highlighted in this special issue, containing contributions of experts in fields such as glycochemistry, molecular biology, computational chemistry, and materials science, that address the roles of carbohydrates to understand biological processes and to develop new approaches for disease diagnosis and treatment.

Kuttel and Ravenscroft describe a molecular modeling study with the capsular polysaccharides of *Streptococcus agalactiae* serotype III and *Streptococcus pneumoniae* serotype 14, leading to a conformational rationale for the antigenic epitopes identified for these polysaccharides. Based on their discovery they suggest a strategy for bacterial evasion of the host immune system by infection with these bacteria.

Chitosan-based films loaded with chitosan microparticles, that contain a bioactive peptide with antihypertensive properties, have been developed by Pintado and coworkers, consisting of an innovative approach to increase peptide efficiency and bioavailability.

McReynolds and coworkers established a new microwave-assisted oxime-based chemoselective methodology to prepare trivalent glycoclusters. The reaction is completed in 30 min, with the additional advantage of using unprotected sugars, and may be a step forward for the synthesis of more complex glycoconjugates and glycoclusters, multivalent molecules relevant for a number of biomedical uses.

Iminosugars are among the most relevant groups of glycomimetics for therapeutic applications. Among their variety of biological properties, their ability to mimic the transition state species in glycosidase catalysis and thus their propensity to inhibit these enzymes, which play a role in a variety of diseases, has led to some compounds which are used in clinics for the treatment of diabetes or Gaucher's disease.

Two original articles in this special issue are devoted to the synthesis of new iminosugar derivatives and the evaluation of their glycosidase inhibitory properties.

Carvalho and coworkers investigated a small library of synthesized iminosugars differing in stereochemistry, ring size, and N-substitution and found two potent β-glucosidase inhibitors bearing

D-*gluco* and L-*ido* configurations with six-membered and seven-membered ring iminosugars, in which the endocyclic amino group was derivatized with the hydroxyethyl group.

The contribution of Ramón Estevez and coworkers is based on the development of new synthetic routes to polyhydroxyoctahydroindoles, iminosugars with potential as pharmacological chaperones for lysosomal storage disorders, caused by mutations in the lysosomal β-galactosidase, and frequently related to misfolding. Resulting from abnormal metabolism of glycosphingolipids, glycogen, mucopolysaccharides or glycoproteins, they may generate neurodegenerative disorders, amongst others. The developed small molecules may act as ligands of the mutant enzyme, promoting the correct folding and preventing its degradation at the endoplasmic reticulum, a novel approach for disease treatment.

Alzheimer's disease (AD) is also a neurodegenerative disorder, and drugs able to prevent disease progression are not yet available. Rauter and coworkers disclose the structure of C-glycosyl flavones as neuroprotective agents able to fully rescue human neuroblastoma cells from both H_2O_2 and Aβ1-42-induced cell death, a step forward to lead structures for further development against AD.

Another approach to treat AD patients is based on the cholinergic approach. Xavier and coworkers describe elegant syntheses of new purine and uracil isonucleosides embodying xylosyl or glucosyl groups, and the discovery of a potent and selective acetylcholinesterase inhibitor bearing a theobromine ring and an octyl chain linked to the glucosyl group.

Cell-surface glycans are recognized as therapeutic targets, as their composition changes in many diseases (e.g., in cancer). The review, authored by Rachel Hevey, covers approaches to develop glycomimetics that improve binding affinities and pharmacokinetic properties towards more drug-like compounds addressing therapies for carbohydrate-binding targets.

Hossain and Andreana revised the progress made in synthetic carbohydrate-based antitumor vaccines that improve immune responses by targeting specific antigens, in a beautiful work that also covers other developments in carbohydrate-based cancer treatments, including glycoconjugate prodrugs, glycosidase inhibitors, and early diagnosis.

We hope the readers enjoy this Special Issue and get inspired to unveil the secrets of life with carbohydrate sciences!

Author Contributions: Amélia Pilar Rauter and Nuno Manuel Xavier contributed equally to this Editorial. All authors have read and agreed to the published version of the manuscript.

Funding: The authors are gratefully acknowledged to Fundação para a Ciência e a Tecnologia for the support of the strategic project UID/MULTI/00612/2019 of Centro de Química e Bioquímica.

Conflicts of Interest: The authors declare no conflicts of interest.

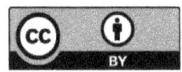

© 2019 by the authors. Licensee MDPI, Basel, Switzerland. This article is an open access article distributed under the terms and conditions of the Creative Commons Attribution (CC BY) license (http://creativecommons.org/licenses/by/4.0/).

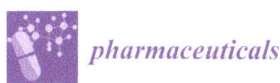

Article

Iminosugars: Effects of Stereochemistry, Ring Size, and *N*-Substituents on Glucosidase Activities

Luís O. B. Zamoner, Valquiria Aragão-Leoneti and Ivone Carvalho *

School of Pharmaceutical Sciences of Ribeirão Preto, University of São Paulo, Av. do Café s/n, Monte Alegre, CEP14040-903 Ribeirão Preto, Brazil
* Correspondence: carronal@usp.br; Tel.: +55-16-33154709

Received: 15 June 2019; Accepted: 10 July 2019; Published: 12 July 2019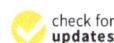

Abstract: *N*-substituted iminosugar analogues are potent inhibitors of glucosidases and glycosyltransferases with broad therapeutic applications, such as treatment of diabetes and Gaucher disease, immunosuppressive activities, and antibacterial and antiviral effects against HIV, HPV, hepatitis C, bovine diarrhea (BVDV), Ebola (EBOV) and Marburg viruses (MARV), influenza, Zika, and dengue virus. Based on our previous work on functionalized isomeric 1,5-dideoxy-1,5-imino-D-gulitol (L-*gulo*-piperidines, with inverted configuration at C-2 and C-5 in respect to glucose or deoxynojirimycin (DNJ)) and 1,6-dideoxy-1,6-imino-D-mannitol (D-*manno*-azepane derivatives) cores *N*-linked to different sites of glucopyranose units, we continue our studies on these alternative iminosugars bearing simple *N*-alkyl chains instead of glucose to understand if these easily accessed scaffolds could preserve the inhibition profile of the corresponding glucose-based *N*-alkyl derivatives as DNJ cores found in miglustat and miglitol drugs. Thus, a small library of iminosugars (14 compounds) displaying different stereochemistry, ring size, and *N*-substitutions was successfully synthesized from a common precursor, D-mannitol, by utilizing an S_N2 aminocyclization reaction via two isomeric bis-epoxides. The evaluation of the prospective inhibitors on glucosidases revealed that merely D-*gluco*-piperidine (miglitol, **41a**) and L-*ido*-azepane (**41b**) DNJ-derivatives bearing the *N*-hydroxylethyl group showed inhibition towards α-glucosidase with IC_{50} 41 μM and 138 μM, respectively, using DNJ as reference (IC_{50} 134 μM). On the other hand, β-glucosidase inhibition was achieved for glucose-inverted configuration (C-2 and C-5) derivatives, as novel L-*gulo*-piperidine (**27a**) and D-*manno*-azepane (**27b**), preserving the *N*-butyl chain, with IC_{50} 109 and 184 μM, respectively, comparable to miglustat with the same *N*-butyl substituent (**40a**, IC_{50} 172 μM). Interestingly, the seven-membered ring L-*ido*-azepane (**40b**) displayed near twice the activity (IC_{50} 80 μM) of the corresponding D-*gluco*-piperidine miglustat drug (**40a**). Furthermore, besides α-glucosidase inhibition, both miglitol (**41a**) and L-*ido*-azepane (**41b**) proved to be the strongest β-glucosidase inhibitors of the series with IC_{50} of 4 μM.

Keywords: iminosugars; polyhydroxypiperidines; polyhydroxyazepanes; glucosidase inhibition; miglustat; miglitol

---

1. Introduction

The major groups of glucosidase inhibitors that have been discovered are polyhydroxylated alkaloids containing piperidines, pyrrolidines, nor-tropanes, pyrrolizidines, and indolizidines as mono and bicyclic systems [1]. A great variety of these compounds, named iminosugars, have been isolated from natural sources, such as plants (*Morus alba*, *Commelina communis*), bacteria (*Bacillus*, *Streptomyces*), and fungi (*Zygosaccharomyces rouxii* for mulberry leaf fermentation) [2], and produced by synthetic strategies with potential inhibition properties not only over α- and β-glucosidases but also glycosyltransferases, glycogen phosphorylase [3–5], nucleoside phosphorylases [6], and sugar-nucleotide mutases (UDP-Galp mutase) [7]. High activity and specificity of iminosugars are associated with the ability of the nitrogen ring to mimic the transition state of pyranosidic or furanosidic units of natural glucosidase substrates that positively influence their shape and charge for enzyme binding.

Access to iminosugar analogues with N-substituted side chains has led to a variety of potent glucosidase and glycosyltransferases inhibitors with broad therapeutic applications, such as treatment of diabetes [8] and Gaucher disease [9], and even immunosuppressive activities [10] and antibacterial [11] and antiviral effects [12,13] against HIV [14], HPV [15], hepatitis C [16], bovine diarrhea (BVDV) [17], Ebola (EBOV) [18] and Marburg viruses (MARV) [19], influenza [20], Zika [21], and dengue virus [22,23]. Despite the α- and β-glucosidase inhibition promoted by nojirimycin itself (**1**), it was achieved a better profile for the corresponding 1-deoxynojirimycin (DNJ, **2**) due to better stability and potency. Furthermore, a combination of these structural features can promote the cellular uptake of N-alkylated DNJ analogues, as shown by those containing long and linear alkyl chains, which displayed better activity in whole cells (human hepatoblastoma cells, HepG2) than purified pork glucosidase I [24]. Conversely, N-alkyl-less lipophilic N-alkyl groups, or even containing an oxygen atom, displayed lower cytotoxicity and significant activity against α-glucosidase, as described for N-methyl- (**3**) [25], N-butyl- (N-Bu-DNJ, miglustat, **4**) [26], N-hydroxyethyl- (N-EtOH-DNJ, miglitol, **5**), N-7-oxadecyl- (N-7-oxadecyl-DNJ, **6**) [27,28], and N-glycyl-deoxynojirimycin (**7**) [29]. In fact, miglustat is particularly useful in the control of type I Gaucher disease [9] and Niemann–Pick type C (NPC) lysosomal storage diseases, via "substrate reduction therapy", as well as miglitol in the treatment of non-insulin-dependent diabetes (type II) (Figure 1) to impair carbohydrate processing in the gut [30]. In addition, inhibition of the target human acid β-glucosidase (glucocerebrosidase, GCase) has been achieved by a set of derived iminosugars as new pharmacological chaperones for the treatment of Gaucher disease [31,32].

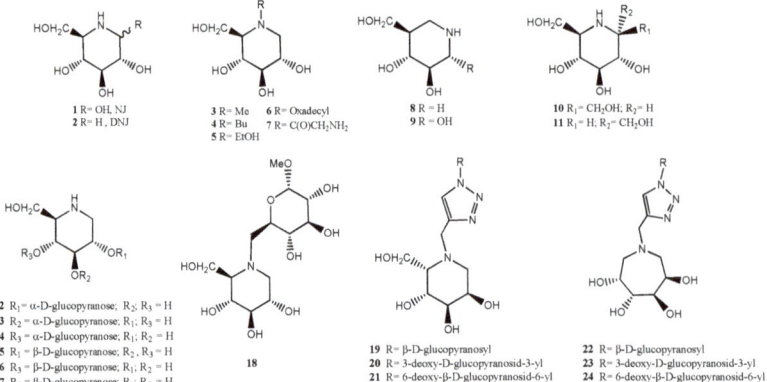

Figure 1. Examples of polyhydroxylated piperidine and azepane iminosugars reported, some of them displaying glucosidase inhibition.

Besides the N-alkyl variations, several studies have pointed to the impact of the modification of DNJ hydroxyl groups involving C-2 to C-6 positions, assessing the influence of both stereochemistry and substituent variations on glycosidase activities. In general, the loss of α-glucosidase (I and II) and ceramide glycosyltransferase activities was evident by modifying C-2, C-3, and C-4, with the exception of N-butyl-1-deoxy-galactonojirimycin (migalastat, used for the treatment of Fabry disease) [30]. On the other hand, changes at C-1 and the ring nitrogen were allowed, based on the high inhibition revealed by DNJ and 1-azasugars (isofagomine (**8**), for instance), the latter obtained by replacing the anomeric carbon and the ring oxygen of glucose by nitrogen and carbon, respectively, with significant activity only against β-glucosidase. Interestingly, introduction of a hydroxyl group at the carbon (C-2) neighboring the nitrogen afforded a potent α-glucosidase inhibitor (noeuromycin, **9**) that preserved the original β-glucosidase activity. Additionally, the extra hydroxymethylene group at the anomeric position of DNJ gave rise to α-homonojirimycin (**10**) and β-homonojirimycin (**11**) with the ability to inhibit α-glucosidase, which was even higher whilst bearing *N*-methyl or *N*-butyl substituents (Figure 1) [1]. Furthermore, seven-membered ring iminosugar have shown potential glucosidase inhibition [33–35]. Comprehensive studies on iminosugar derivatives can be found in literature reviews [36–39].

Inspired by a series of reported deoxynojirimycin disaccharides that were decorated with equal α- or β-glucopyranose units at C-2, C-3, and C-4 DNJ positions (**12-17**) [40,41], along with *N*-glycosylated deoxynojirimycin, MDL 73,945 (**18**) [42], we had reported an alternative approach, using functionalized isomeric 1,5-dideoxy-1,5-imino-D-gulitol (L-*gulo*-piperidines, with inverted configurations at C-2 and C-5 with respect to glucose or DNJ, **19-21**) and 1,6-dideoxy-1,6-imino-D-mannitol (D-*manno*-azepane derivatives, **22-24**) cores *N*-linked to different sites of glucopyranose units, such as C-1, C-3, and C-6 positions [43]. To reach this goal, we used a CuAAC reaction (copper azide alkyne cycloaddition reaction), as a click chemistry strategy, to connect six- and seven-membered iminosugars to glucose in different arrangements through triazole bridges to produce the most active α-glucosidase inhibitor (**21**) of the pseudo-disaccharide series, L-gulopiperidine attached to glucose C-6 position, with IC_{50} approximately three-fold lower than that of DNJ (Figure 1) [43].

Despite the reported loss of α-glucosidase activity under modification at the C-5 position of the iminosugar, such as displayed by 1-deoxy-L-*ido*-nojirimycin (with an inverted configuration at C-5 with respect to DNJ) [24] and for 1,5-dideoxy-1,5-iminoxylitol (lacking the C-5 hydroxymethyl group of DNJ) [27,28], we have been encouraged to continue our studies on L-*gulo*-piperidines based on the remarkable α-glucosidase inhibition previously obtained for pseudo-disaccharides with simultaneous inverted configurations at C-2 and C-5 positions in relation to glucose stereochemistry [43]. Thus, to understand the relative contribution of the ring size, stereochemistry, and *N*-alkyl substitution on glycosidase inhibition, we proceeded with the synthesis of a small library of *N*-substituted 1-deoxy-L-*gulo*-nojirimycin and D-*manno*-azepane derivatives and compared them with the corresponding classical *N*-substituted of 1-deoxy-D-*gluco*-piperidine (DNJ) and L-*ido*-azepane counterparts as glucose-type carbohydrate mimetics. To reach this goal, *N*-hydroxyethyl and *N*-butyl groups of miglitol and miglustat drugs, respectively, were investigated as highly important *N*-alkyl substitutions for glucosidase inhibition, besides *N*-phenethyl [44], and *N*-propynyl [43] as a less-active counterpart.

2. Results and Discussion

2.1. Chemistry

Initially, target 1-deoxy-L-*gulo*-nojirimycin (**26-29a**) and D-*manno*-azepane derivatives (**26-29b**) were synthesized by a regiospecific C_2-symmetric unprotected bis-epoxide opening strategy in the presence of primary amines, followed by an S_N2 aminocyclization reaction to give a mixture of both six- and seven-membered iminosugar isomers [45–47]. As previously reported, the synthesis of unprotected bis-epoxide **25** was promptly achieved from the simple and commercially available starting material, D-mannitol, in two steps, by tosylation of both D-mannitol primary alcohols (71%), followed by a base-promoted intramolecular S_N2 reaction to give 1,2:5,6-dianhydro-D-mannitol **25** (29%), Scheme 1A [43]. Opening of the homochiral C_2-symmetric bis-epoxide **25** by alkylamines (at the less-hindered position of one epoxy function) led to the formation of secondary amines, which promoted an S_N2 aminocyclization reaction to give a mixture of polyhydroxy-piperidine and -azepane by 6-exo-tet or 7-endo-tet processes, respectively. In this series, azepane was isolated in a slightly higher proportion than DNJ, indicating the free 3,4 diol in bis-epoxide **25** did not affect the regioselectivity. Conversely, higher yields of DNJ than azepane derivatives were previously reported using benzyl protecting groups at C-3 and C-4 of bis-epoxide in the presence of several amines (benzylamine, for instance) [46]. Interestingly, this ratio can be reversed in the presence of a

Lewis acid (perchloric acid), which catalyzes epoxide opening to mainly give azepane derivatives. Furthermore, the exclusive formation of seven-membered azasugars using a more rigid *trans*-acetonide protecting group, as observed in 1,2:5,6-dianhydro-3,4-O-isopropylidene-D-mannitol or L-iditol, led to the conclusion that formation of both polyhydroxy-piperidine and -azepane regioisomers can be achieved by an aminocyclization of a flexible bis-epoxide bearing a free or acyclic hydroxyl protecting groups at C-3 and C-4, and the ratio varies according to the experimental conditions [46].

Therefore, the microwave-assisted aminocyclization reaction of bis-epoxide 25 was carried out with four different primary amines (propargylamine, butylamine, ethanolamine, or phenethylamine), which resulted in a mixture of N-alkyl substituted polyhydroxypiperidine 26-29a and azepane 26b-29b regioisomers, being iminosugars 27a,b and 28a,b novel compounds. To prevent laborious separation of a and b regioisomers, some mixtures were treated with acetic anhydride and pyridine for prompt separation of the per-O-acetylated 1-deoxy-L-*gulo*-nojirimycin and D-*manno*-azepane by column chromatography, isolated in different ratio and yields over two steps, as depicted in Table 1. However, the separation of protected regioisomers 31a,b was more demanding and required HPLC purification, mainly because the deprotected products 28a,b were inseparable by chromatographic column or even HPLC under test conditions. Lastly, deprotection of the regioisomers in the presence of sodium methoxide gave products 26-29a and 26-29b in quantitative yields. Eventually, derivatives 27a,b and 29a,b bearing a more lipophilic side chain (butyl and phenethyl, respectively) were separated without the need of previous protection by using chromatography column eluted with DCM/MeOH (4:1). However, the yields of pure polyhydroxy-piperidines and -azepanes were much lower (approximately 10%, 0.8:1 ratio, respectively) than using protection/deprotection strategies (Table 1).

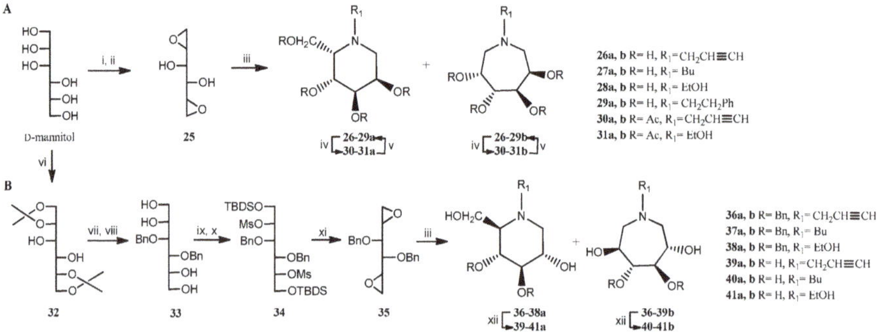

Scheme 1. (A) Synthesis of iminosugars 26-29a and 26-29b from D-mannitol, via bis-epoxide 25. Reagents and conditions: (i) TsCl, py, 71%; (ii) NaOH, $CH_3CN:H_2O$, 40 °C, 29%; (iii) Primary amine: propargylamine, butylamine, ethanolamine, or phenethylamine, MeOH, MW, 90 °C; (iv) Ac_2O, Py; for yields over two steps see Table 1; (v) NaOMe, MeOH (quant). (B) Synthesis of iminosugars 39-41a and 39-41b from D-mannitol, via bis-epoxide 35; (vi) 2,2-dimethoxypropane, TsOH, 96%; (vii) NaH, BnBr, *n*-Bu_4NI, THF, 93%; (viii) HCl, MeOH, 0 °C, (quant); (ix) TBDMS chloride, imidazole, DMF, 0 °C, 88%; (x) MsCl, NEt_3, DCM, 92%; (xi) HCl, MeOH, then NaOH, H_2O, 70%; and (xii) TMSI, DCM, rt, then MeOH, 45–100%.

Table 1. Yields obtained from microwave-assisted aminocyclization reaction of bis-epoxides 25 and 35.

Primary Amine for Aminocyclization Reaction	Yield (%)			
	Polyhydroxy-Piperidine		Polyhydroxy-Azepane	
	1-deoxy-L-*gulo*-nojirimycin 26-29a	1-deoxy-D-*gluco*-nojirimycin (DNJ) 39-41a	D-*manno*-azepane 26-29b	L-*ido*-azepane 39-41b
Propargylamine	32	40	35	37
Butylamine	20	33	24	38
Ethanolamine	17	22	21	28
Phenethylamine*	4	-	5	-

* Low yields obtained when the reaction mixture was purified directly by chromatographic column, without previous acetylation.

In order to keep the stereo-control during the reaction and obtain the iminosugars with the same stereochemistry of glucose, we pursued the classical procedure based on the protection of 1,2- and 5,6- positions of D-mannitol to produce the diisopropylidene intermediate **32** [48], which was benzylated at 3,4- positions and then deprotected under acid catalysis to give compound **33** (Scheme 1B) [47]. Briefly, selective protection of primary hydroxyl functions with bulk groups, followed by activation of the O-2 and O-5 with mesyl chloride and treatment of **34** in MeOH with concentrated HCl allowed the preparation of bis-epoxide **35** because of the intramolecular attack of the released primary hydroxyl functions that displaces the leaving mesyl groups. Then, bis-epoxide **35**, comprising inverted configurations at C-2 and C-5 comparatively to **25**, was converted to the corresponding mixture of N-substituted 1-deoxy-D-*gluco*-nojirimycin (**36-38a**) and 1,6-dideoxy-1,6-imino-L-*ido*-azepane derivatives (**36-38b**) in approximately 1:1 ratio under treatment with propargylamine, butylamine, ethanolamine, or phenethylamine for the aminocyclization reaction, as described for bis-epoxide **25**. Attempts to generate the N-phenethyl derivative of this series were unsuccessful since D-glucitol was isolated as a major product, possibly because phenethylamine promoted a regioselective opening of partially protected 1,2-epoxide (**35**) and then an O-cyclization leading to glucitol, as reported using ammonium formate [49].

After chromatographic separation of regioisomers, removal of the benzyl groups was better achieved under treatment with trimethylsilyl iodide [50] rather than hydrogenation conditions [47] to give final products **39-41a-b** in moderate to quantitative yields (45–100%).

2.2. Biological Assays

Initially, the small library of iminosugar derivatives (**26-29a,b** and **39-41a,b**) was screened for α-glucosidase inhibition (from *Saccharomyces cerevisiae*) activities using *p*-nitrophenyl α-D-glucopyranoside as substrate and prospective inhibitors at 1.0 mM concentration. To broaden the scope of the analysis, β-glucosidase (almond) activity of the same set of compounds was conducted using the corresponding *p*-nitrophenyl β-D-glucopyranoside.

2.2.1. Yeast α-glucosidase Activities

Based on the IC_{50} values using α-glucosidase, the greatest inhibition was verified for both piperidine and azepane DNJ derivatives bearing the N-hydroxylethyl group, D-*gluco*-piperidine (miglitol, **41a**, IC_{50} 41 μM) and L-*ido*-azepane (**41b**, IC_{50} 138 μM), using the DNJ as the reference (IC_{50} 134 μM) (Table 2). The α-glucosidase inhibition promoted by L-*ido*-azepane **41b** was significant and related to DNJ, although with a three-fold lower activity than D-*gluco*-piperidine (**41a**). In spite of finding a patent for azepane **38b**, the data were inaccessible [51], and mixed results were found for nonsubstituted L-*ido*-azepane with inhibition properties (K_i 4.8 μM) lower than the corresponding D-*gluco*-piperidine (DNJ, K_i 0.44 μM) assayed on *Bacillus stearothermophilus* α-glucosidase [46] and high (K_i 29.4 μM) [52] to weak activity (IC_{50} 772 μM [33] or 35% inhibition at 1 mM [53]) using yeast α-glucosidase. In addition, weak or no α-glucosidase inhibition was observed for N-propynyl (**39a,b**) and N-butyl (**40a,b**) DNJ and azepane derivatives in these assays, confirming reported data for **39a** and miglustat (**40a**) [54] and **40b** (14% inhibition at 1 mM) [33] both using yeast α-glucosidase.

In respect to L-*gulo*-piperidine and D-*manno*-azepane series, with inverted configurations at C-2 and C-5, derivatives (**26-29a,b**) bearing N-hydroxyethyl, N-butyl, N-propynyl [43], or N-phenethyl chains on the endocyclic nitrogen proved to be inactive against yeast α-glucosidase at the tested concentration (15–2000 μM), leading to loss of activity even for the N-hydroxyethyl derivatives (**28a,b**) when compared to **41a,b**. Reported α-glucosidase inhibition data for nonsubstituted L-*gulo*-piperidine and D-*manno*-azepane were found as weak as 30% and 55%, respectively, tested at 1 mM in *Bacillus stearothermophilus* [46] or 21% in yeast α-glucosidase at 240 μM [52]. Thus, it was evident that α-glucosidase activities were considerably affected by iminosugar stereochemistry, ring size, and N-substitutions, and inversion of configuration was detrimental for activity regardless of the

N-substituents here described, suggesting the wrong orientation of at least two hydroxyl groups attached at C-2 and C-5, which led to reduced binding affinity at yeast α-glucosidase active sites.

2.2.2. Almond β-glucosidase Activities:

Conversely, the assessment of the series on β-glucosidase revealed that novel L-*gulo*-piperidine (**27a**) and D-*manno*-azepane (**27b**) derivatives (inverted configurations at C-2 and C-5 related to glucose) preserving the *N*-butyl chain showed significant activity, IC$_{50}$ 109 and 184 µM, respectively, comparable to miglustat (**40a**, IC$_{50}$ 172 µM), although three- to five-fold lower than DNJ (IC$_{50}$ 33 µM) (Table 2). In this particular case, the *N*-butyl chain seems to play an important role in β-glucosidase inhibition since the reported data for nonsubstituted was low for both L-*gulo*-piperidine (13% at 1 mM) and D-*manno*-azepane (1% at 1 mM) or no inhibition at 240 µM on the same enzyme [46,52]. Interestingly, for the same set that preserve the *N*-butyl chain but display glucose stereochemistry, the seven-membered ring derivative L-*ido*-azepane **40b** displayed nearly twice the activity (IC$_{50}$ 80 µM) of the corresponding D-*gluco*-piperidine drug (**40a**), which resembled the stronger β-glucosidase inhibition achieved for nonsubstituted L-*ido*-azepane (K_i 17 µM [46], 12.8 µM [52], or IC$_{50}$ 38 µM [53]) than nonsubstituted D-*gluco*-piperidine (K_i 1700 µM) [46]. Furthermore, both derivatives bearing the *N*-hydroxyethyl chain, as occurs in miglitol (**41a**) and L-*ido*-azepane **41b**, proved to be the strongest β-glucosidase inhibitors with IC$_{50}$ of 4 µM. Based on all these findings, it was possible to infer that almond β-glucosidase active sites can accept and interact with a wider range of iminosugars than yeast α-glucosidase.

See dose-response curves obtained from Yeast α-Glucosidase and Almond β-Glucosidase assays in Supplementary Materials.

Table 2. α- and β-Glucosidase activities of synthesized iminosugars having alternative stereochemistry, ring size, and *N*-alkyl and *N*-arylalkyl chains on the endocyclic nitrogen.

	Iminosugars with Inverted Configuration at C-2 and C-5 with Respect to Glucose				Iminosugars Preserving Glucose Stereochemistry			
		Inhibition (µM)					Inhibition (µM)	
		α-Glucosidase	β-Glucosidase				α-Glucosidase	β-Glucosidase
-	-	-	-	DNJ	(structure)		134.4 ± 2.1	33.1 ± 3.1
26a	(structure)	NI	1716 ± 12.8	39a	(structure)		2527 ± 82.2	635.7 ± 8.5
26b	(structure)	NI	NI	39b	(structure)		NI	3437 ± 70.6
27a	(structure)	NI	109.7 ± 9.3	40a	(structure)		NI	172.8 ± 1.7
27b	(structure)	2031 ± 17.1	184.6 ± 2.6	40b	(structure)		NI	80.0 ± 4.9
28a	(structure)	NI	NI	41a	(structure)		41.3 ± 10.1	4.0 ± 1.5
28b	(structure)	NI	NI	41b	(structure)		138.8 ± 1.2	4.0 ± 1.4

Table 2. Cont.

	Iminosugars with Inverted Configuration at C-2 and C-5 with Respect to Glucose			Iminosugars Preserving Glucose Stereochemistry		
		Inhibition (µM)			Inhibition (µM)	
		α-Glucosidase	β-Glucosidase		α-Glucosidase	β-Glucosidase
29a		NI	NI	-	-	-
29b		NI	NI	-	-	-

Enzyme inhibition: IC$_{50}$ in µM, α-Glucosidase from *Saccharomyces cerevisiae* and β-Glucosidase from almonds. NI: no inhibition. DNJ; deoxynojirimycin

3. Conclusions

In summary, a series of iminosugars were successfully synthesized from a common precursor, D-mannitol, to produce two alternative bis-epoxides, further modified by an S$_N$2 aminocyclization reaction to give a mixture of both N-substituted six- and seven-membered iminosugar isomers. Besides the ring size, two additional structural variations were also pursued to broaden the scope of reported strategies, as stereochemistry (maintenance of glucose stereochemistry or inversion of configuration at C-2 and C-5 positions) and N-chain of the endocyclic nitrogen (N-propynyl, -butyl, -hydroxyethyl, and -phenethyl). Classical polyhydroxypiperidines, miglustat and miglitol drugs that maintain glucose configuration (D-*gluco*-nojirimycin, DNJ) and bear N-butyl and N-hydroxyethyl chains, respectively, were synthesized and used as reference for evaluation of the series towards α- and β-glucosidases. Assessment of α-glucosidase activity of iminosugars revealed solely miglitol as the most active of the series, followed by the corresponding L-*ido*-azepane isomer. All other iminosugars proved to not be inhibitors of yeast α-glucosidase. On the other hand, all N-butyl iminosugars having either glucose stereochemistry, D-*gluco*-piperidine miglustat drug and L-*ido*-azepane, or inverted configurations at C-2 and C-5 related to glucose, L-*gulo*-piperidine and D-*manno*-azepane derivatives, displayed significant inhibition of almond β-glucosidase. In spite of that, the strongest inhibition was achieved for D-*gluco*-piperidine miglitol drug and the corresponding L-*ido*-azepane iminosugars containing N-hydroxyethyl chains, but, in these tests, no activity was accomplished for inverted configuration counterparts. Thus, we observed that glucosidase inhibition promoted by some polyhydroxypiperidines was accompanied by proportional inhibition of the corresponding polyhydroxyazepane isomers bearing the same N-chain regardless of the ring stereochemistry. In addition, the findings of this study on β-glucosidase inhibition by L-*gulo*-piperidine and D-*manno*-azepane series are relevant considering their straightforward synthesis compared to DNJ series.

4. Material and Methods

^{1}H (300 MHz) and ^{13}C (75 MHz) NMR spectra were recorded on a Bruker® Ultrashield 300 NMR spectrometer. ^{1}H (400 MHz) and ^{13}C (100 MHz) NMR spectra were recorded on a Bruker® Avance 400 MHz NMR spectrometer. ^{1}H (500 MHz) and ^{13}C (125 MHz) NMR spectra were recorded on a Bruker® Avance 500 MHz NMR spectrometer. All spectra were recorded at room temperature (~20 °C) in Sigma Aldrich® deuterated solvents. Chemical shifts (δ) were expressed in parts per million (ppm) relative to the reference peak. Coupling constants (J) were expressed in Hertz (Hz). Splitting patterns in ^{1}H NMR spectra were designated as s (singlet), br s (broad singlet), d (doublet), br d (broad doublet), t (triplet), q (quartet), dd (doublet of doublets), dt (doublet of triplets), ddd (doublet of doublet of doublets), and m (multiplet). Optical rotations were measured on a Jasco P-2000 polarimeter at 22.5 nd using a sodium lamp and wavelength of 589 nm at 22.5 °C. HPLC purifications were designed in a Shimadzu® SCL-10A HPLC system, Diode Array Detector Shimadzu® SPD-M10A, and processed on Class-VP software. Purification of the compounds **31a** and **31b** was performed in HPLC using a Macherey–Nagel CLC-ODS semiprep column, Methanol 40%, flowrate 4.0 mL/min, and 200 nm. High-resolution mass spectra (HRMS) were obtained on a Bruker Daltonics MicrOTOF-Q II ESI-TOF mass spectrometer, and an Exactive Plus Orbitrap mass spectrometer (Thermo Scientific, Germany) was equipped with an electrospray (H-ESI-II) probe and operated in negative ionization mode. The system was controlled by Xcalibur and Tune (Thermo Scientific). For biological assays, absorbance at 405 nm was measured using SpectraMax M2 Molecular Devices®.

1,2:5,6-di-anhydro-D-mannitol (25) [43]: D-Mannitol (5.05 g, 27.4 mmol) was solubilized in pyridine (25.0 mL) and heated to 120 °C for 15 min. After that, the solution was refrigerated to 0 °C, treated dropwise with tosyl chloride solution (13.10 g, 68.7 mmol/10 mL pyridine) for 1 h, and stirred at 0 °C for 3 h then at r.t. for 1 h. The mixture was coevaporated with toluene, and the solid was diluted in dichloromethane and washed with HCl 1 mol·L^{-1} and saturated NaHCO$_3$. The organic layer was dried over MgSO$_4$ and concentrated. The crude mixture of 1,6-di-O-tosyl-D-mannitol was solubilized in a mixture of acetonitrile and water (38.0 mL, 2:1, v/v), and a small portion of phenolphthalein was added to it. The mixture was stirred at 35–40 °C and titrated with NaOH 5 mol·L^{-1} until the solution remained pink. After that, a mixture of Na$_2$CO$_3$ (87.4 g) in ethyl acetate (324 mL) was added and stirred vigorously. The solid was filtrated and washed with ethyl acetate. The organic solution was dried over MgSO$_4$, filtered, and concentrated. The resulting mixture was purified by flash chromatography (hexane and ethyl acetate, 7:3, v/v) to yield **1** (1.12 g, 7.70 mmol, 28%). ^{1}H NMR (400 MHz, CD$_3$OD): δ 2.77 (2H, dd, J 2.7 Hz, 5.3 Hz, H-1a, H-6a); 2.82 (2H, dd, J 4.0 Hz, 5.3 Hz, H-1b, H-6b); 3.11–3.17 (2H, m, H-2, H-5); 3.46–3.52 (2H, m, H-3, H-4). ^{13}C NMR (100 MHz, CDCl$_3$): δ 46.1 (C-1, C-6); 52.8 (C-2, C-5); 73.3 (C-3, C-4).

1,2:5,6-Di-*O*-isopropilidene D-mannitol (32) [48]

1,2:5,6-Dianhydro-3,4-di-*O*-benzyl-L-iditol (35): prepared as described by Wilkinson et al. [47]

General procedure for the synthesis of L-*gulo*-piperidine and D-*manno*-azepane derivatives (26a,b-31a,b): 1,2:5,6-dianhydro-D-glucitol was solubilized in methanol and 2.5 eq of primary amine (propargylamine, ethanolamine, butylamine, or phenethylamine) was added to the solution. The mixture was heated to 90 °C in a microwave for 5 min (150 W) in a sealed vessel. The solvents were evaporated in vacuum. Compounds **27a,b** and **29a,b** were separated in a flash column (dichloromethane and methanol, 8:2 v/v). Compounds **26a,b** and **28a,b** were acetylated by the addition of pyridine (8.0 mL) and acetic anhydride (22.8 mL) and stirred at r.t. After 3 h, ice was added to the mixture, the product was extracted with ethyl ether, and the organic layer was evaporated and dried with MgSO$_4$. Compounds **30a,b** were separated by column chromatography (toluene and ethyl acetate, 3:7, v/v). Compounds **31a,b** were purified in a HPLC C-18 semiprep column in methanol/water 40% and flow rate 4.0 mL/min.

See ^{1}H, ^{13}C and bidimensional NMR and ESI HRMS spectra of compounds **26-31a,b** and **36-41a,b** in Supplementary Materials.

General procedure for removal of Acetyl groups: Compounds **30a,b** and **31a,b** were dissolved in methanol (1.0 mL), and sodium methoxide 1 M was added dropwise to the solution until pH 9.0 and checked with Tornassol. After half an hour, TLC showed total consumption of starting material, then it was neutralized with ion exchange resin DOWEX® 50WX4-50. After that, the mixture was filtered through a Celite® pad and concentrated in vacuo.

General procedure for removal o Benzyl groups [50]: The corresponding product was solubilized in dichloromethane, and Me$_3$SI (4 eq) was added slowly. The reaction was allowed to stir at r.t. for 15 min. TLC showed total consumption of starting material, then the reaction was quenched with methanol. The product was purified in a SPE-C18 silica pad with methanol/water 1:1 v/v.

***N*-Propynyl-1,5-dideoxy-1,5-imino-L-gulitol (26a)** [43]: 80% (0.0082 g, 0.041 mmol): ^{1}H NMR (500 MHz, D$_2$O): δ 2.71–2.77 (2H, m, H-1a, ≡CH); 2.85 (1H, t, *J* 10.9 Hz, H-1b); 2.88–2.93 (1H, m, H-5);

3.46 (1H, d, *J* 17.6 Hz, H-7a); 3.68 (1H, d, *J* 17.6 Hz, H-7b); 3.83 (1H, dd, *J* 5.4 Hz, 11.7 Hz, H-6a); 3.89 (1H, dd, *J* 3.9 Hz, 11.7 Hz, H-6b); 3.91–3.94 (1H, m, H-3); 4.05–4.14 (2H, m, H-2, H-4). ESI HRMS: [M+H]$^+$ calculated for C$_9$H$_{15}$NO$_4$ 202.1074; found 202.1076.

***N*-Propynyl-1,6-dideoxy-1,6-imino-D-mannitol (26b)** [43]: 86% (0.0088 g, 0.044 mmol): ^{1}H NMR (500 MHz, D$_2$O): δ 2.66 (1H, t, *J* 2.2 Hz, ≡CH); 2.85 (4H, m, H-1a; H-1b; H-6a; H-6b); 3.37 (1H, d, *J* 17.0 Hz, H-7a); 3.41 (1H, d, *J* 17.0 Hz, H-7b); 3.89–3.91 (2H, m, H-3, H-4); 4.12 (2H, t, *J* 4.8 Hz, H-2, H-5). ESI HRMS: [M+H]$^+$ calculated for C$_9$H$_{15}$NO$_4$ 202.1074; found 202.1073.

***N*-Butyl-1,5-dideoxy-1,5-imino-L-gulitol (27a)**: $[\alpha]_D^{22.5}$ 29.5 (*c* 1.8, MeOH), ^{1}H NMR (500 MHz, D$_2$O): δ 0.83 (3H, t, *J* 7.4 Hz, H-10); 1.17–1.28 (2H, m, H-9); 1.37–1.50 (2H, m, H-8); 2.50–2.92 (5H, m, 2×H-1, H-5, 2×H-7); 3.75 (1H, dd, *J* 5.6. 11.8, H-6a); 3.78–3.85 (2H, m, H-3, H-6b); 3.94–4.00 (1H, m, H-2); 4.05–4.11 (1H, m, H-4). ^{13}C NMR (125 MHz, D$_2$O): δ 13.3 (C-10); 20.0 (C-9); 27.4 (C-8); 53.1 (C-1 or C-7); 55.1 (C-1 or C-7); 58.5 (C-6); 68.2 (C-4); 70.1 (C-3); 70.4 (C-3); 72.8 (C-2). ESI HRMS: [M+H]$^+$ calculated for C$_{10}$H$_{22}$NO$_4$ 220.1544; found 220.1538.

***N*-Butyl-1,6-dideoxy-1,6-imino-D-mannitol (27b)**: $[\alpha]_D^{22.5}$ −62.0 (*c* 2.2, MeOH), ^{1}H NMR (500 MHz, D$_2$O): δ 0.76 (3H, t, *J* 7.3 Hz, 3×H-10); 1.07–1.25 (2H, m, 2×H-9); 1.30–1.44 (2H, m, 2×H-8); 2.47–2.57 (2H, m, 2×H-7); 2.65–2.85 (4H, m, 2×H-1, 2×H-6); 3.73–3.79 (2H, m, H-3, H-4); 3.94–4.04 (2H, m, H-2, H-5). ^{13}C NMR (125 MHz, D$_2$O): δ 13.2 (C-10); 20.0 (C-9); 27.5 (C-8); 55.2 (C-1, C-6); 58.4 (C-7); 68.3 (C-2; C-5); 72.8 (C-4; C-3). ESI HRMS: [M+H]$^+$ calculated for C$_{10}$H$_{22}$NO$_4$ 220.1544; found 220.1543.

***N*-Hydroxyethyl-1,5-dideoxy-1,5-imino-L-gulitol (28a)**: $[\alpha]_D^{22.5}$ 16.1 (*c* 0.6, MeOH), ^{1}H NMR (400 MHz, CD$_3$OD): δ 2.53–2.71 (2H, m, H-1a, H-7a); 2.78–2.89 (2H, m, H-5, H-7b); 2.97 (1H, ddd, *J* 4.9; 7.0; 13.5 Hz, H-1b); 3.55–3.98 (7H, m, H-2, H-3, H-4, H-6a, H-6b, H-8a, H-8b). ^{13}C NMR (100 MHz, CD$_3$OD): δ 51.9 (C-7); 55.1 (C-1); 58.6 (C-8); 60.0 (C-6); 61.0 (C-5); 66.5, 70.9, 71.3 (C-2, C-3, C-4). ESI HRMS: [M+H]$^+$ calculated for C$_8$H$_{18}$NO$_5$ 208.1180; found 208.1177.

***N*-Hydroxyethyl-1,6-imino-D-mannitol (28b)**: $[\alpha]_D^{22.5}$ −15.3 (*c* 0.5, MeOH), ^{1}H NMR (400 MHz, CD$_3$OD): δ 2.58–2.80 (4H, m, H-1a; H-6^a; 2×H-7); 2.89 (2H, dd, *J* 4.3; 13.2 Hz, H-1b, H-6b); 3.59 (2H, dd, *J* 6.0; 12.5 Hz, 2×H-8); 3.86–3.92 (2H, m, H-3, H-4); 4.00–4.08 (2H, m, H-2, H-5). ^{13}C NMR (100 MHz, CD$_3$OD): δ 58.4 (C-1; C-6); 60.4 (C-8); 61.8 (C-7); 70.9 (C-2; C-5); 74.0 (C-3; C-4). ESI HRMS: [M+H]$^+$ calculated for C$_8$H$_{18}$NO$_5$ 208.1180; found 208.1182.

***N*-Phenethyl-1,5-dideoxy-1,5-imino-L-gulitol (29a)** [46]

***N*-Phenethyl-1,6-dideoxy-1,6-imino-D-mannitol (29b)** [46]

***N*-Propynyl-2,3,4,6-tetra-*O*-acetyl-1,5-dideoxy-1,5-imino-L-gulitol (30a)** [43]: ^{1}H NMR (400 MHz, CDCl$_3$): δ 2.03, 2.09, 2.13, 2.14 (12H, 4s, 4×CH$_3$); 2.33 (1H, t, *J* 2.3 Hz, ≡CH); 2.80 (1H, dd, *J* 4.7 Hz, 11.2 Hz, H-1a); 2.97 (1H, dd, *J* 9.6 Hz, 11.2 Hz, H-1b); 3.28 (1H, ddd, *J* 3.3 Hz, 5.8 Hz, 10.0 Hz, H-5); 3.44 (1H, dd, *J* 2.3 Hz, 17.8 Hz, H-7a); 3.67 (1H, dd, *J* 2.3 Hz, 17.8 Hz, H-7b); 4.20 (1H, dd, *J* 5.8 Hz, 11.6 Hz, H-6b); 4.24 (1H, dd, *J* 3.3 Hz, 11.6 Hz, H-6a); 5.20–5.27 (3H, m, H-2, H-3, H-4). ^{13}C NMR (100 MHz, CDCl$_3$): δ 20.8; 20.9 (CH$_3$); 43.9 (C-1); 49.6 (C-7); 55.5 (C-5); 61.4 (C-6); 66.5 (C-3, C-4); 68.7 (C-2); 77.2 (≡CH); 169.3; 169.7; 170.5 (C=O). ESI HRMS: [M+H]$^+$ calculated for C$_{17}$H$_{24}$NO$_8$ 370.1496; found 370.1496.

***N*-Propynyl-2,3,4,6-tetra-*O*-acetyl-1,6-dideoxy-1,6-imino-D-mannitol (30b)** [43]: ^{1}H NMR (400 MHz, CDCl$_3$): δ 2.05, 2.12 (12H, 2s, 4×CH$_3$); 2.25 (t, *J* 2.3 Hz, ≡CH); 2.91 (2H, dd, *J* 5.6 Hz, 13.8 Hz, H-1a, H-6a); 2.99 (2H, dd, *J* 4.4 Hz, 13.8 Hz, H-1b, H-6b); 3.39 (1H, dd, *J* 2.3 Hz, 17.3 Hz, H-7a); 3.45 (1H, dd, *J* 2.3 Hz, 17.3 Hz, H-7b); 5.40 (2H, dt, *J* 1.2 Hz, 4.6 Hz, H-2, H-5); 5.48 (2H, t, *J* 1.2 Hz, H-3, H-4). ^{13}C NMR (100 MHz, CDCl$_3$): δ 20.8; 21.0 (CH$_3$); 47.9 (C-7); 54.1 (C-1, C-6); 69.9 (C-2, C-5); 70.9 (C-3 e C-4); 77.2 (≡CH); 169.9; 170.1 (C=O). ESI HRMS: [M+H]$^+$ calculated for C$_{17}$H$_{24}$NO$_8$ 370.1496; found 370.1535.

***N*-Acetoxyethyl-2,3,4,6-tetra-*O*-acetyl-1,5-dideoxy-1,5-imino-L-gulitol (31a)**: ^{1}H NMR (400 MHz, CDCl$_3$): δ 2.06; 2.08; 2.10 (18H, 3s, 5×CH$_3$); 2.89 (1H, dd, *J* 5.0, 13.7 Hz, H-1a); 2.96 (2H, t, H-7, *J* 5.9 Hz, H-7); 3.04 (1H, dd, *J* 2.6; 13.7 Hz, H-1b); 3.45 (1H, dd, *J* 4.8; 11.4 Hz, H-5); 4.05 (1H, dd, *J* 5.6; 11.3 Hz, H-6a); 4.10–4.21 (2H, m, 2×H-8); 4.37 (1H, dd, *J* 7.0; 11.8 Hz, H-6b); 5.15 (1H, dd, *J* 3.3; 9.0 Hz, H-3); 5.20–5.25 (1H, m, H-2); 5.20–5.25 (1H, m, H-2); 5.28 (1H, dd, *J* 4.9; 9.0 Hz, H-4). ^{13}C NMR (100 MHz,

CDCl$_3$): δ 20.8, 20.9, 21.0 (5xCH$_3$); 48.9 (C-1); 52.7 (C-7); 58.2 (C-5); 59.9 (C-6); 68.0 (C-3); 68.1, 68.3 (C-2, C-4).

N-Acetoxyethyl-2,3,4,6-tetra-O-acetyl-1,6-dideoxy-1,6-imino-D-mannitol (31b): ^{1}H NMR (400 MHz, CDCl$_3$): δ 2.03; 2.07; 2.10 (18H, 3s, 5xCH$_3$); 2.85 (2H, t, J 5.8 Hz, H-4, H-4′); 2.91 (2H, dd, J 5.6; 14.0 Hz, H-1a, H-1′a); 3.04 (2H, dd, J 4.3; 14.0 Hz, H-1b, H-1′b); 4.11 (2H, dd, J 5.7; 9.1 Hz, H-5, H-5′); 5.29-5.37 (2H, m, H-2, H-2′); 5.43-5.47 (2H, m, H-3, H-3′). ^{13}C NMR (100 MHz, CDCl$_3$): δ 20.8; 20.9; 21.0 (5xCH$_3$); 54.8 (C-1, C-1′); 56.4 (C-4); 62.2 (C-5); 70.2 (C-2, C-2′); 70.6 (C-3, C-3′).

N-Propynyl-2,3,4,6-tetra-O-acetyl-1,5-dideoxy-1,5-imino-D-glucitol (36a): ^{1}H NMR (400 MHz, CDCl$_3$): δ 2.27 (1H, t, J 2.2 Hz, ≡CH); 2.50 (1H, d, J 9.5 Hz, H-5); 2.60 (1H, t, J 10.7 Hz, H-1a); 2.92 (1H, dd, J 4.9; 10.9 Hz, H-1b); 3.31–3.44 (2H, m, 2xH-7); 3.62–3.91 (5H, m, H-2, H-3, H-4, 2xH-6); 4.77 (2H, dd, J 3.8; 11.2 Hz, CH$_2$Ph); 4.98 (2H, dd, J 11.2; 13.4 Hz, CH$_2$Ph); 7.29–7.45 (10H, m, H-Ph). ^{13}C RMN (100 MHz, CDCl$_3$): δ 42.1 (C-1); 56.1 (C-7); 57.3 (C-6); 63.1 (C-2 or C-5); 69.4 (C-2 or C-5); 74.6 (C≡CH); 75.2 (CH$_2$Ph); 87.3 (C-3; C-4); 127.9, 128.6, 128.7 (Ar); 138.1 (C$_q$). ESI HRMS: [M+H]$^+$ calculated for C$_{23}$H$_{28}$NO$_4$ 382.2013; found 382.2002.

N-Propynyl-2,3,4,6-tetra-O-acetyl-1,6-dideoxy-1,6-imino-L-iditol (36b): ^{1}H NMR (400 MHz, CDCl$_3$): δ 2.31 (1H, t, J 2.3 Hz, ≡CH); 2.77 (2H, dd, J 8.2; 12.3 Hz, H-1a, H-6a); 2.98 (2H, dd, J 1.1; 12.7, H-1b, H6b); 3.40–3.56 (2H, m, 2xH-7); 3.63–3.70 (2H, m, H-3, H-4); 3.80–3.93 (2H, m, H-2, H-5); 4.67 (2H, d, J 11.2 Hz, CH$_2$Ph); 4.81 (2H, d, J 11.2 Hz, CH$_2$Ph); 7.29–7.42 (10H, m, H-Ph). ^{13}C RMN (100 MHz, CDCl$_3$): δ 48.8 (C-7); 56.9 (C-1, C-6); 68.0 (C-2, C-5); 73.8 (CH$_2$Ph); 78.2 (C≡CH); 86.5 (C-3, C-4); 127.9, 128.0, 128.6 (Ar); 137.9 (C$_q$). ESI HRMS: [M+H]$^+$ calculated for C$_{23}$H$_{28}$NO$_4$ 382.2013; found 382.2001.

N-Butyl-2,3,4,6-tetra-O-acetyl-1,5-dideoxy-1,5-imino-D-glucitol (37a): ^{1}H NMR (400 MHz, CDCl$_3$): δ 0.94 (3H, t, J 6.9 Hz, 3xH-10); 1.21–1.38 (2H, m, 2xH-9); 1.39–1.56 (2H, m, 2xH-8); 2.26 (1H, t, J 10.6Hz, H-5); 2.32–2.54 (3H, m, H-1a, H-1b, H-7a); 2.70–2.82 (1H, m, H-7b); 3.13 (1H, dd, J 4.6; 11.2 Hz, H-6a); 3.38 (1H, t, J 8.8 Hz, H-3); 3.60–3.73 (2H, m, H-4, H-6b); 3.77–3.93 (2H, m, H-2, H-XX); 4.75 (2H, dd, J 5.6; 11.2 Hz, CH$_2$Ph); 4.96 (2H, t ap., J 11.0 Hz, CH$_2$Ph); 7.29–7.48 (10H, m, Ar). ^{13}C RMN (100 MHz, CDCl$_3$): δ 14.0 (C-10); 20.6 (C-9); 27.3 (C-8); 52.1 (C-1 or C-7); 55.1 (C-1 or C-7); 57.5 (C-6); 64.9 (C-2 or C-5); 69.3(C-2 or C-5); 74.9 (CH$_2$Ph); 75.1 (CH$_2$Ph); 78.1 (C-3 or C-4); 86.8 (C-3 or C-4); 127.8, 127.9, 128.0, 128.5, 128.7 (C-Ar); 138.1 (C$_q$); 138.5 (C$_q$). ESI HRMS: [M+H]$^+$ calculated for C$_{24}$H$_{34}$NO$_4$ 400.2483; found 400.2477.

N-Butyl-2,3,4,6-tetra-O-acetyl-1,6-dideoxy-1,6-imino-L-iditol (37b): ^{1}H NMR (400 MHz, CDCl$_3$): δ 0.93 (3H, t, J 7.2 Hz, 3xH-10); 1.25–1.40 (2H, m, 2xH-9); 1.42–1.58 (2H, m, 2xH-8); 2.52–2.69 (4H, m, H-1a, H-6a, 2xH-7); 2.92 (2H, d, J 12.5 Hz, H-1b, H-6b); 3.60–3.70 (2H, m, H-3, H-4); 3.78–3.89 (2H, m, H-2, H-5); 4.66 (2H, d, J 11.2 Hz, CH$_2$Ph); 4.79 (2H, d, J 11.2 Hz, CH$_2$Ph); 7.29–7.43 (10H, m, H-Ph). ^{13}C RMN (100 MHz, CDCl$_3$): δ 13.9 (C-10); 20.4 (C-9); 29.3 (C-8); 57.6 (C-7); 59.0 (C-1; C-6); 67.7 (C-2, C-5); 73.6 (CH$_2$Ph); 87.0 (C-3, C-4); 127.9, 128.6 (Ar); 137.0 (C$_q$). ESI HRMS: [M+H]$^+$ calculated for C$_{24}$H$_{34}$NO$_4$ 400.2483; found 400.2475.

N-Hydroxyethyl-2,3,4,6-tetra-O-acetyl-1,5-dideoxy-1,5-imino-D-glucitol (38a): ^{1}H NMR (400 MHz, CDCl$_3$): δ 2.29 (1H, dd, J 9.7, 11.3 Hz, H-1a); 2.37–2.51 (2H, m, H-5, H-7a); 2.94–3.08 (1H, m, H-7b); 3.16 (1H, dd, J 4.4; 11.5 Hz, H-1b); 3.43 (1H, t, J 8.3 Hz, H-3); 3.54–3.77 (4H, m, H-2, H-4, H-8a, H-8b); 3.88 (2H, qd, J 2.8; 12.3 Hz, H-6a, H-6b); 4.67–4.81 (2H, m, CH$_2$Ph); 4.84–4.97 (2H, m, CH$_2$Ph); 7.29–7.45 (10H, m, Ph-H). ^{13}C RMN (100 MHz, CDCl$_3$): δ 53.2 (C-7); 55.3 (C-1); 57.8 (C-6); 59.6 (C-8); 65.7 (C-5); 69.0 (C-2 or C-4); 74.8 (CH$_2$Ph); 78.0 (C-2 or C-4); 85.9 (C-3); 128.0, 128.6 (Ar); 138.4 (C$_q$). ESI HRMS: [M+H]$^+$ calculated for C$_{22}$H$_{30}$NO$_5$ 388.2119; found 388.2120.

N-Hydroxyethyl-2,3,4,6-tetra-O-acetyl-1,6-dideoxy-1,6-imino-L-iditol (38b): ^{1}H NMR (400 MHz, CDCl$_3$): δ 2.66–2.80 (4H, m, 2xH-1, 2xH-2); 2.99 (2H, dd, J 2.8; 13.1 Hz, 2xH-7); 3.62–3.72 (4H, m, H-2, H-5, 2xH-8); 3.80–3.90 (2H, m, H-3, H-4); 4.65 (2H, d, J 11.3 Hz, CH$_2$Ph); 4.84 (2H, d, J 11.3 Hz, CH$_2$Ph); 7.28–7.42 (10H, m, H-Ph). ^{13}C RMN (100 MHz, CDCl$_3$): δ 59.0 (C-7); 59.7 (C-8); 60.7 (C-1; C-6); 70.0 (C-3; C-4); 74.2 (CH$_2$Ph); 85.4 (C-2; C-5); 127.9, 128.0, 128.6, 137.9 (Ar). ESI HRMS: [M+H]$^+$ calculated for C$_{22}$H$_{30}$NO$_5$ 388.2119; found 388.2102.

N-Propynyl-1,5-dideoxy-1,5-imino-D-glucitol (39a) [47]
N-Propynyl-1,6-dideoxy-1,6-imino-L-iditol (39b) [47]
N-Butyl-1,5-dideoxy-1,5-imino-D-glucitol (40a) [55]
N-Butyl-1,6-dideoxy-1,6-imino-L-iditol (40b):** $[\alpha]_D^{22.5}$ 1.3 (*c* 1.1, MeOH), ^{1}H NMR (400 MHz, D$_2$O): δ 0.86 (3H, t, *J* 8.0 Hz, 3xH-10); 1.24–1.36 (2H, m, 2xH-9); 1.56–1.74 (2H, m, 2xH-8); 3.14–3.23 (2H, m, H-7); 3.26–3.37 (4H, m, 2xH-1, 2xH-6); 3.58–3.67 (2H, m, H-2, H-5); 4.01–4.08 (2H, m, H-3, H-4). ^{13}C RMN (100 MHz, D$_2$O): δ 12.9 (C-10); 19.3 (C-9); 25.6 (C-8); 58.6 (C-1; C-6; C-7) 67.1 (C-3 or C-4); 67.7 (C-3 or C-4); (C-2; C-5). ESI HRMS: [M+H]$^+$ calculated for C$_{10}$H$_{22}$NO$_4$ 220.1544; found 220.1545.

**N-Hydroxyethyl-1,5-dideoxy-1,5-imino-D-glucitol (41a) [55]
N-Hydroxyethyl-1,6-dideoxy-1,6-imino-L-iditol (41b):** $[\alpha]_D^{22.5}$ −9.1 (*c* 0.6, MeOH), ^{1}H NMR (400 MHz, D$_2$O): δ 2.62–2.77 (4H, m, H-1a; H-1b; H-6a; H-6b); 2.91 (2H, dd, *J* 3.8;13.7 Hz, H-7a, H-7b); 3.40–3.48 (2H, m, H-2, H-3); 3.69 (4H, m, H-4, H-5, H-8a, H-8b,). ^{13}C RMN (100 MHz, D$_2$O): δ 58.4 (C-7), 59.3 (C-1, C-6, C-8); 70.8 (C-4, C-5), 75.6 (C-2, C-3). ESI HRMS: [M+H]$^+$ calculated for C$_8$H$_{18}$NO$_5$ 208.1185; found 208.1176.

Biological assays [43]: Yeast α-glucosidase (EC 3.2.1.20) and almond β-glucosidase (EC 3.2.1.21) activity was assessed using a 96-well plate assay. Assays contained 20 mM NaOAc at pH 6.8 (α-glucosidase) and pH 6.2 (β-glucosidase), 10 mM PIPES (piperazine-N,N′-bis(2-ethanesulfonic acid), 0.1 mM EDTA, α-glucosidase (5 μg/mL), β-glucosidase (6 μg/mL), and inhibitor (0.1–2 mM). Enzyme and inhibitor were equilibrated at 37 °C for 30 min. The reaction was initiated by the addition of *p*-nitrophenyl α-D-glucopyranoside (200 μM) or *p*-nitrophenyl β-D-glucopyranoside (200 μM), and then it was quenched with 100 μL of sodium carbonate 3.0 M after 25 min incubation at 37 °C. Assays were repeated in duplicate and data averaged.

Supplementary Materials: The following are available online at http://www.mdpi.com/1424-8247/12/3/108/s1, ^{1}H, ^{13}C and bidimensional NMR and ESI HRMS spectra of compounds 26-31a,b and 36-41a,b; Table: IC$_{50}$ of final compounds and Dose-response curves obtained from Yeast α-Glucosidase and Almond β-Glucosidase assays.

Author Contributions: Conceptualization, I.C.; methodology, L.O.B.Z., V.A.-L.; software, L.O.B.Z.; validation, L.O.B.Z. and I.C.; formal analysis, L.O.B.Z. and I.C.; investigation, L.O.B.Z., Valquiria Aragão-Leoneti and I.C.; resources, L.O.B.Z., Valquiria Aragão-Leoneti and I.C.; data curation, L.O.B.Z. and I.C.; writing—original draft preparation, I.C.; writing—review and editing, L.O.B.Z. and I.C.; visualization, L.O.B.Z. and I.C.; supervision, I.C.; project administration, I.C.; funding acquisition, I.C.

Funding: This research was funded by Fundação de Amparo à Pesquisa do Estado de São Paulo (FAPESP), grant number 2007/00910-6, Conselho Nacional de Desenvolvimento Científico e Tecnológico (CNPq,), grant number 503709/2011-5, and Coordenação de Aperfeiçoamento de Pessoal de Nível Superior (CAPES).

Acknowledgments: We acknowledge financial support from Fundação de Amparo à Pesquisa do Estado de São Paulo (FAPESP, Proc. n. 2007/00910-6), Conselho Nacional de Desenvolvimento Científico e Tecnológico (CNPq, Proc. n. 503709/2011-5), and Coordenação de Aperfeiçoamento de Pessoal de Nível Superior (CAPES).

Conflicts of Interest: The authors declare no conflict of interest. The funders had no role in the design of the study; in the collection, analyses, or interpretation of data; in the writing of the manuscript, or in the decision to publish the results.

References

1. Melo, E.B.; Gomes, A.S.; Carvalho, I. α-and β-Glucosidase inhibitors: Chemical structure and biological activity. *Tetrahedron* **2006**, *62*, 10277–10302.
2. Gao, K.; Zheng, C.; Wang, T.; Zhao, H.; Wang, J.; Wang, Z.; Zhai, X.; Jia, Z.; Chen, J.; Zhou, Y.; et al. Review 1-Deoxynojirimycin: Occurrence, Extraction, Chemistry, Oral Pharmacokinetics, Biological Activities and In Silico Target Fishing. *Molecules* **2016**, *21*, 1600. [CrossRef] [PubMed]
3. Schuster, M.; Blechert, S. Inhibition of fucosyltransferase V by a GDP-azasugar. *Bioorg. Med. Chem. Lett.* **2001**, *11*, 1809–1811. [CrossRef]
4. Jakobsen, P.; Lundbeck, J.M.; Kristiansen, M.; Breinholt, J.; Demuth, H.; Pawlas, J.; Candela, M.P.T.; Andersen, B.; Westergaard, N.; Lundgren, K.; et al. Imino sugars: Potential inhibitors of liver glycogen phosphorylase. *Bioorg. Med. Chem.* **2001**, *9*, 733–744. [CrossRef]

5. Compain, P.; Martin, O.R. Carbohydrate mimetics-based glycosyltransferase inhibitors. *Bioorg. Med. Chem.* **2001**, *9*, 3077–3092. [CrossRef]
6. Fedorov, A.; Shi, W.; Kicska, G.; Fedorov, E.; Tyler, P.C.; Furneaux, R.H.; Hanso, J.C.; Gainsford, G.J.; Larese, J.Z.; Schramm, V.L.; et al. Transition state structure of purine nucleoside phosphorylase and principles of atomic motion in enzymatic catalysis. *Biochemistry* **2001**, *40*, 853–860. [CrossRef] [PubMed]
7. Lee, R.E.; Smith, M.D.; Pickering, L.; Fleet, G.W.J. An approach to combinatorial library generation of galactofuranose mimics as potential inhibitors of mycobacterial cell wall biosynthesis: Synthesis of a peptidomimetic of uridine 5′-diphosphogalactofuranose (UDP-galf). *Tetrahedron Lett.* **1999**, *40*, 8689–8692. [CrossRef]
8. Campo, V.L.; Aragão-Leoneti, V.; Carvalho, I. Glycosidases and diabetes: Metabolic changes, mode of action and therapeutic perspectives. In *Carbohydrate Chemistry*; Amélia Pilar, R., Thisbe, L., Eds.; Royal Society of Chemistry: Cambridge, UK, 2013; Volume 9, pp. 181–203.
9. Rosenbloom, B.E.; Weinreb, N.J. Gaucher disease: A comprehensive review. *Crit. Rev. Oncog.* **2013**, *18*, 163–175. [CrossRef] [PubMed]
10. Yang, X.; Xiong, D.; Song, C.; Tai, G.; Ye, X. Synthesis of N-dialkylphosphoryl iminosugar derivatives and their immunosuppressive activities. *Org. Biomol. Chem.* **2015**, *13*, 9364–9368. [CrossRef] [PubMed]
11. Warfield, K.; Ramstedt, U. Iminosugars as Antibacterial Compounds and Uses Thereof for Treating Bacterial Infections. PCT Int. App. WO 2014143999 A1, 18 September 2014.
12. Alonzi, D.S.; Scott, K.A.; Dwek, R.A.; Zitzmann, N. Iminosugar antivirals: The therapeutic sweet spot. *Biochem. Soc. Trans.* **2017**, *45*, 571–582. [CrossRef]
13. Chang, J.; Block, T.M.; Guo, J. Antiviral therapies targeting host ER alpha-glucosidases: Current status and future directions. *Antivir. Res.* **2013**, *99*, 251–260. [CrossRef] [PubMed]
14. Fowler, P.A.; Haines, A.H.; Taylor, R.J.K.; Chrystal, E.J.T.; Gravestock, M.B. Synthesis and biological activity of acyclic analogues of nojirimycin. *J. Chem. Soc. Perkin Trans.* **1994**, *1*, 2229–2235. [CrossRef]
15. Wetherilla, L.F.; Wassona, C.W.; Swinscoea, G.; Kealya, D.; Fosterb, R.; Griffinc, S.; Macdonald, A. Alkyl-imino sugars inhibit the pro-oncogenic ion channel function of humanpapillomavirus (HPV) E5. *Antivir. Res.* **2018**, *158*, 113–121. [CrossRef] [PubMed]
16. Jacob, J.R.; Mansfield, K.; You, J.E.; Tennant, B.C.; Kim, Y.H. Natural iminosugar derivatives of 1-deoxynojirimycin inhibit glycosylation of hepatitis viral envelope proteins. *J. Microbiol.* **2007**, *45*, 431–440. [PubMed]
17. Ouzounov, S.; Mehta, A.; Dwek, R.A.; Block, T.M.; Jordan, R. The combination of interferon α-2b and n-butyl deoxynojirimycin has a greater than additive antiviral effect upon production of infectious bovine viral diarrhea virus (BVDV) in vitro: Implications for hepatitis C virus (HCV) therapy. *Antivir. Res.* **2002**, *55*, 425–435. [CrossRef]
18. Miller, J.L.; Spiro, S.G.; Dowall, S.D.; Taylor, I.; Rule, A.; Alonzi, D.S.; Sayce, A.C.; Wright, E.; Bentley, E.M.; Thom, R.; et al. In Vivo Efficacy of Iminosugars in a Lethal Ebola Virus Guinea Pig Model. *PLoS ONE* **2016**, *11*, 1–18. [CrossRef] [PubMed]
19. Warfield, K.L.; Warren, T.K.; Qiu, X.; Wells, J.; Mire, C.; Geisbert, J.B.; Stuthman, K.S.; Garza, N.L.; Tongeren, S.A.V.; Shurtleff, A.C.; et al. Assessment of the potential for host-targeted iminosugars UV-4 and UV-5 activity against filovirus infections in vitro and in vivo. *Antivir. Res.* **2017**, *138*, 22–31. [CrossRef] [PubMed]
20. Tyrrell, B.E.; Sayce, A.C.; Warfield, K.L.; Miller, J.L.; Zitzmann, N. Iminosugars: Promising therapeutics for influenza infection. *Crit. Rev. Microbiol.* **2017**, *43*, 521–545. [CrossRef] [PubMed]
21. Treston, A.M.; Warfield, K.L. Methods of Treating Zika Virus Infection. PCT Int. App. WO 2017201052 A1, 23 November 2017.
22. Miller, J.L.; Tyrrell, B.E.; Zitzmann, N. Mechanisms of Antiviral Activity of Iminosugars Against Dengue Virus. In *Dengue and Zika: Control and Antiviral Treatment Strategies*; Rolf Hilgenfeld, R., Vasudevan, S.G., Eds.; Springer: Berlin/Heidelberg, Germany, 2018; Volume 1062, pp. 277–301.
23. Sayce, A.C.; Alonzi, D.S.; Killingbeck, S.S.; Tyrrell, B.E.; Hill, M.L.; Caputo, A.T.; Iwaki, R.; Kinami, K.; Ide, D.; Kiappes, J.L.; et al. Iminosugars Inhibit Dengue Virus Production viaInhibition of ER Alpha-Glucosidases Not Glycolipid Processing Enzymes. *PLoS Negl. Trop. Dis.* **2010**, *3*, e0004524. [CrossRef]
24. Tan, A.; Broek, L.V.D.; Boeckel, S.V.; Ploegh, H.; Bolscher, J.J. Chemical modification of the glucosidase inhibitor 1-deoxynojirimycin. Structure-activity relationships. *Biol. Chem.* **1991**, *266*, 14504–14510.

25. Collins, P.; Ferrier, R. *Monosaccharides: Their Chemistry and Their Roles in Natural Products*; Wiley: New York, NY, USA, 1995; pp. 37–38.
26. Sorbera, L.A.; Castaner, J.; Bayes, M. Miglustat. *Drugs Fut.* **2003**, *28*, 229–236. [CrossRef]
27. Asano, N.; Oseki, k.; Kizu, H.; Matsui, K. Nitrogen-in-the-Ring Pyranoses and Furanoses: Structural Basis of Inhibition of Mammalian Glycosidases. *J. Med. Chem.* **1994**, *37*, 3701–3706. [CrossRef] [PubMed]
28. Van den Broek, L.A.G.M.; Vermaas, D.J.; van Kemenade, F.J.; Tan, M.C.C.A.; Rotteveel, F.T.M.; Zandberg, P.; Butters, T.D.; Miedema, F.; Ploegh, H.L.; van Boeckel, C.A.A. Synthesis of oxygen-substituted N-alkyl 1-deoxynojirimycin derivatives: Aza sugar α-glucosidase inhibitors showing antiviral (HIV-1) and immunosuppressive activity. *Recl. Trav. Chim. Pays-Bas* **1994**, *113*, 507–516. [CrossRef]
29. Hines, J.; Chang, H.; Gerdeman, M.S.; Warn, D.E. Isotope edited NMR studies of glycosidases: Design and synthesis of a novel glycosidase inhibitor. *Bioorg. Med. Chem. Lett.* **1999**, *9*, 1255–1260. [CrossRef]
30. Horne, G.; Wilson, F.X.; Tinsley, J.; Williams, D.H.; Storer, R. Iminosugars past, present and future: Medicines for tomorrow. *Drug Discov. Today* **2011**, *16*, 107–118. [CrossRef]
31. Parmeggiani, C.; Catarzi, S.; Matassini, C.; D'Adamio, G. Human Acid β-Glucosidase Inhibition by Carbohydrate Derived Iminosugars: Towards New Pharmacological Chaperones for Gaucher Disease. *ChemBioChem* **2015**, *16*, 2054–2064. [CrossRef]
32. Trapero, A.; Llebaria, A. Glucocerebrosidase inhibitors for the treatment of Gaucher disease. *Future Med. Chem.* **2013**, *5*, 573–590. [CrossRef]
33. Désiré, J.; Mondon, M.; Fontelle, N.; Nakagawa, S.; Hirokami, Y.; Adachi, I.; Iwaki, R.; Fleet, G.W.J.; Alonzi, D.S.; Twigg, G.; et al. N-and C-alkylation of seven-membered iminosugars generates potent glucocerebrosidase inhibitors and F508del-CFTR correctors. *Org. Biomol. Chem.* **2014**, *12*, 8977–8996. [CrossRef]
34. Shih, T.L.; Liang, M.T.; Wu, K.D.; Lin, C.H. Synthesis of polyhydroxy 7-and N-alkyl-azepanes as potent glycosidase inhibitors. *Carbohydr. Res.* **2011**, *346*, 183–190. [CrossRef]
35. Taghzouti, H.; Goumain, S.; Harakat, D.; Portella, C.; Behr, J.B.; Plantier-Royon, R. Synthesis of 2-carboxymethyl polyhydroxyazepanes and their evaluation as glycosidase inhibitors. *Bioorg. Chem.* **2015**, *58*, 11–17. [CrossRef]
36. Nash, R.J.; Kato, A.; Yu, C.Y.; Fleet, G.W. Iminosugars as therapeutic agents: Recent advances and promising trends. *Future Med. Chem.* **2011**, *2011 3*, 513–521. [CrossRef]
37. Brás, N.F.; Cerqueira, N.M.; Ramos, M.J.; Fernandes, P.A. Glycosidase inhibitors: A patent review (2008–2013). *Expert Opin. Ther. Pat.* **2014**, *24*, 857–874. [CrossRef] [PubMed]
38. Asano, N. Iminosugars: The Potential of Carbohydrate Analogs. In *Carbohydrate Chemistry: State of the Art and Challenges for Drug Development*; Cipolla, L., Ed.; University of Milano-Bicocca: Milano, Italy, 2015; Chapter 11; pp. 279–301. [CrossRef]
39. Wadood, A.; Ghufran, M.; Khan, A.; Azam, S.S.; Jelani, M.; Uddin, R. Selective glycosidase inhibitors: A patent review (2012–present). *Int. J. Biol. Macromol.* **2018**, *111*, 82–91. [CrossRef] [PubMed]
40. Asano, N.; Oseki, K.; Kaneko, E.; Matsui, K. Enzymic synthesis of alpha- and beta-D-glucosides of 1-deoxynojirimycin and their glycosidase inhibitory activities. *Carbohydr. Res.* **1994**, *258*, 255–266. [CrossRef]
41. Yoshikuni, Y.; Ezure, Y.; Seto, T.; Mori, K.; Watanabe, M.; Enomoto, H. Synthesis and alpha-glucosidase-inhibiting activity of a new alpha-glucosidase inhibitor, 4-O-alpha-D-glucopyranosylmoranoline and its N-substituted derivatives. *Chem. Pharm. Bull.* **1989**, *37*, 106–109. [CrossRef] [PubMed]
42. Robinson, K.M.; Begovic, M.E.; Rhinehart, B.L.; Heineke, E.W.; Ducep, J.B.; Kastner, P.R.; Marshall, F.N.; Danzin, C. New potent α-glucohydrolase inhibitor MDL 73945 with long duration of action in rats. *Diabetes* **1991**, *40*, 825–830. [CrossRef]
43. Zamoner, L.O.B.; Aragão-Leoneti, V.; Mantoani, S.P.; Rugen, M.D.; Nepogodiev, S.A.; Field, R.A.; Carvalho, I. CuAAC click chemistry with N-propargyl 1,5-dideoxy-1,5-imino-Dgulitol and N-propargyl 1,6-dideoxy-1,6-imino-D-mannitol provides access to triazole-linked piperidine and azepane pseudo-disaccharide iminosugars displaying glycosidase inhibitory properties. *Carbohydr. Res.* **2016**, *429*, 29–37. [CrossRef] [PubMed]
44. Alonzi, D.S.; Dwek, R.A.; Butters, T.D. Improved cellular inhibitors for glycoprotein processinga-glucosidases:biological characterisation of alkyl-and arylalkyl-N-substituted deoxynojirimycins. *Tetrahedron Asymmetry* **2009**, *20*, 897–901. [CrossRef]

45. Poitout, L.; Le Merrer, Y.; Depezay, J.C.L. Polyhydroxylated piperidines and azepanes from D-mannitol synthesis of 1-deoxynojirimycin and analogues. *Tetrahedron Lett.* **1994**, *35*, 3293–3296. [CrossRef]
46. Le Merrer, Y.; Poitout, L.; Depezay, J.C.; Dosbaa, I.; Geoffroy, S.; Foglietti, M. Synthesis of azasugars as potent inhibitors of glycosidases. *Bioorg. Med. Chem.* **1997**, *5*, 519–533. [CrossRef]
47. Wilkinson, B.L.; Bornaghi, L.F.; Lopez, M.; Healy, P.C.; Poulsen, S.; Houston, T.A. Synthesis of N-Propargyl Imino-Sugar Scaffolds for Compound Library Generation using Click Chemistry. *Aust. J. Chem.* **2010**, *63*, 821–829. [CrossRef]
48. Jurczak, J.; Bauer, T.; Chmielewski, M.A. general approach to the synthesis of 2,3-di-O-protected derivatives of D-glyceraldehyde. *Carbohydr. Res.* **1987**, *164*, 493–498. [CrossRef]
49. Aragão-Leoneti, V.; Carvalho, I. Simple and efficient synthesis of 2,5-anhydro-D-glucitol. *Tetrahedron Lett.* **2013**, *54*, 1087–1089. [CrossRef]
50. Jung, M.E.; Lyster, M.A. Quantitative dealkylation of alkyl ethers via treatment with trimethylsilyl iodide. A new method for ether hydrolysis. *J. Org. Chem.* **1977**, *42*, 3761–3764. [CrossRef]
51. Kasai, K.; Okada, K.; Saito, S.; Tokutake, M.; Tobe, K. Preparation of N-substituted-hexahydro-3,4,5,6-tetrahydroxyazepine as Glycosidase Inhibitors. Jpn. Kokai Tokkyo Koho JP 2001002648 A, 9 January 2001.
52. Qian, X.; Morís-Varas, F.; Fitzgerald, M.C.; Wong, C.-H. C_2-Symmetrical Tetrahydroxyazepanes as Inhibitors of Glycosidases and HIV/FIV Proteases. *Bioorg. Med. Chem.* **1996**, *4*, 2055–2069. [CrossRef]
53. Li, H.; Liu, T.; Zhang, Y.; Favre, S.; Pierre, C.B.; Vogel, T.D.B.; Oikonomakos, N.G.; Marrot, J.; Blériot, Y. New Synthetic Seven-Membered 1-Azasugars Displaying Potent Inhibition Towards Glycosidases and Glucosylceramide Transferase. *ChemBioChem* **2008**, *9*, 253–260. [CrossRef] [PubMed]
54. Cendret, V.; Legigan, T.; Mingot, A.; Thibaudeau, S.; Adachi, I.; Forcella, M.; Parenti, P.; Bertrand, J.; Becq, F.; Norez, C.; et al. Synthetic deoxynojirimycin derivatives bearing a thiolated, fluorinated or unsaturated N-alkyl chain: Identification of potent α-glucosidase and trehalase inhibitors as well as F508del-CFTR correctors. *Org. Biomol. Chem.* **2015**, *13*, 10734–10744. [CrossRef]
55. Zhang, Z.X.; Wu, B.; Wang, B.; Li, T.H.; Zhang, P.F.; Guo, L.N.; Wang, W.J.; Zhao, W.; Wang, P.G. Facile and stereo-controlled synthesis of 2-deoxynojirimycin, Miglustat and Miglitol. *Tetrahedron Lett.* **2011**, *52*, 3802–3804. [CrossRef]

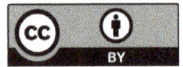

© 2019 by the authors. Licensee MDPI, Basel, Switzerland. This article is an open access article distributed under the terms and conditions of the Creative Commons Attribution (CC BY) license (http://creativecommons.org/licenses/by/4.0/).

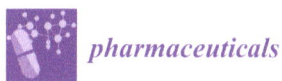

Article

Synthesis and Biological Evaluation of Structurally Varied 5′-/6′-Isonucleosides and Theobromine-Containing *N*-Isonucleosidyl Derivatives

Nuno M. Xavier [1,2,*], Eduardo C. de Sousa [1], Margarida P. Pereira [1,2], Anne Loesche [3], Immo Serbian [3], René Csuk [3] and M. Conceição Oliveira [4]

[1] Centro de Química e Bioquímica, Faculdade de Ciências, Universidade de Lisboa, Ed. C8, 5º Piso, Campo Grande, 1749-016 Lisboa, Portugal
[2] Centro de Química Estrutural, Faculdade de Ciências, Universidade de Lisboa, Ed. C8, 5º Piso, Campo Grande, 1749-016 Lisboa, Portugal
[3] Bereich Organische Chemie, Martin-Luther-Universität Halle-Wittenberg, Kurt-Mothes-Str. 2, D-06120 Halle (Saale), Germany
[4] Centro de Química Estrutural, Instituto Superior Técnico, Universidade de Lisboa, Av. Rovisco Pais, 1049-001 Lisboa, Portugal
* Correspondence: nmxavier@fc.ul.pt; Tel.: +351-217500853

Received: 15 May 2019; Accepted: 27 June 2019; Published: 2 July 2019

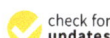

Abstract: Isonucleosides are rather stable regioisomeric analogs of nucleosides with broad therapeutic potential. We have previously demonstrated the ability of 5′ and 6′-isonucleosides to inhibit the activity of acetylcholinesterase, a major target for Alzheimer's disease therapy. Continuing with our research on this topic, we report herein on the synthesis and biological evaluation of a variety of novel terminal isonucleosides and theobromine isonucleotide analogs. Xylofuranose-based purine or uracil 5′-isonucleosides and xylofuranos-5′-yl or glucos-6′-yl theobromine derivatives were accessed via Mitsunobu coupling between partially protected xylofuranose or glucofuranose derivatives with a nucleobase using conventional or microwave-assisted heating conditions. Theobromine-containing *N*-isonucleosidyl sulfonamide and phosphoramidate derivatives were synthesized from isonucleosidyl acetate precursors. The most active compounds in the cholinesterase inhibition assays were a glucopyranose-based theobromine isonucleosidyl acetate, acting as a dual inhibitor of acetylcholinesterase (AChE, K_i = 3.1 μM) and butyrylcholinesterase (BChE, K_i = 5.4 μM), and a 2-*O*,4-*O*-bis-xylofuranos-5′-yl uracil derivative, which displayed moderate inhibition of AChE (K_i = 17.5 μM). Docking studies revealed that the active molecules are positioned at the gorge entrance and at the active site of AChE. None of the compounds revealed cytoxic activity to cancer cells as well as to non-malignant mouse fibroblasts.

Keywords: isonucleosides; theobromine; Mitsunobu reaction; cholinesterase inhibitors

1. Introduction

Isonucleosides are regioisomers of nucleosides in which a nucleobase or an analogous nitrogeneous hetereoaromatic motif is linked to the sugar moiety at a non-anomeric position. This group of structures has attracted significant interest in the search of new nucleos(t)ide analogs, owing to the therapeutic potential of these groups of compounds, especially as anticancer and antiviral agents [1,2]. The lack of an *N*-glycosidic bond in isonucleosides linking the sugar and nucleobase moieties confers them a higher chemical and enzymatic stability than that of nucleosides. Most of the reported isonucleosides possess the nucleobase linked to furanose systems at C-2 or at C-3 [3–11], among which some molecules exhibited anticancer [4,5] or antiviral [6–9,11] activities. Pyranosyl isonucleosides have been relatively less exploited and the few reported examples include 2′-fluoroarabino-2′-yl pyrimidine derivatives [12], which displayed anticancer activities, and pyranos-6′-yl isonucleosides [13,14], which resulted from our previous investigations and showed selective and moderate to good inhibition of acetylcholinesterase (AChE). This enzyme hydrolyses the neurotransmitter acetylcholine and is a main therapeutic target for the symptomatic treatment of Alzheimer's disease (AD) [15,16]. Isonucleosides comprising 2-acetamido-6-chloropurine or theobromine units linked to methyl glucoside moieties and a bis-glucopyranosid-6-yl thymine derivative were the most significant inhibitors with K_i values ranging from 7.1 µM to 4.3 µM. The good inhibitory effect of the theobromine 6′-isonucleoside (**A**, Figure 1) motivated the synthesis of furanosyl analogs, which included an N-isonucleosidyl sulfonamide derivative (**B**, Figure 1) [17]. This isonucleotide analog, in which a sulfonamide is a neutral surrogate and a potential mimetic of a phosphate group, also showed micromolar and selective inhibition of AChE, besides revealing low toxicity in normal fibroblasts and in a neuronal cell, indicating therefore the interest of this type of skeleton in the search for new lead molecules for AD.

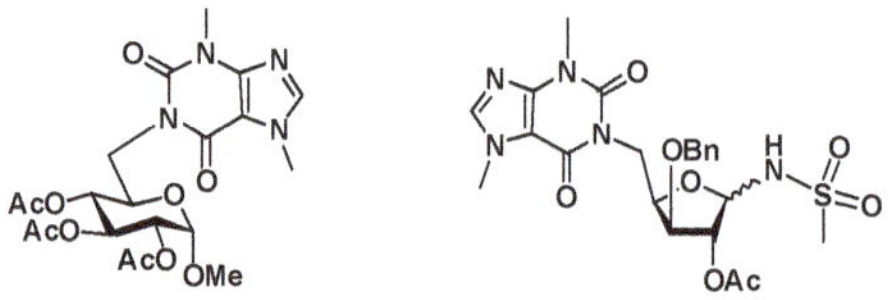

Figure 1. Terminal theobromine isonucleosides, including a glucopyranosid-6′-yl derivative (**A**) and a furanos-5′-yl-based N-isonucleosidyl sulfonamide (**B**), as selective AChE inhibitors.

Encouraged by our previous results, we further explored the synthesis and biological potential of terminal isonucleosides, focusing on furanosyl derivatives and giving further emphasis to theobromine derivatives. We report herein on the synthesis of various xylofuranos-5′-yl purine and uracil derivatives, furanosyl or pyranosyl xylo/gluco-configured terminal theobromine isonucleosides and theobromine N-isonucleosidyl analogs of compound **B** comprising anomeric sulfonamide and phosphoramidate moieties. Molecules possessing a long O-alkyl chain at C-3 (octyl, dodecyl groups), instead of an O-benzyl group present in the previous reported theobromine furanosyl derivatives (such as **B**), were accessed. The presence of the long hydrocarbon chain may enhance the aptitude of the compounds to cross the blood brain barrier, which is a relevant property to consider when planning anti-AD agents [18], particularly if brain AChE is targeted. The ability of the synthesized compounds to inhibit cholinesterases (ChEs) was further evaluated. Moreover, in view of the anticancer potential of nucleos(t)ide analogs, the cytotoxicity of the new isonucleosides on cancer cells was assessed.

2. Results

2.1. Chemistry

The synthesis of 3′-O-dodecyl xylofuranos-5′-yl isonucleosides was based on the Mitsunobu coupling between the 3′-O-dodecyl-1,2-O-isopropylidene xylofuranose precursor (**2**), which was prepared from 3′-O-dodecyl-1,2-O-isopropylidene glucofuranose (**1**) [19], with purine derivatives and uracil in the presence of diethyl azodicarboxylate (DEAD) and triphenylphosphine (Scheme 1). The reaction with the purine alkaloid theobromine in THF at 50 °C during 2 days led to the desired isonucleoside **3** in a low yield (16%). The conversion was significantly improved when performing the reaction under microwave irradiation (MW, 150 W, Pmax 250 Psi) at 65 °C in a mixture of tetrahydrofuran/N,N-dimethylformamide (THF/DMF), conducting to **3** in a satisfactory yield of 44% after only 30 min. The coupling of **2** with adenine was carried out using the above mentioned

MW-assisted protocol, since we have previously observed low conversions even after long reaction times (16–96 h) in the Mitsunobu reaction between this nucleobase and partially protected glucosides under conventional heating [14]. The N^9-xylofuranos-5′-yl adenine **4** was obtained in moderate yield (33%) within 50 min as the sole heterocoupling product, whose N^9-C-5 linkage was determined by HMBC correlations between protons H-5′ and C-4/C-8 of the purine moiety. N^9-regioselectivity also occurred in the coupling between **2** and 2-acetamido-6-chloropurine, which was performed under conventional heating conditions leading to the isonucleoside **5** in 51% yield. Similarly, as for **4**, the HMBC spectra of **5** showed the key correlations between H-5′ and both C-4/C-8 which comproved the regiochemistry of the isonucleosidic bond. In contrast with purines, the Mitsunobu reaction involving uracil afforded different regiosomeric products of both mono- and bis-coupling, an outcome previously found when using pyrimidines in analogous reactions performed under conventional heating [14]. The isonucleosides comprising the uracil moiety linked by N^1 (**6**) and by N^3 (**7**) were obtained in identical yields (12%–13%) and were assigned based on the HMBC correlations of the protons H-5′ with C-2/C-6 or with C-2/C-4, respectively. The distinct chemical shifts for C-5′ in the ^{13}C NMR spectra of **6** and **7**, at 48.1 ppm and at 40.1 ppm, respectively, were additional indicative spectral features for their regiochemical elucidation. The uracil-linked disaccharides N^1,N^3- and 2-*O*,4-*O*-xylofuran-5-yl uracils (**8**, **9**) were formed in yields of 29% and 5%, respectively. Assignment of the N^1,N^3-bis-xylofuranos-5-yl uracil (**8**) was based on its NMR spectral data, which combined the features of both N^1- and N^3-linked isonucleosides, namely through the HMBC correlations between H-5′ protons with C-2/C-6 and between H-5″ with C-2/C-4 as well as the C-5′ and C-5″ resonances at 49.0 ppm and 40.8 ppm, respectively. In the case of the 2,4-bis-*O*-xylofuranos-5-yl uracil derivative (**9**), the ^{1}H NMR and ^{13}C NMR signals of the uracil moiety are deshielded relatively to those of the N^1,N^3-linked regioisomer **8**. The differences between the signals of H-6 and H-5 of the uracil ring are particularly notorious, appearing at 8.18 ppm and 6.41 ppm in **9**, whereas in the case of **8** these protons resonate at 7.24 ppm and 5.69 ppm, respectively. In addition, the signals of C-5′ and C-5″ of the sugar moiety at 64.4 and 64.7 ppm further confirmed their connection to the 2-O and 4-O atoms of the uracil unit.

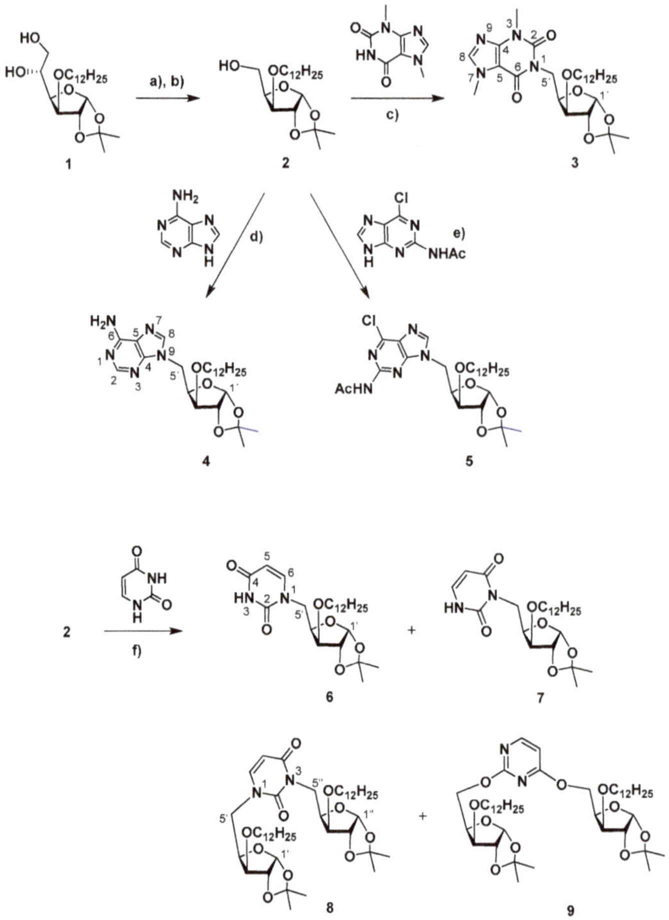

Scheme 1. Reagents and conditions: (**a**) NaIO₄, THF (60 % aq. soln.), room temp., 2.5 h, 79% [19]; (**b**) NaBH₄, EtOH/H₂O, room temp., 1 h, 81% [19]; (**c**) theobromine, PPh₃, diethyl azodicarboxylate (DEAD), THF, 50 °C, 48 h, 16% or THF/DMF, MW, max. 150 W, 65 °C, 30 min, 44%; (**d**) adenine, PPh₃, DEAD, THF/DMF, MW, max. 150 W, 65 °C, 50 min, 31%; (**e**) 2-NHAc-6-Cl-purine, PPh₃, DEAD, THF, 50 °C, 16 h, 51%; (**f**) uracil, PPh₃, DEAD, THF, 50 °C, 18 h, 12% (**6**), 13% (**7**), 29% (**8**), 5% (**9**).

Motivated by our previous studies, which revealed the interest of theobromine isonucleosides as promising lead molecules for AD (Figure 1) [14,17], we further focused our synthetic work on a variety of theobromine derivatives. The theobromine xylofuranosyl isonucleoside **3** was the precursor for the synthesis of isonucleotide analogs via derivatization at the anomeric center (Scheme 2). Thus, **3** was subjected to acid-mediated hydrolysis of the acetonide moiety (aq. trifluoroacetic acid (TFA) 60%), leading to diol **10**. Further acetylation (Ac₂O/pyridine) afforded the isonucleosidyl acetate **11**, which was subsequently converted into *N*-isonucleosidyl derivatives containing polar anomeric moieties capable of hydrogen bond interactions as potential isosteres of a phosphate group. *N*-isonucleosidation of methanesulfonamide with **11** in the presence of BF₃·Et₂O provided the *N*-isonucleosidyl sulfonamide **12** in 81% yield, as a 3-*O*-dodecyl analog of isonucleoside **B** (Figure 1). An anomeric mixture (β/α ratio, 1:0.4) was obtained, which may be a result from the α and β-directing effects exerted by the neighboring acetate group participation and by the remote participation of theobromine carbonyl group, respectively, as well as from anomerization via the acyclic *N*-sulfonyl imine intermediate, as previously described in the synthesis of **B** (Figure 1) [17]. On the other hand, the isonucleosidyl acetate **11** was subjected to MW-assisted anomeric azidation with trimethylsilyl azide (TMSN$_3$), mediated by trimethylsilyl triflate (TMSOTf), leading to the α- and β-isonucleosidyl azides **13** in a 1:0.8 ratio and 86% yield. The formation of the α-anomer is likely to arise also from the above mentioned remote group participation in assisting the isonucleosidyl cation intermediate, an effect already described to influence the stereochemical outcome of the anomeric azidation of glucuronamide derivatives [17,20]. Moreover, the xylonolactone-containing theobromine isonucleoside **14** was formed as a secondary product in 14% yield and was obtained in a mixture containing the β-isonucleosyl azide, the separation of which could not be achieved by column chromatography. The structure of lactone **14** was identified based on its NMR and high resolution mass spectrometry (HRMS) data. HMBC experiments showed correlations between H-2′, which appeared at rather low field (δ = 5.59 ppm), H-3′ and H-4′ with C-1′ (δ = 170 ppm). The mechanism leading to the lactone **14** probably involves the formation of an isonucleosidyl imine intermediate, through nitrogen elimination from the anomeric azide moiety, and subsequent hydrolysis during the workup. The azide **13-α** was engaged in a Staudinger-type reaction with trimethylphosphite to furnish the N-isonucleosidyl phosphoramidate **15** in 56% yield as a 1:0.3 mixture of α- and β-anomers. Despite the α-anomeric configuration of the isonucleosidyl azide precursor, the β-configured product likely arises from anomerization via acyclic N-phosphoryl imine/iminium intermediates.

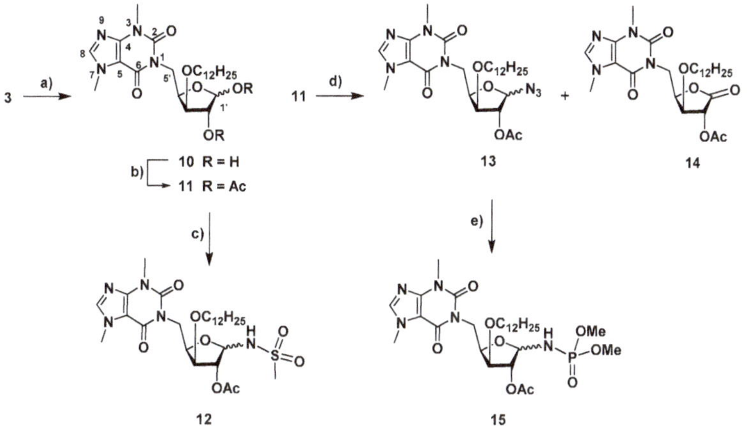

Scheme 2. Reagents and conditions: (**a**) trifluoroacetic acid (TFA) (60% aq. soln.), room temp., 2 h, 83% (α/β = 1:0.9; (**b**) Ac$_2$O, py, room temp., 1.5 h, 69% (α/β = 1:0.5); (**c**) CH$_3$SO$_2$NH$_2$, BF$_3$·Et$_2$O, CH$_2$Cl$_2$/CH$_3$CN, room temp., 2 h, 81% (β/α = 1:0.4); (**d**) trimethylsilyl azide (TMSN$_3$), trimethylsilyl triflate (TMSOTf), CH$_3$CN, 65 °C, MW, max. 150 W, 1 h 40 min, 86% (**13**, β/α ratio, 1:0.8) and 14% (**14**); (**e**) P(OMe)$_3$, CH$_2$Cl$_2$, room temp., 23 h, 56% (α/β = 1:0.3).

Furanosyl and pyranosyl theobromine isonucleosides containing a 3-O-octyl moiety were also synthesized. The 3-O-octyl-1,2-O-isopropylidene glucofuranose precursor (**16**, Scheme 3) was accessed through 3-O-octylation of diacetone-D-glucose with octyl bromide in the presence of sodium hydride and subsequent selective hydrolysis of the primary acetonide (aq. acetic acid 70%). The diol **16** was then subjected to oxidative cleavage with sodium periodate and the resulting aldehyde was reduced (NaBH$_4$) to afford the xylofuranose derivative **17**. The reaction of **17** with theobromine under the MW-assisted Mitsunobu conditions, which was followed by removal of the isopropylidene moiety, gave the xylofuranos-5′-yl theobromine **18**, as an anomeric mixture, in 20% overall yield.

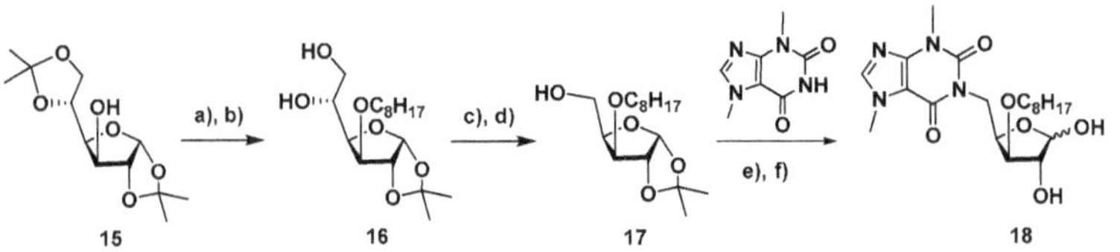

Scheme 3. Reagents and conditions: (**a**) $C_8H_{17}Br$, NaH, DMF, room temp., 22 h; (**b**) AcOH (70% aq. soln.), room temp., 26 h, 88%; 2 steps; (**c**) $NaIO_4$, THF (60% aq. soln.), room temp., 4 h; (**d**) $NaBH_4$, $EtOH/H_2O$, room temp., 1.5 h, 65%, 2 steps; (**e**) theobromine, PPh_3, DEAD, DMF, 65 °C, MW, max. 150 W, 30 min; (**f**) TFA (60% aq. soln.), room temp., 4 h, 20%, 2 steps.

The direct regioselective Mitsunobu coupling of diol **16** with theobromine at C-6 could also be achieved, although in low yield (16%), when carrying out the reaction in refluxing DMF (Scheme 4), while the previously mentioned MW-assisted protocol did not enable significant conversion of **16**. Acid hydrolysis of the obtained glucofuranos-6′-yl theobromine **19** led to the pyranos-6′-yl isonucleoside **20**, the acetylation of which provided the tri-O-acetylated derivative **21**. The regiochemistry of the isonucleosidic linkage (N^1-C-6) in **20** was confirmed by the HMBC correlations between the protons H-6′ and both C-2/C-6. The $BF_3·Et_2O$-mediated reaction of **21** with methanesulfonamide gave the N-isonucleosidyl sulfonamide **22** in 38% yield as an anomeric mixture (β/α ratio, 1:0.4).

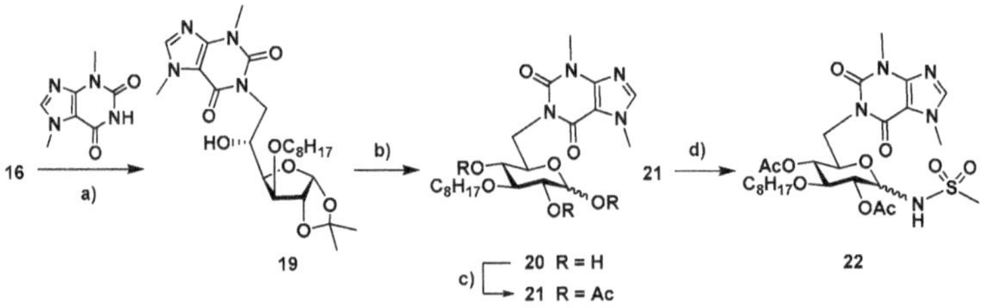

Scheme 4. Reagents and conditions: (**a**) theobromine, PPh_3, DEAD, DMF, reflux, 20 h, 16%; (**b**) TFA (60% aq. soln.), room temp., 5 h, 87% (α/β = 1:0.9); (**c**) Ac_2O, py, room temp., 2.5 h, 84% (α/β = 1:0.7); (**d**) $CH_3SO_2NH_2$, $BF_3·Et_2O$, CH_2Cl_2/CH_3CN, room temp., 3.5 h, 38% (β/α = 1:0.4).

2.2. Biological Evaluation

The newly synthesized xylofuranosyl isonucleosides (**3–10** and **18**), the theobromine-containing isonucleosidyl sulfonamides (**12** and **22**), azide (**13-α**) and phosphoramidate (**15**) and the glucopyranos-6′-yl theobromine derivative **21** were subjected to biological evaluation. Their ability to inhibit the enzymes acetylcholinesterase (AChE, from *Electrophorus electricus*) and butyrylcholinesterase (BChE, from equine serum) was assessed by the Ellman's method. The cholinesterase inhibitor galantamine hydrobromide, which is clinically used for the treatment of AD, was used as a standard. The percent inhibition (at 50 μM) determined for the compounds, the inhibition constants, K_i (for competitive inhibition) or K_i' (for uncompetitive inhibition) for the active molecules, and the respective types of inhibition are compiled in Table 1.

Table 1. Results of the evaluation of the inhibitory activities of the compounds on cholinesterases.

Compound	AChE		BChE	
	% Inhibition [a]	K_i (μM) [K_i' (μM)] (type of inhibition)	% Inhibition [a]	K_i (μM) [K_i' (μM)] (type of inhibition)
Galantamine hydrobromide	96.7	0.2 ± 0.1 (competitive)	86.3	2.4 ± 0.0 (competitive)
Xylofuranos-5′-yl isonucleosides				
Purine derivatives				
4	16.3	n.d.	11.9	n.d.
5	25.3	n.d.	32.5	n.d.
Uracil derivatives				
6	22.5	n.d.	28.5	n.d.
7	17.8	n.d.	7.5	n.d.
8	26.1	n.d.	32.8	n.d.
9	40.3	17.5 ± 0.7 [103.0 ± 4.3] (mixed-type)	29.8	n.d.
Theobromine derivatives				
3	13.8	n.d.	11.7	n.d.
10	2.6	n.d.	22.9	n.d.
13-α	18.9	n.d.	35.0	n.d.
18	14.5	n.d.	19.6	n.d.
Glucopyranos-6′-yl theobromine isonucleoside				
21	66.5	3.1 ± 0.2 [>100] (mixed-type)	75.1	5.4 ± 0.3 [>60] (mixed-type)
Theobromine-containing isonucleotide analogs				
12	1.0	n.d.	4.6	n.d.
15	12.4	n.d.	35.9	n.d.
22	28.3	n.d.	52.6	n.d.

[a] % Inhibition at 50 μM. AChE, acetylcholinesterase; BChE, butyrylcholinesterase.

Among the furanosyl isonucleosides, only the 2-*O*,4-*O*-uracil-linked pseudodisaccharide **9** showed significant effect on the activity of cholinesterases, exhibiting a moderate mixed-type inhibition of AChE, in which the competitive character is more pronounced than the uncompetitive one (K_i = 17.5 μM, K_i' = 103.0 μM, Figure 2). The remaining furanosyl isonucleosides were considered inactive, showing, at 50 μM concentration, less than 40% inhibition of the activity of both enzymes. The theobromine-containing furanosyl isonucleotide analogs (**12**, **15**), containing sulfonamide or phosphoramidate groups, as well the isonucleosidyl azide **13-α**, were also devoid of any inhibitory effects. Given the fact that the previously reported *N*-isonucleosidyl sulfonamide **B** (Figure 1) showed effective inhibition of AChE, the lack of activity of the 3-*O*-dodecylated analog **12** clearly demonstrates that the presence of the 3-*O*-benzyl group in **B** is crucial for its inhibitory activity. In contrast, replacing a 3-*O*-dodecyl by a 3-*O*-octyl group appears not to cause a significant change on the activity of xylofuranos-5′-yl theobromine derivatives, as demonstrated by the similar effects of isonucleosides **10** and **18**.

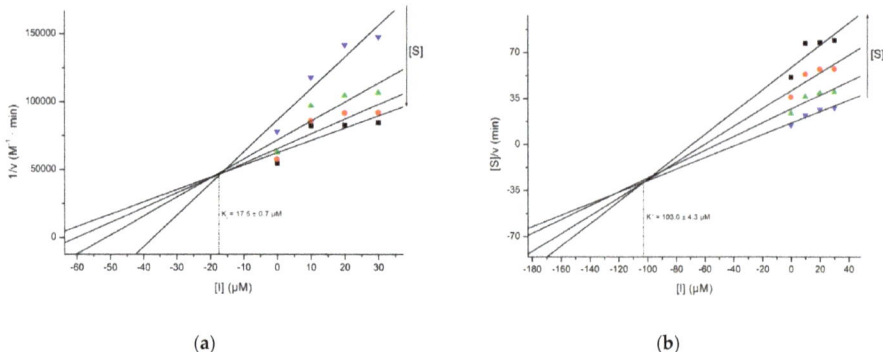

Figure 2. Dixon (**a**) and Cornish–Bowden (**b**) plots for the inhibition of AChE by compound **9**.

With respect to glucopyranos-6′-yl theobromine isonucleosides, the isonucleosidyl acetate **21** displayed noteworthy inhibitory effects on both cholinesterases. It was the most active compound of the series, exhibiting dual inhibition of AChE and BChE by a mixed-type mechanism with a dominant competitive component, with single digit micromolar K_i values (Figure 3) that are at least ca. 32-fold (K_i = 3.1 µM) and 11-fold lower (K_i = 5.4 µM) than their K_i' values, respectively. It was only twice less active than the standard galantamine hydrobromide on BChE. The inhibition of BChE may provide therapeutic benefits in AD, since an increasing activity of this enzyme with accompanying decreasing levels of its congener AChE occurs over the course of the disease. Thus, the brain acetylcholine levels became gradually dependent on BChE [21] and a dual AChE/BChE inhibition or a selective BChE inhibition may provide a more effective treatment in advanced stages of AD. The N-isonucleosidyl sulfonamide **22** was a weaker cholinesterase inhibitor than its precursor **21**, displaying selective effect towards BChE with 53% inhibition of the enzymatic activity at 50 µM.

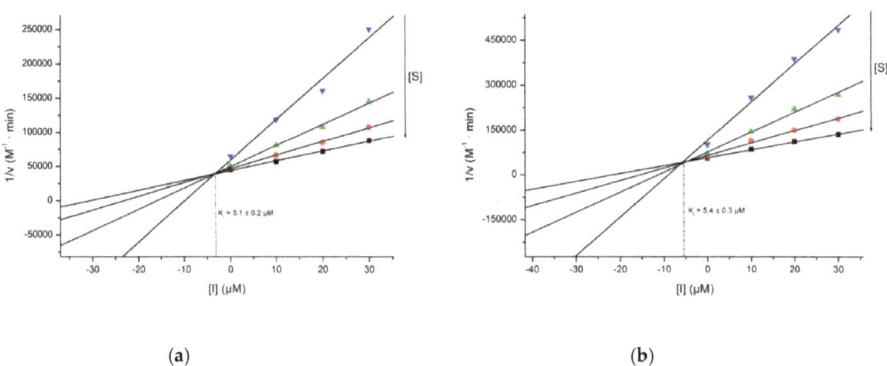

Figure 3. Dixon plots for the inhibition of AChE (**a**) and BChE (**b**) by compound **21**.

The compounds were tested for their cytotoxicity against human cancer cell lines, namely A375 (epithelial melanoma), A2780 (ovarian carcinoma), HT29 (colorectal adenocarcinoma), MCF7 (breast adenocarcinoma) and SW1736 (thyroid carcinoma), as well as towards non-malignant mouse embryonic fibroblasts (NIH 3T3), using the sulforhodamine-B (SRB) colorimetric assay. None of the molecules revealed cytotoxic effects at concentrations below 30 µM (cut-off of the assay) to either cancer or healthy cells, being therefore considered inactive (EC_{50} > 30 µM) against the tested cell lines.

2.3. Molecular Docking Studies

To further understand the binding interactions on a molecular level of compounds **9** and **21**, a molecular docking was performed with Autodock 4 [22]. The crystal structures of AChE (PDB: 1C2O) and BChE (PDB: 6EMI) were retrieved from the RCSB Protein Databank. Due to its anomeric mixture, compound **21** was docked as α and β anomers.

Concerning the AChE docking results, **21-β** outperformed compounds **21-α** and **9** significantly (Figure 4). With respect to the docking positions of **21-β**, this compound seems to fit quite nicely into the entrance of the cavity, where the theobromine moiety is positioned at the entrance of the active site gorge, pointing towards the enzyme's binding pocket (Figure 5). The main interaction of the theobromine unit is with Tyr124 at the peripheral anionic site (PAS), which appears to be based on an O–H···N hydrogen bond with one of the theobromine nitrogen atoms. The tri-*O*-acetylated glucopyranosyl unit is located in front of the binding pocket, where the acetyl groups bind via N–H···O hydrogen bonds to Trp286 at the PAS and Arg296, located between the acyl pocket and the PAS, or Phe295 at the acyl binding pocket, where the N–H···O binding cannot be differentiated between these residues.

AChE			BChE			
9	21-α	21-β	9	21-α	21-β	
−7.86	−7.89	−9.75	−7.82	−7.66	−7.78	Lowest values
−7.24	−7.64	−9.17	−6.85	−7.59	−7.76	
−7.22	−7.38	−8.94	−6.36	−7.42	−7.34	
−7.19	−7.35	−8.93	−6.07	−7.35	−7.2	
−6.26	−7.34	−8.8	−5.98	−7.18	−7.19	
−6.2	−7.33	−8.79	−5.69	−6.89	−7	
−5.29	−7.21	−8.62	−5.59	−6.88	−6.91	
−4.55	−7.21	−8.54	−5.18	−6.71	−6.8	
−4.43	−7.19	−8.54	−5.07	−6.7	−6.78	Highest values
−4.12	−7.1	−8.5	−4.85	−6.7	−6.75	

Figure 4. Binding energies (kcal/mol) of the top docking poses of compounds **9**, **21-α** and **21-β** into AChE and BChE.

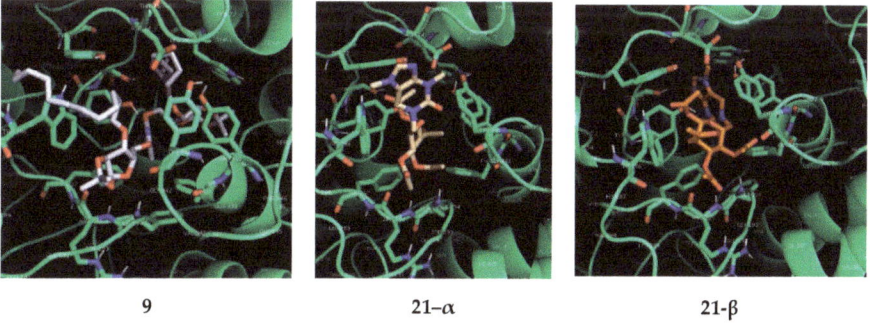

        9   21–α   21–β

Figure 5. Lowest-energy binding poses of compounds **9**, **21-α** and **21-β** to AChE.

In compound **21-α**, the conformation however hinders the theobromine moiety to enter the active site and give a favorable binding position (Figure 5). Therefore, the theobromine system is mainly located outside of the active site of AChE, establishing as key interaction an O–H···Ar π-interaction with Tyr72 at the PAS. Another strong binding occurs with one of the acetyl groups with Phe294.

The docking of compound **9** (Figure 5) shows a strong O–H···N interaction of Tyr124 at the PAS with one of the pyrimidines nitrogens. Herein it seems that compound **9** is able to enter the binding pocket where one half fills the cavity of the AChE active site while the other furanosyl moiety sticks out and blocks the entrance of the binding pocket, where Phe295 shows an O–H···O binding to the furanosyl oxygen.

The docking of **9**, **21-α** and **21-β** in the structure of BChE resulted in quite similar results, whereas the binding interactions of compound **9** in comparison to **21** fall off significantly (see Figure S20, in the Supplementary Materials). The best docking position however shows a strong binding from π-stacking of the pyrimidine moiety of **9** with Tyr332. This also is a major binding mode of **21-β** as this compound also shows a strong π-stacking interaction of the theobromine moiety with Tyr332 and weak interactions of the acetyl groups with sidechains present in the active site of BChE. Compound **21-α** shows an interaction of the theobromine nitrogens with the peptide carbonyl of Leu286 and Ser287. However, for the BChE active site, it is difficult to identify strong interactions between the inhibitors and its amino acid residues.

3. Discussion

A variety of novel terminal isonucleosides embodying purine derivatives or uracil were synthesized using the Mitsunobu coupling as a key step. Microwave irradiation proved to be a useful tool in the Mitsunobu reaction between 3-O-dodecyl/octyl-1,2-O-isopropylidene xylofuranose with theobromine or adenine, enabling the access to 5′-isonucleosides in shorter reaction times (30-50 min) than those needed in conventional stirring for analogous reactions (>16 h) and in moderate yields. In the case of the synthesis of the 3′-O-dodecyl-xylofuranos-5′-yl theobromine derivative **3**, a significant increase on the reaction yield (from 16% to 44%) was achieved using MW-assisted heating. Potential nucleotide mimetics, namely theobromine-based N-isonucleosidyl sulfonamides or an N-isonucleosidyl phosphoramidate, which is a previously unreported type of structure, were synthesized through anomeric functionalization of isonucleosidyl acetates, whose stereochemical outcome was influenced by the remote participating effect of the theobromine carbonyl groups.

Biological evaluation revealed the ability of a theobromine isonucleosidyl acetate possessing a glucopyranose moiety (**21**) to inhibit both AChE and BChE at single-digit micromolar concentrations, reinforcing the potential of theobromine isonucleosides as cholinesterase inhibitors. Since the anomeric mixture was evaluated, it appears that **21-β** accounts more for the detected competitive inhibitory effect on AChE, as indicated by the docking simulations. The theobromine unit in **21-β** as well as the sugar moiety are important for the binding to the enzyme, establishing interactions at the PAS and at the front of the active site, respectively.

The N-isonucleosidyl sulfonamide derivative (**22**) showed significantly weaker effects than its precursor **21**, a result which is in contrast with our previous findings that suggested that an anomerically linked sulfonamide moiety, namely in compound **B** (Figure 1), would lead to an increase on the AChE inhibitory ability of the theobromine isonucleoside. This result as well as the lack of activity of the 3-O-dodecyl theobromine N-isonucleosidyl sulfonamide **12** indicate that the 3-O-substituent and the sugar ring system in these types of molecules also account for their ChE inhibitory abilities. A uracil-linked pseudodisaccharide (**9**) was the only xylofuranose-based isonucleoside which showed significant ChE inhibitory effect, with selective and moderate activity on AChE, which further demonstrate the AChE inhibitory potential of molecules based on this type of skeleton, notwithstanding its large size. Similarly, to a thymine-linked pseudodisaccharide previously described as a competitive AChE inhibitor [14], the interactions between compound **9** and the enzyme seem also to span both the PAS and the active site, with half of the molecule blocking the entrance to the active site gorge and the pyrimidine unit being involved in a key interaction.

The lack of cytotoxicity of the tested molecules to either cancer or non-malignant cells reflects the lower propensity of terminal nucleosides than non-terminal ones to exhibit cytotoxic effects. It is known that 2′-isonucleosides can be, although in a low extend, intracellularly phosphorylated at the primary hydroxyl group by kinases [9,23] and that isonucleoside triphosphates can be recognized by DNA polymerases and be incorporated into the growing DNA chain arresting its elongation [24], similarly to the mechanism of action of the known anticancer nucleosides [1,2]. The absence of a terminal hydroxyl group able for phosphorylation in these newly synthesized 5′-/6′-isonucleosides precludes them to undergo such biological pathway which eventually would lead to cytotoxic effects.

Nevertheless, the non-toxicity of these molecules to healthy cells motivates studies focusing on other biological properties to further explore their therapeutic interest.

4. Materials and Methods

4.1. Chemistry

4.1.1. General Methods

The progress of the reactions was checked by thin layer chromatography (TLC) using silica gel aluminum plates (Merck 60 F_{254}) with visualization under UV light (254 nm) and/or by immersion in a 10% H_2SO_4 solution in ethanol or in a solution of cerium (IV) sulfate (0.2% w/v) and ammonium molybdate (5% w/v) in H_2SO_4 (6% aq.) followed by heating (200 °C). Microwave experiments were carried out in a CEM Discover SP Microwave Synthesizer. Flash column chromatography was performed on silica gel 60 G (0.040–0.063 mm, E. Merck). Optical rotations (589 nm, 20 °C) were measured on a Perkin–Elmer 343 polarimeter. NMR spectra were acquired using a BRUKER Avance 400 spectrometer operating at 400.13 MHz for ^1H or 100.62 MHz for ^{13}C. The chemical shifts are given in parts per million (ppm). The spectra were calibrated with internal TMS (in the case of ^1H NMR spectra in CDCl$_3$) or with the respective solvent residual peak. Coupling constants (J) are given in hertz (Hz). Assignments were made with the help of 2D experiments (COSY, HSQC, HMBC). HRMS spectra were acquired with a QqTOF Impact II mass spectrometer (Bruker Daltonics) equipped with an electrospray ion source (ESI) and were recorded in positive mode.

Synthesis of compound **2** was previously described [19].

4.1.2. General Procedure for the Mitsunobu Coupling of 3-O-Octyl/Dodecyl-1,2-O-isopropylidene-α-D-xylo/glucofuranose (**2**, **17**) with Purine Derivatives/Uracil

To a solution of partially protected 1,2-O-isopropylidene-α-D-xylo/glucofuranose (1 mmol) in THF (28 mL) or DMF (10 mL) under nitrogen atmosphere, PPh$_3$ (2 equiv.), diethyl azodicarboxylate (DEAD, 2 equiv.) and purine derivative/uracil (2 equiv.) were added. The mixture was stirred under the conditions indicated further. The mixture was concentrated under vacuum and the crude residue was subjected to column chromatography.

4.1.3. General Microwave-Assisted Procedure for the Mitsunobu Coupling of 3-O-Octyl/Dodecyl-1,2-O-isopropylidene-α-D-xylofuranose (**2**, **17**) with Theobromine/Adenine

To a solution of partially protected 1,2-O-isopropylidene-α-D-xylofuranose (0.2 mmol) in THF/DMF (1:1, 2 mL) or DMF (2 mL), PPh$_3$ (2 equiv.), diethyl azodicarboxylate (DEAD, 2 equiv.) and theobromine (2 equiv.) were sequentially added. The mixture was stirred under microwave irradiation (150 W max., P max = 250 Psi) at 65 °C for 30–50 min. The solvent was evaporated, and the crude residue was subjected to column chromatography on silica-gel.

4.1.4. 1-(5-Deoxy-3-O-dodecyl-1,2-O-isopropylidene-α-D-xylofuranos-5-yl)-3,7-dimethyl-3,7-dihydro-1H-purine-2,6-dione (3)

Obtained according to the general procedure for Mitsunobu coupling, starting from compound **2** (328 mg, 0.916 mmol), theobromine (340 mg, 1.89 mmol) and using PPh$_3$ (502 mg, 1.91 mmol) and DEAD (40% wt. soln. in toluene, 0.89 mL, 1.95 mmol) in THF (25 mL). The reaction mixture was stirred at 50 °C for 48 h. Purification by column chromatography (from AcOEt/hexane 1:1 to 4:1) afforded **5** (76 mg, 16%) as a yellow oil.

Alternatively, the title compound could be obtained using the MW-assisted procedure, starting from compound **2** (79 mg, 0.219 mmol), theobromine (80 mg, 0.44 mmol) and using PPh$_3$ (115 mg, 0.43 mmol) and DEAD (40% wt. soln. in toluene, 0.2 mL, 0.44 mmol) in THF/DMF (1:1, 2 mL), within a reaction mixture of 30 min and in 44% yield (50 mg). $[\alpha]_D^{20}$ = −5 (c = 1, in CH$_2$Cl$_2$). ^{1}H NMR (CDCl$_3$, 400 MHz): δ 7.49 (s, 1H, H-8), 5.97 (d, 1 H, H-1′, $J_{1',2'}$ = 3.9), 4.74 (dd, 1 H, H-5′a, $J_{4',5'a}$ = 8.8, $J_{5'a,5'b}$ = 14.1), 4.59–4.52 (m, 2 H, H-2′, H-4′), 3.99–3.91 (m, 4 H, CH$_3$, N^7, H-5′b, $J_{4',5'b}$ = 1.8), 3.90 (d, 1 H, H-3′, $J_{3',4'}$ = 3.4), 3.69–3.59 (m, 1 H, H-1″a), 3.56 (s, 3 H, CH$_3$-N^3), 3.48–3.38 (ddd, H-1″b), 1.62–1.51 (m 2 H, CH$_2$-2″), 1.43 (s, 3 H, CH$_3$, i-Pr), 1.38–1.16 (m, 21 H, CH$_2$-3″ to CH$_2$-11″, CH$_3$, i-Pr), 0.86 (t, 3 H, CH$_3$-12″, J = 6.7). ^{13}C NMR (CDCl$_3$, 100 MHz): δ 155.4 (C-6), 151.7 (C-2), 148.9 (C-4), 141.5 (C-8), 111.5 (Cq, i-Pr), 107.9 (C-5), 105.3 (C-1′), 83.5 (C-3′), 82.5 (C-2′), 78.6 (C-4′), 70.5 (CH$_2$-1″), 40.0 (C-5′), 33.7 (CH$_3$, N^7), 32.1 (CH$_2$-2″), 29.8, 29.8, 29.8, 29.8, 29.7, 29.6, 29.5, 26.8 (CH$_3$, N^3, CH$_2$-3″ to CH$_2$-10″), 26.3, 26.3 (2 × CH$_3$, i-Pr), 22.8 (CH$_2$-11″), 14.3 (CH$_3$-12″). HRMS: calcd for C$_{27}$H$_{44}$N$_4$O$_6$ [M + H]$^+$ 521.3334, found 521.3333; calcd for C$_{27}$H$_{44}$N$_4$O$_6$ [M + Na]$^+$ 543.3153, found 543.3149.

4.1.5. 9-(5-Deoxy-3-O-dodecyl-1,2-O-isopropylidene-α-D-xylofuranos-5-yl)adenine (4)

Obtained according to the general MW-assisted procedure for Mitsunobu coupling, starting from compound **2** (80 mg, 0.22 mmol), adenine (60 mg, 0.44 mmol) and using PPh$_3$ (117 mg, 0.44 mmol) and DEAD (40% wt. soln. in toluene, 0.2 mL, 0.44 mmol), in THF/DMF (1:1, 2 mL). The reaction mixture was stirred for 50 min. Purification by column chromatography (from AcOEt/cyclohexane 2:1 to AcOEt) afforded **4** (33 mg, 31%) as a colorless oil. ^{1}H NMR (CDCl$_3$, 400 MHz): δ 8.36 (s, 1 H, H-2), 7.93 (s, 1 H, H-8), 5.96 (d, 1 H, H-1′, $J_{1',2'}$ = 3.6), 5.69 (br.s, 2 H, NH$_2$), 4.52 (d, 1 H, H-1′, $J_{1',2'}$ = 3.2), 4.64–4.50 (m, 3 H, H-2′, H-5′a, H-4′), 4.35 (dd, 1 H, H-5′b, $J_{5'a,5'b}$ = 15.9, $J_{4',5'b}$ = 10.0), 3.87 (d, 1 H, H-3′, $J_{2',3'}$ = 2.8), 3.69–3.60 (m, 1 H, H-1″a), 3.47–3.38 (m, 1 H, H-1″b), 1.62–1.53 (m 2 H, CH$_2$-2″), 1.42–1.20 (m, 26 H, CH$_2$-3″ to CH$_2$-11″, 2 × CH$_3$, i-Pr), 0.87 (t, 4.2 H, CH$_3$-12″, J = 6.7). ^{13}C NMR (CDCl$_3$, 100MHz): δ 155.4 (C-6), 153.0 (C-2), 150.3 (C-4), 141.7 (C-8), 119.6 (C-5), 112.0 (Cq, i-Pr), 105.3 (C-1′), 82.7 (C-3′), 82.2 (C-2′), 78.4 (C-4′), 70.6 (CH$_2$-1″), 42.9 (C-5′), 32.1 (CH$_2$-2″), 29.8, 29.8, 29.8, 29.8, 29.7, 29.6, 29.5, 26.9, 26.3, 26.3, 22.8 (CH$_2$-3″ to CH$_2$-11″, 2 × CH$_3$, i-Pr), 14.3 (CH$_2$-12″). HRMS: calcd for C$_{25}$H$_{41}$N$_5$O$_4$ [M + H]$^+$ 476.3231, found 476.3226. calcd for C$_{25}$H$_{41}$N$_5$O$_4$ [M + Na]$^+$ 498.3051, found 498.3043.

4.1.6. 2-Acetamido-6-chloro-9-(5-deoxy-3-O-dodecyl-1,2-O-isopropylidene-α-D-xylofuranos-5-yl)purine (5)

Obtained according to the general procedure for Mitsunobu coupling, starting from compound **2** (337 mg, 0.94 mmol), 2-acetamido-6-chloropurine (399 mg, 1.88 mmol) and using PPh$_3$ (504 mg, 1.92 mmol) and DEAD (40% wt. soln. in toluene, 0.82 mL, 1.8 mmol) in THF (25 mL). The reaction mixture was stirred at 50 °C for 16 h. Purification by column chromatography (from AcOEt/petroleum ether 1:2) afforded **5** (265 mg, 51%) as a yellow oil.

$[\alpha]_D^{20}$ = −14 (c = 1, in CH$_2$Cl$_2$). ^{1}H NMR (400 MHz, CDCl$_3$) δ 8.11 (s, 1 H, H-8), 5.95 (d, 1 H, H-1′, $J_{1',2'}$ = 3.7), 4.60 (d, 1 H, H-2′), 4.56–4.46 (m, 2 H, H-4′, H-5′a), 4.39 (dd, 1 H, H-5′b, $J_{4',5'b}$ = 9.0, $J_{5'a,5'b}$ = 15.0), 3.85 (d, 1 H, H-3′, $J_{3',4'}$ = 3.0), 3.68–3.58 (m, 1 H, H-1″a), 3.45–3.35 (ddd, H-1″b), 2.54 (s, 3 H, CH$_3$, NHAc), 1.60–1.49 (m 2 H, CH$_2$-2″), 1.40 (s, 3 H, CH$_3$, i-Pr), 1.36–1.16 (m, 21 H, CH$_2$-3″ to CH$_2$-11″, CH$_3$, i-Pr), 0.87 (t, 3 H, CH$_3$-12″, J = 6.7). ^{13}C NMR (100 MHz, CDCl$_3$) δ: 153.0 (C-4), 152.0, 151.3 (C-2, C-6), 145.7 (C-8), 128.0 (C-5), 112.2 (Cq, i-Pr), 105.3 (C-1′), 82.6 (C-3′), 82.0 (C-2′), 77.8 (C-4′), 70.6 (CH$_2$-1″), 43.2 (C-5′), 32.0 (CH$_2$-2″), 29.8, 29.8, 29.8, 29.8, 29.7, 29.6, 29.5, 26.9 (CH$_2$-3″ to CH$_2$-10″), 26.3, 26.2 (2 ×

CH$_3$, i-Pr), 25.3 (CH$_3$, NHAc), 22.8 (CH$_2$-11″), 14.3 (CH$_3$-12″). HRMS: calcd for C$_{27}$H$_{42}$ClN$_5$O$_5$ [M + H]$^+$ 552.2947, found 552.2957; calcd for C$_{27}$H$_{42}$ClN$_5$O$_5$ [M + Na]$^+$ 574.2767, found 574.2778.

4.1.7. 1-(5-Deoxy-3-O-dodecyl-1,2-O-isopropylidene-α-D-xylofuranos-5-yl)uracil (**6**), 3-(5-deoxy-3-O-dodecyl-1,2-O-isopropylidene-α-D-xylofuranos-5-yl)uracil (**7**), 1,3-bis-(5-deoxy-3-O-dodecyl-1,2-O-isopropylidene-α-D-xylofuranos-5-yl)uracil (**8**) and 2,4-bis-O-(5-deoxy-3-O-dodecyl-1,2-O-isopropylidene-α-D-xylofuranos-5-yl)uracil (**9**)

Obtained according to the general procedure for Mitsunobu coupling, starting from compound **2** (286 mg, 0.798 mmol), uracil (182 mg, 1.62 mmol) and using PPh$_3$ (425 mg, 1.62 mmol) and DEAD (40% wt. soln. in toluene, 0.7 mL, 1.54 mmol) in THF (25 mL). The reaction mixture was stirred at 50 °C for 18 h. Purification by column chromatography (from AcOEt/petroleum ether 1:5 to AcOEt) afforded **9** (17 mg, 5%), **8** (91 mg, 29%), **6** (42 mg, 12%) and **7** (46 mg, 13%) as colorless oils.

Compound **6**: $[\alpha]_D^{20}$ = −2 (c = 1, in CH$_2$Cl$_2$). ^{1}H NMR (CDCl$_3$, 400 MHz): δ 8.99 (s, 1 H, NH), 7.30 (d, 1 H, H-6, $J_{5,6}$ = 7.9), 5.91 (d, 1 H, H-1′, $J_{1',2'}$ = 3.7), 5.66 (d, 1 H, H-5), 4.56 (d, 1 H, H-2′), 4.41 (dt, 1 H, H-4′, $J_{4',5'b}$ = 8.8), 4.33 (dd, 1 H, H-5′a, $J_{4',5'a}$ = 2.6, $J_{5'a,5'b}$ = 14.6), 3.85 (d, 1 H, H-3′, $J_{3',4'}$ = 3.2), 3.69–3.57 (m, 2 H, H-1″a, H-5′b), 3.44–3.34 (ddd, H-1″b), 1.60–1.50 (m 2 H, CH$_2$-2″), 1.46 (s, 3 H, CH$_3$, i-Pr), 1.34–1.18 (m, 21 H, CH$_2$-3″ to CH$_2$-11″, CH$_3$, i-Pr), 0.87 (t, 3 H, CH$_3$-12″, J = 6.7). ^{13}C NMR (CDCl$_3$, 100MHz): δ 163.8 (C-4), 151.1 (C-2), 145.7 (C-6), 112.1 (Cq, i-Pr), 105.2 (C-1′), 102.1 (C-5), 82.9 (C-3′), 82.2 (C-2′), 78.1 (C-4′), 70.6 (CH$_2$-1″), 48.1 (C-5′), 32.0 (CH$_2$-2″), 29.8, 29.8, 29.8, 29.7, 29.7, 29.5, 29.5, 26.8 (CH$_2$-3″ to CH$_2$-10″) 26.3, 26.2 (2 × CH$_3$, i-Pr), 22.8 (CH$_2$-11″), 14.3 (CH$_3$-12″). HRMS: calcd for C$_{24}$H$_{40}$N$_2$O$_6$ [M + Na]$^+$ 475.2779, found 475.2782; calcd for C$_{24}$H$_{40}$N$_2$O$_6$ [M + H]$^+$ 453.2959, found 453.2962.

Compound **7**: $[\alpha]_D^{20}$ = +6 (c = 1, in CH$_2$Cl$_2$). ^{1}H NMR (CDCl$_3$, 400 MHz): δ 9.98 (br.d, 1 H, NH), 7.20 (dd, 1 H, H-6, $J_{NH,6}$ = 5.8, $J_{5,6}$ = 7.6), 5.94 (d, 1 H, H-1′, $J_{1',2'}$ = 3.8), 5.72 (dd, 1 H, H-5, $J_{NH,5}$ = 1.2, $J_{5,6}$ = 7.6), 4.59–4.46 (m, 3 H, H-2′, H-4′, H-5′a), 4.00–3.90 (m, 1 H, H-5′b) 3.88 (d, 1 H, H-3′, $J_{3',4'}$ = 2.4), 3.68–3.59 (m, 2 H, H-1″a), 3.47–3.37 (ddd, H-1″b), 1.64–1.51 (m 2 H, CH$_2$-2″), 1.45 (s, 3 H, CH$_3$, i-Pr), 1.37–1.16 (m, 21 H, CH$_2$-3″ to CH$_2$-11″, CH$_3$, i-Pr), 0.86 (t, 3 H, CH$_3$-12″, J = 6.7). ^{13}C NMR (CDCl$_3$, 400 MHz): δ 163.6 (C-4), 153.0 (C-2), 139.1 (C-6), 111.7 (Cq, i-Pr), 105.2 (C-1′), 102.0 (C-5), 83.3 (C-3′), 82.4 (C-2′), 78.2 (C-4′), 70.6 (CH$_2$-1″), 40.1 (C-5′), 32.0 (CH$_2$-2″), 29.8, 29.8, 29.8, 29.8, 29.7, 29.6, 29.5, 26.8 (CH$_2$-3″ to CH$_2$-10″), 26.3, 26.2 (2 × CH$_3$, i-Pr), 22.8 (CH$_2$-11″), 14.3 (CH$_3$-12″). HRMS: calcd for C$_{24}$H$_{40}$N$_2$O$_6$ [M + Na]$^+$ 475.2779, found 475.2788; calcd for C$_{24}$H$_{40}$N$_2$O$_6$ [M + H]$^+$ 453.2959, found 453.2969.

Compound **8**: $[\alpha]_D^{20}$ = −4 (c = 1, in CH$_2$Cl$_2$). ^{1}H NMR (CDCl$_3$, 400 MHz): δ 7.24 (d, 1 H, H-6, $J_{5,6}$ = 7.9), 5.93, 5.90 (2 d, 2 H, H-1′, H-1″, $J_{1',2'}$ = 3.8, $J_{1'',2''}$ = 3.8), 5.69 (d, 1 H, H-5), 4.63–4.46 (m, 4 H, H-5″a, H-2′ H-2″, H-4″), 4.44 (ddd, 1 H, H-4′), 4.31 (dd, 1 H, H-5′a, $J_{5'a,5'b}$ = 14.7, $J_{4',5'a}$ = 2.6), 3.92 (dd, 1 H, H-5″b, $J_{5''a,5''b}$ = 13.8, $J_{4'',5''a}$ = 1.6), 3.86 (d, 1 H, H-3″, $J_{3'',4''}$ = 3.3), 3.82 (d, 1 H, H-3′, $J_{3',4'}$ = 3.1), 3.68–3.55 (m, 3 H, H-5′b, H-1‴a, H-1⁗a), 3.46–3.32 (m, 2 H, H-1‴b, H-1⁗b), 1.60–1.49 (m 4 H, CH$_2$-2‴, CH$_2$-2⁗) 1.45, 1.43 (2 s, 2 × 3 H, 2 × CH$_3$, i-Pr), 1.35–1.16 (m, 42 H, CH$_2$-3‴ to CH$_2$-11‴, CH$_2$-3⁗ to CH$_2$-11⁗, 2 × CH$_3$, i-Pr), 0.86 (t, 3 H, CH$_3$-12‴, CH$_3$-12⁗, J = 6.7). ^{13}C NMR (CDCl$_3$, 100MHz): δ 163.2 (C-4), 151.9 (C-2), 143.4 (C-6), 112.0, 111.5 (Cq, i-Pr), 105.3, 105.3, (C-1′, C-1″), 101.8 (C-5), 83.5 (C-3″), 82.9 (C-3′), 82.4, 82.1 (C-2′, C-2″), 78.3 (C-4′), 78.1 (C-4″), 70.5 (CH$_2$-1‴, CH$_2$-1⁗), 49.0 (C-5′), 40.8 (C-5″), 32.0 (CH$_2$-2‴, CH$_2$-2⁗), 29.8, 29.8, 29.8, 29.7, 29.7, 29.7, 29.7, 29.6, 29.5, 29.5, 29.5, 26.8 (CH$_2$-3‴ to CH$_2$-10‴, CH$_2$-3⁗ to CH$_2$-10⁗), 26.3, 26.3, 26.2, 26.2 (4 × CH$_3$, i-Pr), 22.8 (CH$_2$-11‴, CH$_2$-11⁗), 14.3 (CH$_3$-12‴, CH$_3$-12⁗). HRMS: calcd for C$_{44}$H$_{76}$N$_2$O$_{10}$ [M + Na]$^+$ 815.5392, found 815.5420; calcd for C$_{44}$H$_{76}$N$_2$O$_{10}$ [M + H]$^+$ 793.5573, found 793.5584.

Compound **9**: $[\alpha]_D^{20}$ = −31 (c = 1, in CH$_2$Cl$_2$). ^{1}H NMR (CDCl$_3$, 400 MHz): δ = 8.18 (d, 1H, H-6, J = 5.7), 6.41 (d, 1 H, H-5), 5.97–5.92 (m, 2 H, H-1′, H-1″, J = 3.9, J = 4.2), 4.69 (dd, 1H, H-5′a, $J_{5a,5b}$ = 10.5, $J_{4,5a}$ = 3.9), 4.63–4.42 (m, 7 H, H-2′, H-2″, H-4′, H-4″, H-5′b, H-5″a, H-5″b), 3.95, 3.89 (2 d, 2 × 1 H, H-3′, H-3″, J = 2.2 Hz, J = 2.8), 3.66–3.52 (m, 2 H, H-1‴a, H-1⁗a), 3.48–3.36 (m, 2 H, H-1‴b, H-1⁗b), 1.59–1.45 (m, 10 H, 2 × CH$_3$, i-Pr, CH$_2$-2‴, CH$_2$-2⁗); 1.36–1.14 (m, 42 H, 2 × CH$_3$, i-Pr, CH$_2$-3‴ to CH$_2$-11‴, CH$_2$-3⁗ to CH$_2$-11⁗); 0,87 (t, 6 H, CH$_3$-12‴, CH$_3$-12⁗, J = 6.5) ppm. ^{13}C NMR (CDCl$_3$, 400

MHz): δ 170.9 (C-4), 164.8 (C-2), 158.7 (C-6), 111.9, 111.8 (2 × Cq, *i*-Pr), 105.4, 105.3 (C-1', C-1''), 102.54 (C5), 82.7, 82.6, 82.4, 82.4 (C-2', C-2'', C-3', C3''), 78.4, 78.3 (C-4', C4''), 70.8, 70.7 (CH$_2$-1'''/ CH$_2$-1''''), 64.7, 64.4 (C-5', C-5''), 32.1, 29.8, 29.8, 29.7, 29.7, 29.5, 27.0, 26.5, 26.4, 26.2, 26.1 (4 × CH$_3$, *i*-Pr, CH$_2$-2''' to CH$_2$-10''', CH$_2$-2'''' to CH$_2$-10''''), 22.8 (CH$_2$-11''', CH$_2$-11''''), 14.4 (CH$_3$-12''', CH$_3$-12'''') ppm. HRMS: calcd for C$_{44}$H$_{76}$N$_2$O$_{10}$ [M + H]$^+$ 793.5573, found 793.5592; calcd for C$_{44}$H$_{76}$N$_2$O$_{10}$ [M + Na]$^+$ 815.5392, found 815.5414.

4.1.8. 1-(5-Deoxy-3-*O*-dodecyl-α,β-D-xylofuranos-5-yl)-3,7-dimethyl-3,7-dihydro-1*H*-purine-2,6-dione (**10**)

A solution of 1-(5-deoxy-3-*O*-dodecyl-1,2-*O*-isopropylidene-α-D-xylofuranos-5-yl)-3,7-dimethyl-3,7-dihydro-1*H*-purine-2,6-dione (**3**, 39 mg, 0.075 mmol) in aq. trifluoroacetic acid (TFA, 60%, 3 mL) was stirred at room temp. for 2 h. The solvents were co-evaporated with toluene and the residue was subjected to column chromatography (from AcOEt/hexane, 10:1 to AcOEt/MeOH, 12:1) to afford **10** (30 mg, 83%, anomeric mixture, α/β ratio, 1:0.9) as colorless oil. ^{1}H NMR (400 MHz, CDCl$_3$) δ: 7.54 (s, 1.9 H, H-8 α, β), 5.56 (br.s, 1 H, H-1' α), 5.11 (1, 0.9 H, H-1' β), 4.67–4.38 (m, 3.8 H, H-4' α, H-4' β, H-5'a α, H-5'a β), 4.34–4.19 (m, 1.9 H, H-2' α, H-2' β), 4.08–3.90 (m, 9.5 H, H-3' α, H-3' β, H-5'b α, H-5'b β, CH$_3$-N^7 α, β), 3.71–3.42 (m, 9.5 H, CH$_2$-1'' α, CH$_2$-1'' β, CH$_3$-N^3 α, β) 1.70–1.60 (m 3.8 H, CH$_2$-2'' α, CH$_2$-2'' β), 1.37–1.20 (m, 34.2 H, CH$_2$-3'' to CH$_2$-11''), 0.87 (t, 5.7 H, CH$_3$-12'', *J* = 6.7). ^{13}C NMR (100 MHz, CDCl$_3$) δ: 155.9 (C-6 α, β), 152.0, 151.9 (C-2 α, β), 149.1, 148.9 (C-4 α, β), 142.1 (C-8 α, β), 107.9, 107.8 (C-5 α, β), 103.5 (C-1' β), 96.4 (C-1' α), 84.6 (C-3' β), 84.1 (C-3' α), 80.1 (C-2' α), 76.8 (C-4' α, β), 75.2 (C-2' β), 71.5 (CH$_2$-1'' α), 70.9 (CH$_2$-1'' β), 43.0 (C-5', α, β), 33.8, 33.7 (CH$_3$, N^7, α, β), 32.1 (CH$_2$-2'', α, β), 30.1, 29.9, 29.9, 29.8, 29.8, 29.8, 29.8, 29.7, 29.6, 29.6, 29.5, 26.2, 22.8, (CH$_3$, N^3, CH$_2$-3'' to CH$_2$-11'', α, β), 14.3 (CH$_2$-12'', α, β). HRMS: calcd for C$_{24}$H$_{40}$N$_4$O$_6$ [M + Na]$^+$ 503.2840, found 503.2836; calcd for C$_{24}$H$_{40}$N$_4$O$_6$ [M + H]$^+$ 481.3021, found 481.3018.

4.1.9. 1-(1,2-Di-*O*-acetyl-5-deoxy-3-*O*-dodecyl-α,β-D-xylofuranos-5-yl)-3,7-dimethyl-3,7-dihydro-1*H*-purine-2,6-dione (**11**)

A solution of 1-(5-deoxy-3-*O*-dodecyl-α,β-D-xylofuranos-5-yl)-3,7-dimethyl-3,7-dihydro-1*H*-purine-2,6-dione (**10**, 41 mg, 0.078 mmol) in pyridine (3 mL) and acetic anhydride (1.5 mL) was stirred at room temp. for 1.5 h. After co-evaporation of the solvents with toluene, the residue was subjected to column chromatography (AcOEt/hexane, 5:1) to give **11** (33 mg, 69%, anomeric mixture, α/β ratio, 1:0.5) as a colorless oil. ^{1}H NMR (400 MHz, CDCl$_3$) δ: 7.50, 7.48 (2 s, 1.5 H, H-8 α, β), 6.38 (dd, 1 H, H-1' α, $J_{1',2'\ α}$ = 4.5), 5.99 (1, 0.5 H, H-1' β), 5.27 (t, 1 H, H-2' α), 5.23 (s, 0.5 H, H-2' β), 4.84–4.58 (m, 3 H, H-4' α, H-4' β, H-5'a α, H-5'a β), 4.19 (t, 1 H, H-3, $J_{2',3'\ α}$ ~ $J_{2',4'\ α}$ = 5.5), 4.01 (br.d, 0.5 H, H-3' β, $J_{3',4'\ β}$ = 5.0), 3.99–3.84 (m, 6 H, CH$_3$-N^7 α, β, H-5'b α, H-5'b β), 3.74–3.65 (m, 0.5 H, H-1''a β), 3.65–3.44 (m, 7 H, CH$_2$-1'' α, H-1''b β, CH$_3$-N^3 α, β), 2.18 (s, 1.5 H, CH$_3$, Ac, β), 2.05 (s, 4.5 H, CH$_3$, Ac, α, β), 1.99 (s, 3 H, CH$_3$, Ac, α), 1.63–1.50 (m, 3 H, CH$_2$-2'', α, β), 1.41–1.16 (m, 27 H, CH$_2$-3'' to CH$_2$-11''), 0.85 (t, 4.5 H, CH$_3$-12'', *J* = 6.8). ^{13}C NMR (100 MHz, CDCl$_3$) δ: 170.5, 169.8 (CO, Ac, β), 169.7, 169.4 (CO, Ac, α), 155.3, 155.3 (C-6 α, β), 151.7 (C-2 α, β), 148.9, 148.8 (C-4 α, β), 141.6, 141.4 (C-8 α, β), 107.8 (C-5 α, β), 99.0 (C-1' β), 84.2 (C-1' α), 82.0 (C-3' β), 80.7 (C-3' α), 80.2 (C-4' β), 79.8 (C-2' β), 76.5 (C-2' α), 76.2 (C-4' α), 71.2, 71.0 (CH$_2$-1'', α, β), 41.9 (C-5' β), 41.3 (C-5' α), 33.7, 33.7 (CH$_3$, N^7, α, β), 32.0 (CH$_2$-2'', α, β), 29.9, 29.8, 29.8, 29.8, 29.7, 29.7, 29.6, 29.5, 26.3, 26.2, 22.8, (CH$_3$, N^3, CH$_2$-3'' to CH$_2$-11'', α, β), 21.5, 21.0, 20.9, 20.7 (CH$_3$, Ac, α, β), 14.2 (CH$_2$-12'', α, β).

4.1.10. *N*-[2-*O*-Acetyl-1,5-dideoxy-5-(3,7-dimethyl-3,7-dihydro-2,6-dioxo-1*H*-purin-1-yl)-3-*O*-dodecyl-α,β-D-xylofuranos-1-yl]methanesulfonamide (**12**)

To a solution of 1-(1,2-di-*O*-acetyl-5-deoxy-3-*O*-dodecyl-α,β-D-xylofuranos-5-yl)-3,7-dimethyl-3,7-dihydro-1*H*-purine-2,6-dione (**11**, 22 mg, 0.039 mmol) in CH$_2$Cl$_2$/acetonitrile (1.2 mL, 4:1) under nitrogen and at 0 °C, BF$_3$·Et$_2$O (0.03 mL, 0.24 mmol) and methanesulfonamide (21 mg, 0.22 mmol) were added. The mixture was stirred at room temp. for 2 h. Then, it was diluted with CH$_2$Cl$_2$ and washed with a satd. aq. NaHCO$_3$ soln. The aqueous phase was extracted with CH$_2$Cl$_2$ (2×) and the combined organic layers were dried with anhydrous MgSO$_4$. After filtration and evaporation of the solvent, the residue was subjected to column chromatography (AcOEt/hexane, 15:1) to afford **12** (19 mg, 81%, anomeric mixture, β/α ratio, 1:0.4) as a yellow oil. ^{1}H NMR (400 MHz, CDCl$_3$) δ: 7.52, 7.51 (2 s, 1.4 H, H-8 α, β), 5.73 (d, 1 H, NH, β, $J_{1',\text{NH }\beta}$ = 11.1), 5.61 (dd, 0.4 H, H-1' α, $J_{1',2'\,\alpha}$ = 3.5, $J_{1',\text{NH }\alpha}$ = 11.3), 5.23 (d, 1 H, H-1' β), 5.20 (s, 1 H, H-2' β), 5.14 (dd, 0.4 H, H-2' α, $J_{1',2'\,\alpha}$ = 3.5, $J_{2',3'\,\alpha}$ = 0.9), 5.07 (d, 0.4 H, NH α), 4.72 (dd, 1 H, H-5'a β, $J_{5'a,5'b\,\beta}$ = 13.9, $J_{4',5'a\,\beta}$ = 9.5), 4.63–4.45 (m, 2.2 H, H-5'a α, H-5'b α, H-4' α, H-4' β, $J_{5'a,5'b\,\alpha}$ = 13.8, $J_{4',5'a\,\alpha}$ = 8.7), 4.02–3.91 (m, 6.6 H, H-3' α, H-3' β, H-5'b β, CH$_3$-N^7 α, β), 3.81–3.72 (m, 1.4 H, H-1''a α, H-1''a β), 3.61–3.49 (m, 5.6 H, H-1''b α, H-1''b β, CH$_3$-N^3 α, β), 3.11 (s, 3 H, S-CH$_3$, β), 3.03 (s, 1.2 H, S-CH$_3$, α), 2.11 (s, 1.2 H, CH$_3$, Ac, α), 2.07 (s, 3 H, CH$_3$, Ac, β), 1.70–1.60 (m 2.8 H, CH$_2$-2'' α, CH$_2$-2'' β), 1.37–1.20 (m, 25.2 H, CH$_2$-3'' to CH$_2$-11'', α, β), 0.87 (t, 4.2 H, CH$_3$-12'', α, β, J = 6.7). ^{13}C NMR (100 MHz, CDCl$_3$) δ: 169.6, 168.9 (CO, Ac, α, β) 155.3 (C-6 α, β), 151.7 (C-2 α, β), 149.1, 149.0 (C-4 α, β), 141.8, 141.7 (C-8 α, β), 107.7 (C-5 α, β), 88.0 (C-1' β), 82.9 (C-1' α), 81.5 (C-3' α), 81.0 (C-3' β), 79.4 (C-4' β), 78.9 (C-2' β), 71.8 (CH$_2$-1'', α, β), 43.0 (SCH$_3$, β), 42.3, 41.7 (SCH$_3$ α, C-5' β), 33.8 (CH$_3$-N^7, α, β), 32.0 (CH$_2$-2'', α, β), 29.9, 29.9, 29.8, 29.8, 29.7, 29.7, 29.6, 29.6, 29.5, 26.1, 22.8 (CH$_3$-N^3, CH$_2$-3'' to CH$_2$-11'', α, β) 21.0, 21.0 (CH$_3$, Ac, α, β), 14.3 (CH$_2$-12'', α, β). HRMS: calcd for C$_{27}$H$_{45}$N$_5$O$_8$S [M + H]$^+$ 600.3062, found 600.3058; calcd for C$_{27}$H$_{45}$N$_5$O$_8$S [M + Na]$^+$ 622.2881, found 622.2878.

4.1.11. 1-(2-O-Acetyl-1-azido-1,5-dideoxy-3-O-dodecyl-α-D-xylofuranos-5-yl)-3,7-dimethyl-3,7-dihydro-1H-purine-2,6-dione (**13**) and
1-(2-O-acetyl-5-deoxy-3-O-dodecyl-D-xylono-1,4-lacton-5-yl)-3,7-dimethyl-3,7-dihydro-1H-purine-2,6-dione (**14**)

To a solution of 1-(1,2-di-O-acetyl-5-deoxy-3-O-dodecyl-α,β-D-xylofuranos-5-yl)-3,7-dimethyl-3,7-dihydro-1H-purine-2,6-dione (**11**, 30 mg, 0.053 mmol) in acetonitrile (5 mL), trimethylsilyl azide (TMSN$_3$, 0.06 mL, 0.43 mmol) and trimethylsilyl triflate (TMSOTf, 0.08 mL, 0.044 mmol) were sequentially added. The mixture was stirred at 65 °C under microwave irradion (150 W, Pmax = 250 Psi) for 1 h 40 min. The solution was then diluted with CH$_2$Cl$_2$ and washed with a sat. aq. NaHCO$_3$ soln. The aqueous phase was extracted with CH$_2$Cl$_2$ (3×) and the combined organic phases were dried with anhydrous MgSO$_4$. After filtration and evaporation, the residue was subjected to column chromatography (from AcOEt/cyclohexane, 1:1 to AcOEt) to afford **13-α** (11 mg, 38%) and a mixture (18 mg) containing **13-β** and the xylonolactone derivative **14** in a 3.3:1 ratio (corresponding to 14 mg of **13-β** (48%) and 4 mg of **14** (14%)).

Data for **13-α**: $[\alpha]_D^{20}$ = +74 (c = 1, in CH$_2$Cl$_2$). ^{1}H NMR (400 MHz, CDCl$_3$) δ: 7.52 (s, 1 H, H-8), 5.58 (d, 1 H, H'-1, $J_{1',2'}$ = 4.7), 5.12 (t, 1 H, H'-2, $J_{1',2'}$ ~ $J_{2',3'}$), 4.71–4.56 (m, 2 H, H'-4, H'-5a), 4.12 (t, 1 H, H'-3, $J_{2',3'}$ ~ $J_{3',4'}$ ~ 4.5), 3.99 (s, 3 H, CH$_3$-N^7), 3.91 (d, 1 H, H'-5b, J = 12.2), 3.66–3.53 (m, 4 H, H-1''a, CH$_3$-N^3), 3.54–3.45 (m, 1 H, H-1''b), 2.13 (s, 3 H, CH$_3$, OAc), 1.62–1.52 (m, 2 H, CH$_2$-2''), 1.38–1.18 (m, 18 H, CH$_2$-3'' to CH$_2$-11''), 0.87 (t, 3 H, CH$_3$-12'', J = 6.7). ^{13}C NMR (100 MHz, CDCl$_3$) δ: 170.1 (CO, OAc), 155.4 (C-6), 151.7 (C-2), 149.0 (C-4), 141.7 (C-8), 107.8 (C-5), 89.6 (C-1'), 81.4 (C-3'), 77.7 (C'-2), 76.5 (C'-4); 71.2 (C-1''), 41.2 (C-5'), 33.8 (CH$_3$-N^7), 32.1, 29.9, 29.9, 29.8, 29.8, 29.7, 29.6, 29.5, 26.2, 22.8 (CH$_3$-N^3, CH$_2$-2'' to CH$_2$-11''), 20.8 (CH$_3$, OAc), 14.3 (C-12''). HRMS: calcd for C$_{26}$H$_{41}$N$_7$O$_6$ [M + H]$^+$ 548.3191, found 548.3187; calcd for C$_{26}$H$_{41}$N$_7$O$_6$ [M + Na]$^+$ 570.3011, found 570.3004.

Data for **13-β**: ^{1}H NMR (400 MHz, CDCl$_3$) δ: 7.50 (s, 1 H, H-8), 5.11 (s, 1 H, H'-2), 5.02 (s, 1 H, H'-1) 4.83 (dd, 1 H, H-5'a, $J_{5'a,5'b}$ = 14.3, $J_{5'a,4'}$ = 8.3), 4.59 (ddd, 1 H, H-4'), 4.07 (dd, 1 H, H-5'b, $J_{5'b,4'}$ = 1.9), 3.99 (s, 3 H, CH$_3$-N^7), 3.91 (d, 1 H, H'-3, $J_{3',4'}$ = 4.3), 3.79–3.70 (m, 1 H, H-1''a), 3.58 (s, 3 H, CH$_3$-N^3), 3.54–3.45 (m, 1 H, H-1''b), 2.07 (s, 3 H, CH$_3$, OAc), 1.65–1.56 (m, 2 H, CH$_2$-2''), 1.44–1.17 (m, 18 H, CH$_2$-3'' to CH$_2$-11''), 0.86 (t, 3 H, CH$_3$-12'', J = 6.7)*. ^{13}C NMR (100 MHz, CDCl$_3$) δ: 169,7 (CO, OAc), 155.3 (C-6), 151.8 (C-2), 149.0 (C-4), 141.6 (C-8), 107.8 (C-5), 93.3 (C-1'), 81.9 (C-4'), 81.4 (C'-3), 79.8 (C'-2); 70.9 (C-1''), 41.2 (C-5'), 33.8 (CH$_3$-N^7), 32.1, 29.9, 29.8, 29.8, 29.7, 29.6, 29.5, 26.2, 22.8 (CH$_3$-N^3, CH$_2$-2'' to CH$_2$-11''), 20.8 (CH$_3$, OAc), 14.3 (C-12'')*. HRMS: calcd for C$_{26}$H$_{41}$N$_7$O$_6$ [M + H]$^+$ 548.3191, found 548.3186.

Data for **14**: ^{1}H NMR (400 MHz, CDCl$_3$) δ: 7.51 (s, 1 H, H-8), 5.59 (d, 1 H, H'-2, $J_{2',3'}$ = 6.7), 5.07 (ddd, 1 H, H'-4), 4.83 (dd, 1 H, H-5'a, $J_{5'a,5'b}$ = 14.3, $J_{5'a,4'}$ = 10.9), 4.37 (t, 1 H, H'-3, $J_{2',3'}$ ~ $J_{3',4'}$), 4.07 (dd, 1 H, H-5'b, $J_{5'b,4'}$ = 3.0), 3.97 (s, 3 H, CH$_3$-N^7), 3.65–3.53 (m, 5 H, CH$_3$-N^3, CH$_2$-1''), 2.17 (s, 3 H, CH$_3$, OAc), 1.66–1.54 (m, 2 H, CH$_2$-2''), 1.47–1.15 (m, 18 H, CH$_2$-3'' to CH$_2$-11''), 0.87 (t, 3 H, CH$_3$-12'', J = 6.7)*. ^{13}C NMR (100 MHz, CDCl$_3$) δ: 170.0 (C-1'), 169.4 (CO, Ac), 155.1 (C-6), 151.6 (C-2), 149.1 (C-4), 141.8 (C-8), 107.7 (C-5), 78.7 (C-3'), 75.9 (C-4'), 72.2 (C'-2), 71.3 (C-1''), 40.5 (C-5'), 33.8 (CH$_3$-N^7), 32.1, 29.9, 29.8, 29.8, 29.7, 29.5, 29.5, 26.1, 22.8 (CH$_3$-N^3, CH$_2$-2'' to CH$_2$-11''), 20.7 (CH$_3$, OAc), 14.3 (C-12'')*. HRMS: calcd for C$_{26}$H$_{40}$N$_4$O$_7$ [M + H]$^+$ 521.2970, found 521.2966.

* Data extracted from the spectrum of a mixture containing **13-β/14**.

4.1.12. Dimethyl N-[2-O-acetyl-1,5-dideoxy-3-O-dodecyl-5-(3,7-dimethyl-3,7-dihydro-2,6-dioxo-1H-purin-1-yl)-α,β-D-xylofuranos-1-yl]phosphoramidate (**15**)

To a solution of 1-(2-O-acetyl-1-azido-1,5-dideoxy-3-O-dodecyl-α-D-xylofuranos-5-yl)-3,7-dimethyl-3,7-dihydro-1H-purine-2,6-dione (**13-α**, 11 mg, 0.02 mmol) in CH$_2$Cl$_2$ (2 mL), trimethyl phosphite (0.03 mL, 0.25 mmol) was added. The solution was stirred at room temperature for 23 h. The solution was then concentrated under vacuum and the residue was subjected to column chromatography (from AcOEt/hexane, 15:1 to AcOEt/MeOH, 15:1) to afford **15** (7 mg, 56%, anomeric mixture, α/β ratio, 1:0.3) as a colorless oil. ^{1}H NMR (400 MHz, CDCl$_3$) δ: 7.50 (s, 1.3 H, H-8 α, β), 5.33 (ddd, 1 H, H-1' α, $J_{1',2'\,α}$ = 3.9 Hz, $J_{1',P\,α}$ = 7.5 Hz, $J_{1',NH\,α}$ = 11.6), 5.14 (s, 0.3 H, H-2' β), 5.06 (d, 1 H, H-2' α, $J_{1',2'\,α}$ = 3.4 Hz), 4.96 (dd, 0.3 H, H-1' β, $J_{1',P\,β}$ = 7,8 Hz, $J_{1',NH\,β}$ = 11.2), 4.73–4.57 (m, 1.3 H, H-5'a, α, β, $J_{5'a,5'b\,α}$ = 13.9, $J_{4',5'a\,α}$ = 9.1, $J_{5'a,5'b\,β}$ = 13.8, $J_{4',5'a\,β}$ = 8.9), 4.54–4.42 (m, 1.3 H, H-4', α, β), 4.15 (t, 0.3 H, NH, β, $J_{1',NH\,β}$ ~ $J_{NH,P\,β}$ = 11.2 Hz), 4.05–3.85 (m, 6.5 H, H-5'b α, β, H-3' α, β, CH$_3$-N^7 α, β), 3.77–3.46 (m, 15.6 H, 2 × OCH$_3$ α, 2 × OCH$_3$ β, CH$_2$-1'' α, β, H-3' α, β, CH$_3$-N^7 α, β), 2.11 (s, 3 H, CH$_3$, Ac, α), 2.06 (s, 0.9 H, Ac, β), 1.66–1.54 (m, 2.6 H, CH$_2$-2'' α, β), 1.38–1.17 (m, 23.4 H, CH$_2$-3'' to CH$_2$-11'' α, β), 0,87 (t, 3.9 H, CH$_2$-12'' α, β, J = 6.7). ^{13}C NMR (100 MHz, CDCl$_3$) δ: 169.9, 169.7 (CO, Ac α, β), 155.4 (C-6 α, β), 151.7 (C-2 α, β); 149.0, 148.9 (C-4 α, β), 141.6, 141.5 (C-8 α, β), 107.8 (C-5 α, β), 87.4 (C-1' β), 82.4 (C-1' α), 82.2, 81.5 (C-3' α, β), 79.9 (C-2' β); 78.4 (C-4' α or β), 76.2, 76.0, 76.0 (C-2' α, C-4' α or β), 71.4, 71.3 (CH$_2$-1'' α, β); 53.4, 53.4, 53.3, 53.2 (4 d, 2 × OCH$_3$ α, β, $J_{C,P}$ = 4.8), 41.7, 40-8 (C-5' α, β), 33.7 (CH$_3$-N^7 α, β), 32.1, 29.8, 29.8, 29.8, 29.6, 29.5, 26.2, 26.2, 22.8 (CH$_3$-N^3 α, β, CH$_2$-2'' to CH$_2$-11''), 21.1, 21.0 (CH$_3$, Ac, β), 14.3 (CH$_3$-12'' α, β). ^{31}P NMR (162 MHz, CDCl$_3$) δ: 8.49. HRMS: calcd for C$_{28}$H$_{48}$N$_5$O$_9$P [M + H]$^+$ 630.3262, found 630.3270; calcd for C$_{28}$H$_{48}$N$_5$O$_9$P [M + Na]$^+$ 652.3082, found 652.3090.

4.1.13. 3-O-Octyl-1,2-O-isopropylidene-α-D-glucofuranose (**16**)

To a solution of 1,2:5,6-di-O-isopropylidene-α-D-glucofuranose (**15**, 3.0 g, 11.53 mmol) in anhydrous DMF (30 mL) under nitrogen atmosphere and at 0 °C and, NaH (60%, 0.69 g, 17.25 mmol) was added. The suspension was stirred at 0 °C for 10 min. Then, octyl bromide (2.38 mL, 13.79 mmol) was added and the mixture was stirred at room temperature for 22 h. It was then diluted with CH$_2$Cl$_2$ and washed with water and brine solution. The aqueous phase was extracted with CH$_2$Cl$_2$ (3×) and the combined organic layers were dried with anhydrous MgSO$_4$, filtered and concentrated. To the resulting residue, aq. acetic acid (70% soln., 38 mL) was added and the resulting solution was stirred at room temperature for 26 h. After co-evaporation with toluene, the residue was subjected to column chromatography (EtOAc/hexane, 1:3) to afford 16 (3.37 g, 88%, 2 steps) as a colorless oil. ^{1}H NMR (CDCl$_3$, 400 MHz): 5.82 (d, 1 H, H-1, $J_{1,2}$ = 3.7), 4.47 (d, 1 H, H-2), 4.03 (dd, 1 H, H-4, $J_{3,4}$ = 3.2, $J_{4,5}$ = 7.8), 3.95–3.85 (m, 2 H, H-3, H-5), 3.73 (dd, part A of AB system, H-6a, $J_{5,6a}$ = 3.0, $J_{6a,6b}$ = 11.6), 3.63 (dd, part B of AB system, H-6b, $J_{5,6b}$ = 5.6), 3.59–3.49 (m, 1 H, H-1'a), 3.49–3.14 (m, 3 H, H-1'b, OH-5, OH-6), 1.57–1.44 (m, 2 H, CH$_2$-2'), 1.41 (s, 3 H, CH$_3$, i-Pr), 1.31–1.12 (m, 13 H, CH$_2$-3' to CH$_2$-7', CH$_3$, i-Pr), 0.81 (t, 3 H, CH$_3$-8', J = 6.6). ^{13}C NMR (CDCl$_3$, 100 MHz): 111.6 (Cq, i-Pr), 105.0 (C-1), 82.6 (C-3), 82.1 (C-2), 79.7 (C-4), 70.6 (C-1'), 69.3 (C-5), 64.2 (C-6), 31.8, 29.7, 29.3, 29.2, 26.7, 26.2, 26.0, 22.6

(C-2' to C-7', 2 × CH_3, i-Pr), 14.1 (C-8'). HRMS: calcd for $C_{17}H_{32}O_6$ [M + H]$^+$ 333.2272, found 333.2266; calcd for $C_{17}H_{32}O_6$ [M + Na]$^+$ 355.2091, found 355.2081.

4.1.14. 3-O-Octyl-1,2-O-isopropylidene-α-D-xylofuranose (17)

To a solution of 3-O-octyl-1,2-O-isopropylidene-α-D-glucofuranose (16, 3.14 g, 9.45 mmol) in 60% aq. THF (22 mL), at 0 °C, sodium metaperiodate (4.85 g, 22.68 mmol) was added. The mixture was stirred for 4 h at room temperature. Then, it was diluted with EtOAc and washed with water and brine solution. The aqueous phase was extracted with EtOAc (3×) and the combined organic layers were dried with anhydrous $MgSO_4$. After filtration and concentration under vacuum, the residue was dissolved in $EtOH/H_2O$ (57 mL, 2:1). To the resulting solution at 0 °C, $NaBH_4$ (0.461 g, 12 mmol) was added and the mixture was stirred at room temperature for 1.5 h. Then, EtOAc was added. The mixture was washed with brine soln. and the aqueous phase was extracted with EtOAc (2×). The combined organic layers were dried with anhydrous $MgSO_4$, filtered and concentrated. The residue was subjected to column chromatography (EtOAc/petroleum ether, 2:1) to afford 17 (1.85 g, 65%, 2 steps) as a colorless oil. ^{1}H NMR (CDCl$_3$, 400 MHz): 5.98 (d, 1 H, H-1, $J_{1,2}$ = 3.8), 4.57 (d, 1 H, H-2), 4.27 (br. q, 1 H, H-4), 4.00–3.85 (m, 2 H, H-3, H-5a, H-5b, $J_{3,4}$ = 3.3, $J_{4,5a}$ = 4.6, $J_{4,5b}$ = 4.4, $J_{5a,5b}$ = 12.3), 3.68–3.58 (m, 1 H, H-1'a), 3.47–3.38 (m, 1 H, H-1'b), 1.61–1.51 (m, 2 H, CH_2-2'), 1.49 (s, 3 H, CH_3, i-Pr), 1.38–1.19 (m, 13 H, CH_2-3' to CH_2-7', CH_3, i-Pr), 0.88 (t, 3 H, CH_3-8', J = 6.6). ^{13}C NMR (CDCl$_3$, 100 MHz): 111.8 (Cq, i-Pr), 105.2 (C-1), 84.5 (C-3), 82.5 (C-2), 79.9 (C-4), 70.6 (C-1'), 61.3 (C-5), 31.9, 29.8, 29.5, 29.3, 27.0, 26.5, 26.2, 22.8 (C-2' to C-7', 2 × CH_3, i-Pr), 14.2 (C-8'). HRMS: calcd for $C_{16}H_{30}O_5$ [M + H]$^+$ 303.2166, found 303.2156; calcd for $C_{16}H_{30}O_5$ [M + Na]$^+$ 325.1985, found 325.1974.

4.1.15. 1-(5-Deoxy-3-O-dodecyl-α-D-xylofuranos-5-yl)-3,7-dimethyl-3,7-dihydro-1H-purine-2,6-dione (18)

A solution of 3-O-octyl-1,2-O-isopropylidene-α-D-xylofuranose (17, 80 mg, 0.26 mmol) in DMF (2 mL) was subjected to the MW-assisted protocol for Mitsunobu coupling, according to the general procure, using PPh$_3$ (138 mg, 0.526 mmol), DEAD (40 % wt soln in toluene, 0.2 mL, 0.44 mmol) and theobromine (95 mg, 0.527 mmol). The mixture was stirred for 30 min. Column chromatography was performed using (AcOEt/petroleum ether, 2:1 as eluent. To the obtained residue, aq. TFA (60% soln., 3 mL) was added and the resulting solution was stirred at room temperature for 4 h. After co-evaporation of the solvents with toluene, the residue was subjected to column chromatography (from AcOEt/petroleum ether, 20:1 to AcOEt/MeOH, 12:1) to afford 10 (22 mg, 20%, 2 steps, anomeric mixture, α/β ratio, 1:1) as a colorless oil. ^{1}H NMR (400 MHz, CDCl$_3$) δ: 7.54, 7.51 (s, 2 H, H-8 α, β), 5.56 (d, 1 H, H-1' α, $J_{1',2'\alpha}$ = 4.0), 5.11 (d, 1 H, H-1' β, $J_{1',2'\beta}$ = 1.5), 4.68–4.41 (m, 4 H, H-4' α, H-4' β, H-5'a α, H-5'a β), 4.30 (dd, 1 H, H-2' β, $J_{2',3'\beta}$ = 3.6), 4.22 (br.t, 1 H, H-2' α), 4.08–3.91 (m, 10 H, H-3' α, H-3' β, H-5'b α,H-5'b β, CH_3-N^7 α, β), 3.71–3.61 (m, 2 H, H-1"a α, H-1"a β), 3.60–3.43 (m, 8 H, H-1"b α, H-1"b β, CH_3-N^3 α, β) 1.66–1.50 (m 4 H, CH_2-2" α, CH_2-2" β), 1.41–1.16 (m, 20 H, CH_2-3" to CH_2-7"), 0.87 (t, 6 H, CH_3-8", J = 6.6). ^{13}C NMR (100 MHz, CDCl$_3$) δ: 155.9, 155.5 (C-6 α, β), 152.0, 151.9 (C-2 α, β), 149.2, 149.0 (C-4 α, β), 142.0, 141.8 (C-8 α, β), 107.9, 107.8 (C-5 α, β), 103.4 (C-1' β), 96.2 (C-1' α), 84.6 (C-3' β), 84.2 (C-3' α), 80.3 (C-2' β), 77.1 (C-4' α, β), 75.3 (C-2' α), 71.5 (CH$_2$-1" α), 70.9 (CH$_2$-1" β), 43.1, 41.5 (C-5', α, β), 33.8, 33.8 (CH$_3$, N^7, α, β), 32.0 (CH$_2$-2", α, β), 30.0, 30.0, 29.9, 29.6, 29.4, 29.4, 26.2, 26.2, 22.8, (CH$_3$, N^3, CH$_2$-3" to CH$_2$-7", α, β), 14.3 (CH$_2$-8", α, β). HRMS: calcd for $C_{20}H_{32}N_4O_6$ [M + H]$^+$ 425.2395, found 425.2390; calcd for $C_{20}H_{32}N_4O_6$ [M + Na]$^+$ 447.2214, found 447.2208.

4.1.16. 1-(6-Deoxy-3-O-dodecyl-1,2-O-isopropylidene-α-D-glucofuranos-6-yl)-3,7-dimethyl-3,7-dihydro-1H-purine-2,6-dione (19)

A solution of 3-O-octyl-1,2-O-isopropylidene-α-D-glucofuranose (16, 80 mg, 0.241 mmol) in DMF (2 mL) was subjected to the protocol for Mitsunobu coupling, according to the general procure, using PPh$_3$ (138 mg, 0.526 mmol), DEAD (40 % wt soln in toluene, 0.24 mL, 0.526 mmol) and theobromine (95 mg, 0.527 mmol). The mixture was stirred under reflux for 20 h. Purification by column chromatography (from AcOEt/petroleum ether 3:1 to 4:1) afforded **19** (19 mg, 16%; isolated yield: 11 mg, 9%) as a colorless oil. ^{1}H NMR (CDCl$_3$, 400 MHz): 7.51 (s, 1 H, H-8), 5.97 (d, 1 H, H-1′, $J_{1,2}$ = 3.7), 4.54 (d, 1 H, H-2′), 4.43 (dd, part A of AB system, H-6′a, $J_{5',6'a}$ = 7.3, $J_{a,b}$ = 17.4), 4.29–4.19 (m, 2 H, H-5′, H-6′b), 4.11 (dd, 1 H, H-4′, $J_{3',4'}$ = 3.2, $J_{4',5'}$ = 6.3), 4.03 (d, 1 H, H-3′), 3.98 (s, 3 H, CH$_3$-N^7), 3.67–3.47 (m, 5 H, CH$_2$-1″, CH$_3$-N^3), 1.72–1.52 (m, 2 H, CH$_2$-2″), 1.50 (s, 3 H, CH$_3$, *i*-Pr), 1.36–1.16 (m, 13 H, CH$_2$-3″ to CH$_2$-7″, CH$_3$, *i*-Pr), 0.86 (t, 3 H, CH$_3$-8″, *J* = 6.6). ^{13}C NMR (CDCl$_3$, 100 MHz): 153.4 (C-6), 149.9 (C-4), 141.7 (C-8), 111.7 (Cq, *i*-Pr), 105.5 (C-1′), 83.1 (C-3′), 82.4 (C-2′), 81.3 (C-4′), 70.9 (C-1″), 69.0 (C-5′), 45.2 (C-6′), 33.8 (CH$_3$, N^7), 31.9, 30.0, 29.9, 29.8, 29.6, 29.5, 29.3, 27.0, 26.5, 26.2, 22.8 (CH$_3$, N^3, C-2″ to C-7″, 2 × CH$_3$, *i*-Pr), 14.2 (C-8″). HRMS: calcd for C$_{24}$H$_{38}$N$_4$O$_7$ [M + H]$^+$ 495.2813, found 495.2808; calcd for C$_{24}$H$_{38}$N$_4$O$_7$ [M + Na]$^+$ 517.2633, found 517.2626.

4.1.17. 1-(6-Deoxy-3-*O*-dodecyl-α-D-glucopyranos-6-yl)-3,7-dimethyl-3,7-dihydro-1*H*-purine-2,6-dione (**20**)

A solution of 1-(6-deoxy-3-*O*-dodecyl-1,2-*O*-isopropylidene-α-D-glucofuranos-6-yl)-3,7-dimethyl-3,7-dihydro-1*H*-purine-2,6-dione (**19**, 20 mg, 0.04 mmol) in aq. trifluoroacetic acid (TFA, 60%, 3 mL) was stirred at room temp. for 5 h. The solvents were co-evaporated of with toluene and the residue was subjected to column chromatography (from AcOEt/petroleum ether 15:1 to AcOEt/MeOH, 20:1) to afford **20** (16 mg, 87%, anomeric mixture, α/β ratio, 1:0.9) as colorless oil. ^{1}H NMR (CDCl$_3$, 400 MHz): 7.62, 7.61 (2 s, 1.9 H, H-8, α, β), 5.28 (br.s, 1 H, H-1′α), 4.61 (d, 0.9 H, H-1′β, $J_{1',2'\,β}$ = 7.5), 4.52 (dd, 0.9 H, H-6′a β, $J_{5',6'a\,β}$ = 2.1, $J_{6a,6b\,β}$ = 14.0), 4.45 (dd, 1 H, H-6′a α, $J_{5',6'a\,α}$ = 3.5, $J_{6a,6b\,α}$ = 14.4), 4.38–4.28 (m, 1.9 H, H-26′b α, H-6′b β), 4.13 (dt, 1 H, H-5′α, $J_{4',5'\,α}$ = 9.7, $J_{5',6'a\,α}$ = $J_{5',6'b\,α}$ = 3.5), 4.01, 4.00 (2 s, 5.7 H, CH$_3$-N^7), 3.95–3.73 (m, 3.8 H, CH$_2$-1″, α, β), 3.67–3.57 (s, 7.6 H, H-3′ β, H-4′ β, CH$_3$-N^3), 3.54–3.49 (m, 2.9 H, H-2′ α, H-3′ α, H-5 β), 3.46–3.01 (m, 7.6 H, H-′ β, H-4′ α, OH-1, OH-2, OH-4), 1.66–1.55 (m, 3.8 H, CH$_2$-2″, α, β), 1.39–1.20 (m, 19 H, CH$_2$-3″ to CH$_2$-7″, α, β), 0.86 (t, 5.7 H, CH$_3$-8″, α, β, *J* = 6.5). ^{13}C NMR (CDCl$_3$, 100 MHz): 156.0 (C-6 α, β), 152.4 (C-2 α, β), 149.0 (C-4 α, β), 142.1 (C-8 α, β), 107.7 (C-5 α, β), 107.7 (C-5 α, β), 97.2 (C-1′ β), 92.6 (C-1′ α), 83.5 (C-3′ β), 81.2 (C-3′ α), 75.1 (C-4′ β), 74.8 (C-2′ β), 73.8 (C-1″), 73.7 (C-5′ β), 72.2 (C-2′ α), 72.1 (C-2′ β), 72.1 (C-4′ α), 71.3 (C-5′ α), 41.6 (C-6′ α, β), 33.9 (CH$_3$, N^7, α, β), 32.0, 31.0, 30.2, 29.9, 29.6, 29.4, 26.2, 22.8 (CH$_3$, N^3, C-2″ to C-7″, α, β), 14.3 (C-8″, α, β). HRMS: calcd for C$_{21}$H$_{34}$N$_4$O$_7$ [M + H]$^+$ 455.2500, found 455.2494; calcd for C$_{21}$H$_{34}$N$_4$O$_7$ [M + Na]$^+$ 477.2320, found 477.2313.

4.1.18. 1-(1,2,4-Tri-*O*-acetyl-6-deoxy-3-*O*-dodecyl-α-D-glucopyranos-6-yl)-3,7-dimethyl-3,7-dihydro-1*H*-purine-2,6-dione (**21**)

A solution of 1-(6-deoxy-3-*O*-dodecyl-α-D-glucopyranos-6-yl)-3,7-dimethyl-3,7-dihydro-1*H*-purine-2,6-dione (**20**, 27 mg, 0.059 mmol) in pyridine (1.6 mL) and acetic anhydride (1 mL) was stirred at room temp. for 2.5 h. After co-evaporation with toluene, the residue was subjected to column chromatography (AcOEt/hexane, 15:1 to AcOEt) to give **21** (29 mg, 84%, anomeric mixture, β/α ratio, 1:0.7) as a yellow oil. ^{1}H NMR (CDCl$_3$, 400 MHz): 7.53, 7.52 (2 s, 1.7 H, H-8, α, β), 6.24 (br.s, 0.7 H, H-1′α, $J_{1',2'\,α}$ = 3.6), 5.51 (d, 1 H, H-1′β, $J_{1',2'\,β}$ = 8.1), 5.16–4.97 (m, 3.4 H, H-2′α, H-2′β, H-4′α, H-4′β, $J_{2',3'\,α}$ = 9.9, $J_{3',4'\,α}$ = 9.8, $J_{2',3'\,β}$ ~ $J_{3',4'\,β}$ ~ $J_{4',5'\,β}$ ~ 9.5), 4.63–4.49 (m, 1.7 H, H-6′a α, H-6′a β, $J_{6a,6b\,β}$ = 13.8, $J_{6a,6b\,α}$ = 14.0, $J_{5,6a\,α}$ = 9.8, $J_{5,6a\,β}$ = 9.3), 4.33 (td, 0.7 H, H-5′ α, $J_{4',5'\,α}$ = $J_{5',6'a\,α}$ = 9.8, $J_{5',6'b\,α}$ = 2.1), 4.04–3.94 (m, 6.1 H, CH$_3$-N^7, H-5′ β), 3.90–3.75 (m, 2.4 H, H-6′b α, H-6′b β, H-3 α), 3.66–3.50 (m, 9.5 H, CH$_2$-1″, α, β, H-3′ β, CH$_3$-N^3), 2.18, 2.16, 2.08, 2.07, 2.04, 2.04 (6 s, 15.3 H, 3 x CH$_3$, 3 × Ac, α, β), 1.55–1.42 (m, 3.4 H, CH$_2$-2″, α, β), 1.37–1.19 (m, 17 H, CH$_2$-3″ to CH$_2$-7″, α, β), 0.86 (t, 5.1 H, CH$_3$-8″, α, β, *J* = 6.7). ^{13}C NMR (CDCl$_3$, 100 MHz): 169.9, 169.6, 169.4. 169.1, 169.0 (CO, Ac, α, β), 155.2, 155.1 (C-6 α, β), 151.6, 151.6 (C-2 α, β), 149.0, 148.9 (C-4 α, β), 141.7, 141.7 (C-8 α, β), 107.7, 107.7 (C-5 α, β), 92.3 (C-1′ β), 89.6 (C-1′ α), 80.4 (C-3′ β), 77.0 (C-3′ α), 73.1, 72.9 (C-1″ α, β), 72.6 (C-5′ β), 72.0, 72.0, 71.6, 71.5 (C-2′, C-4′, α, β), 69.6 (C-5′ α), 42.0, 41.9 (C-6′ α, β), 33.8, 33.7 (CH$_3$, N^7, α, β), 32.0, 31.1, 30.4, 30.3, 29.9, 29.8, 29.6, 29.5, 29.4, 29.4, 26.1, 26.1, 22.8 (CH$_3$, N^3, C-2″ to C-7″, α, β), 21.1, 21.1,

20.9, 20.8 (CH$_3$, Ac, α, β), 14.2 (C-8″, α, β). HRMS: calcd for C$_{27}$H$_{40}$N$_4$O$_{10}$ [M + H]$^+$ 581.2817, found 581.2819; calcd for C$_{27}$H$_{40}$N$_4$O$_{10}$ [M + Na]$^+$ 603.2637, found 603.2633.

4.1.19. *N*-[2,4-Di-*O*-acetyl-1,6-dideoxy-6-(3,7-dimethyl-3,7-dihydro-2,6-dioxo-1*H*-purin-1-yl)-3-*O*-dodecyl-α,β-D-glucopyranos-1-yl]methanesulfonamide (**22**)

To a solution of 1-(1,2,4-tri-*O*-acetyl-6-deoxy-3-*O*-dodecyl-α-D-glucopyranos-6-yl)-3,7-dimethyl-3,7-dihydro-1*H*-purine-2,6-dione (**21**, 20 mg, 0.034 mmol) in CH$_2$Cl$_2$/acetonitrile (1.2 mL, 4:1) under nitrogen and at 0 °C, BF$_3$·Et$_2$O (0.02 mL, 0.16 mmol) and methanesulfonamide (19 mg, 0.19 mmol) were added. The mixture was stirred at room temp. for 3.5 h. Then, it was diluted with CH$_2$Cl$_2$ and washed with a satd. aq. NaHCO$_3$ soln. The aqueous phase was extracted with CH$_2$Cl$_2$ (2×) and the combined organic layers were dried with anhydrous MgSO$_4$. After filtration and evaporation of the solvent, the residue was subjected to column chromatography (AcOEt/petroleum ether, 10:1) to afford **22** (8 mg, 38%, anomeric mixture, β/α ratio, 1:0.4) as a yellow oil. ^{1}H NMR (400 MHz, CDCl$_3$) δ: 7.53 (s, 1.4 H, H-8 α, β), 6.21 (br.s, 0.4 H, N*H* α), 5.52 (d, 1 H, NH, β, $J_{1',NH\,β}$ = 9.6), 5.06–4.89 (m, 1.8 H, H-4′ α, H-4′ β, H-1 α), 4.82 (t,1 H, H-2′ β, $J_{1',2'\,β}$ ~$J_{2',3'\,α}$ ~ 9.3), 4.61–4.51 (m, 1.4 H, H-1′ β, H-2 α), 4.46 (dd, 1 H, H-6′a β, $J_{6a,6b\,β}$ = 13.8, $J_{5,6a\,β}$ = 9.8), 4.37–4.25 (m, 0.8 H, H-5′ α, H-6′a α), 3.89 (d, 1 H, H-6′b β), 3.98, 3.95 (2 s, 4.2 H, CH$_3$-N^7 α, β), 3.82–3.73 (m, 1.8 H, H-5′ β, H-6′b α, H-3′ α), 3.66–3.47 (m, 8 H, H-3′ β, CH$_3$-N^3 α, β, CH$_2$-1″, α, β), 2.85 (s, 4.2 H, S-CH$_3$, α, β), 2.18, 2.11, 2.06, 2.01 (s, 8.4 H, CH$_3$, Ac, α), 1.52–1.42 (m 2.8 H, CH$_2$-2″ α, CH$_2$-2″ β), 1.36–1.14 (m, 14 H, CH$_2$-3″ to CH$_2$-7″, α, β), 0.88 (t, 4.2 H, CH$_3$-8″, α, β, *J* = 6.6). ^{13}C NMR (100 MHz, CDCl$_3$) δ: 171.0, 170.1, 169.0 (CO, Ac, α, β), 155.1 (C-6 α, β), 151.5 (C-2 α, β), 149.2 (C-4 α, β), 142.1 (C-8 α, β), 107.6 (C-5 α, β), 83.1 (C-1′ β), 80.4 (C-3′ β), 74.3 (C-5′ β), 73.4 (CH$_2$-1″, α, β), 72.0 (C-2′ β), 71.8 (C-4′ β), 43.2 (SCH$_3$, β), 42.1, 42.1 (C-6′ β, C-6′ α), 42.0 (SCH$_3$, α), 33.7 (CH$_3$, N^7, α, β), 32.0, 30.3, 29.9, 29.9, 29.8, 29.6, 29.4, 26.1, 22.8 (CH$_3$, N^3, C-2″ to C-7″, α, β), 21.1, 21.0 (CH$_3$, Ac, α), 14.2 (C-8″, α, β). HRMS: calcd for C$_{26}$H$_{41}$N$_5$O$_{10}$S [M + H]$^+$ 616.2647, found 616.2645; calcd for C$_{26}$H$_{41}$N$_5$O$_{10}$S [M + Na]$^+$ 638.2466, found 638.2464.

^{1}H NMR and ^{13}C NMR Spectra for compounds **3–12**, **13-α**, **15–22** can be found in the Supplementary Materials.

4.2. Biological Assays

4.2.1. Cholinesterase Inhibition Assays

A TECAN Spectra-FluorPlus working on the kinetic mode and measuring the absorbance at λ = 415 nm was used for the enzymatic studies. Acetylcholinesterase (from *Electrophorus electricus*), 5,5′-dithiobis-(2-nitrobenzoic acid) (DTNB) and acetylthiocholine iodide were purchased from Fluka. Butyrylcholinesterase (from equine serum) was bought from Sigma. Experimental details for preparation of the solutions and the procedures for the enzyme assays can be found in the Supplementary Materials.

4.2.2. Cytotoxicity Assays

The cytotoxicity of the compounds was evaluated using the sulforhodamine-B (SRB) colorimetric assay. The EC$_{50}$ values in μM from SRB assays were determined after 96 h of treatment and were averaged from three independent experiments performed each in triplicate; confidence interval CI = 95%, cut-off the assay 30 μM. Compounds with EC$_{50}$ > 30 μM are considered inactive. The cell lines were kindly provided by Th. Müller (Dep. of Haematology/Oncology, Martin Luther Universität Halle-Wittenberg). Human cancer cell lines: A375 (epithelial melanoma), A2780 (ovarian carcinoma), HT29 (colorectal adenocarcinoma), MCF7 (breast adenocarcinoma), SW1736 (thyroid carcinoma); non-malignant: NIH 3T3 (mouse embryonic fibroblasts).

4.3. Molecular Docking Studies

From the RCSB Protein Databank the crystal structures of AChE (PDB: 1C2O) and BChE (PDB: 6EMI) were selected. The compounds were built using Datawarrior and geometry optimized using MMFF94 force field. For the enzyme preparation, water and co-crystallized ligands were removed, gasteiger charges were added and non-polar hydrogens were merged with into the corresponding heavy atom.

The search space consisted of a 126 × 126 × 126 grid with 0.2 angstrom spacing centered on either the binding site of AChE or BChE. Dockings were executed with Lamarckian GA (200 population size; 25,000,000 evaluations; 15 runs). The pose showing the best binding energy (pose 1, ranked by energy) is shown in the manuscript.

5. Conclusions

In conclusion, purine/uracil 5′-isonucleosides and theobromine-containing 5′/6′-isonucleosides and isonucleotide analogs were synthesized in few steps from easily available *xylo*- or *gluco*-configured furanose precursors. A theobromine 6′-isonucleoside was shown to act as a dual AChE/BChE inhibitor at single-digit micromolar concentration range, with a K_i value for BChE being only ca. two-fold lower than that of galantamine hydrobromide. This finding, along with the rather short synthetic pathway for theobromine terminal isonucleosides, encouraging structural optimization, points to the interest of this type of scaffold in the search for stable and non-cytotoxic cholinesterase inhibitor lead compounds.

Supplementary Materials: The following are available online at http://www.mdpi.com/1424-8247/12/3/103/s1.

Author Contributions: Conceptualization, N.M.X.; methodology, N.M.X. (synthesis), R.C. (biological evaluation, docking studies); investigation, N.M.X, E.C.d.S., M.P.P. (synthesis), A.L., R.C. (biological evaluation), I.S., R.C. (docking studies), M.C.O. (HRMS analysis); supervision, N.M.X. (synthesis), R.C. (biological evaluation, docking studies); writing—original draft preparation, N.M.X.; writing—review and editing, N.M.X., R.C.; project administration and funding acquisition, N.M.X.

Funding: This research was funded by 'Fundação para a Ciência e Tecnologia' (FCT), grant number IF/01488/2013, the exploratory project IF/01488/2013/CP1159/CT0006 and the strategic projects UID/MULTI/00612/2013 and UID/MULTI/00612/2019.

Acknowledgments: The authors thank the IAESTE student trainee R. Joshi for support in compound synthesis and Lucie Fischer and Sophie Hoenke for collaborating in the cytotoxicity assays.

Conflicts of Interest: The authors declare no conflict of interest.

References

1. Jordheim, L.P.; Durantel, D.; Zoulim, F.; Dumontet, C. Advances in the development of nucleoside and nucleotide analogues for cancer and viral diseases. *Nat. Rev. Drug Discov.* **2013**, *12*, 447–464. [CrossRef] [PubMed]
2. Shelton, J.; Lu, X.; Hollenbaugh, J.A.; Cho, J.H.; Amblard, F.; Schinazi, R.F. Metabolism, biochemical actions, and chemical synthesis of anticancer nucleosides, nucleotides, and base analogs. *Chem. Rev.* **2016**, *116*, 14379–14455. [CrossRef] [PubMed]
3. Montgomery, J.A.; Clayton, S.D.; Thomas, H.J. Isonucleosides. I. Preparation of methyl 2-deoxy-2-(purin-9-yl) arabinofuranosides and methyl 3-deoxy-3-(purin-9-yl) xylofuranosides. *J. Org. Chem.* **1975**, *40*, 1923–1927. [CrossRef] [PubMed]
4. Yu, H.W.; Zhang, L.R.; Zhuo, J.C.; Ma, L.T.; Zhang, L.H. Studies on the synthesis and biological activities of 4′-(R)-hydroxy-5′-(S)-hydroxymethyl-tetrahydrofuranyl purines and pyrimidines. *Bioorg. Med. Chem.* **1996**, *4*, 609–614. [CrossRef]
5. Yu, H.W.; Zhang, H.Y.; Yang, Z.J.; Min, J.M.; Ma, L.T.; Zhang, L.H. Studies on the syntheses and biological activities of isonucleosides. *Pure Appl. Chem.* **1998**, *70*, 435–438. [CrossRef]
6. Huryn, D.M.; Sluboski, B.C.; Tam, S.Y.; Weigele, M.; Sim, I.; Anderson, B.D.; Mitsuya, H.; Broder, S. Synthesis and anti-HIV activity of isonucleosides. *J. Med. Chem.* **1992**, *35*, 2347–2354. [CrossRef]

7. Tino, J.A.; Clark, J.M.; Field, A.K.; Jacobs, G.A.; Lis, K.A.; Michalik, T.L.; McGeever-Rubin, B.; Slusarchyk, W.A.; Spergel, S.H. Synthesis and antiviral activity of novel isonucleoside analogs. *J. Med. Chem.* **1993**, *36*, 1221–1229. [CrossRef]
8. Solke, K.F.; Huang, J.L.; Russell, J.W.; Whiterock, V.J.; Sundeen, J.E.; Stratton, L.W.; Clark, J.M. Pharmacokinetics and antiviral activity of a novel isonucleoside, BMS-181165, against simian varicella virus infection in African green monkeys. *Antivir. Res.* **1994**, *23*, 219–224. [CrossRef]
9. Nair, V.; St. Clair, M.H.; Reardon, J.E.; Krasny, H.C.; Hazen, R.J.; Paff, M.T.; Boone, L.R.; Tisdale, M.; Najera, I.; Dornsife, R.E.; et al. Antiviral, metabolic, and pharmacokinetic properties of the isomeric dideoxynucleoside 4(*S*)-(6-amino-9*H*-purin-9-yl) tetrahydro-2(*S*)-furanmethanol. *Antimicrob. Agents Chemother.* **1995**, *39*, 1993–1999. [CrossRef]
10. Purdy, D.F.; Zintek, L.B.; Nair, V. Synthesis of isonucleosides related to AZT and AZU. *Nucleosides Nucleotides* **1994**, *13*, 109–126. [CrossRef]
11. Nair, V.; Piotrowska, D.G.; Okello, M.; Vadakkan, J. Isonucleosides: Design and synthesis of new isomeric nucleosides with antiviral potential. *Nucleosides Nucleotides Nucleic. Acids* **2007**, *26*, 687–690. [CrossRef]
12. Bobek, M.; An, S.H.; Skrincosky, D.; De Clercq, E.; Bernacki, R.J. 2′-Fluorinated isonucleosides. 1. Synthesis and biological activity of some methyl 2′-deoxy-2′-fluoro-2′-pyrimidinyl-D-arabinopyranosides. *J. Med. Chem.* **1989**, *32*, 799–807. [CrossRef] [PubMed]
13. Xavier, N.M.; Lucas, S.D.; Jorda, R.; Schwarz, S.; Loesche, A.; Csuk, R.; Oliveira, M.C. Synthesis and evaluation of the biological profile of novel analogues of nucleosides and of potential mimetics of sugar phosphates and nucleotides. *Synlett* **2015**, *26*, 2663–2672. [CrossRef]
14. Batista, D.; Schwarz, S.; Loesche, A.; Csuk, R.; Costa, P.J.; Oliveira, M.C.; Xavier, N.M. Synthesis of glucopyranos-6′-yl purine and pyrimidine isonucleosides as potential cholinesterase inhibitors. Access to pyrimidine-linked pseudodisaccharides through Mitsunobu reaction. *Pure Appl. Chem.* **2016**, *88*, 363–379. [CrossRef]
15. Čolović, M.B.; Krstić, D.Z.; Lazarević-Pašti, T.D.; Bondžić, A.M.; Vasić, V.M. Acetylcholinesterase inhibitors: Pharmacology and toxicology. *Curr. Neuropharmacol.* **2013**, *11*, 315–335. [CrossRef] [PubMed]
16. McHardy, S.F.; Wang, H.L.; McCowen, S.V.; Valdez, M.C. Recent advances in acetylcholinesterase inhibitors and reactivators: An update on the patent literature (2012–2015). *Expert Opin. Ther. Pat.* **2017**, *27*, 455–476. [CrossRef] [PubMed]
17. Pereira, R.G.; Pereira, M.P.; Serra, S.G.; Loesche, A.; Csuk, R.; Silvestre, S.; Costa, P.J.; Oliveira, M.C.; Xavier, N.M. Furanosyl nucleoside analogs embodying triazole or theobromine units as potential lead molecules for Alzheimer's disease. *Eur. J. Org. Chem.* **2018**, *2018*, 2667–2681. [CrossRef]
18. Pardridge, W.M. Alzheimer's disease drug development and the problem of the blood-brain barrier. *Alzheimer's Dement.* **2009**, *5*, 427–432. [CrossRef]
19. Xavier, N.M.; Goncalves-Pereira, R.; Jorda, R.; Hendrychová, D.; Oliveira, M.C. Novel dodecyl-containing azido and glucuronamide-based nucleosides exhibiting anticancer potential. *Pure Appl. Chem.* **2019**. [CrossRef]
20. Xavier, N.M.; Porcheron, A.; Batista, D.; Jorda, R.; Řezníčková, E.; Kryštof, V.; Oliveira, M.C. Exploitation of new structurally diverse D-glucuronamide-containing *N*-glycosyl compounds: Synthesis and anticancer potential. *Org. Biomol. Chem.* **2017**, *15*, 4667–4680. [CrossRef]
21. Mushtaq, G.; Greig, N.H.; Khan, J.A.; Kamal, M.A. Status of acetylcholinesterase and butyrylcholinesterase in Alzheimer's disease and type 2 diabetes mellitus. *CNS Neurol. Disord. Drug Targets* **2014**, *13*, 1432–1439. [CrossRef] [PubMed]
22. Morris, G.M.; Huey, R.; Lindstrom, W.; Sanner, M.F.; Belew, R.K.; Goodsell, D.S.; Olson, A.J. AutoDock4 and AutoDockTools4: Automated docking with selective receptor flexibility. *J. Comput. Chem.* **2009**, *30*, 2785–2791. [CrossRef] [PubMed]
23. Nair, V.; Sharma, P.K. Synthesis of the 5′-phosphonate of 4(*S*)-(6-amino-9*H*-purin-9-yl) tetrahydro-2(*S*)-furanmethanol [*S*, *S*-IsoddA]. *ARKIVOC* **2003**, *15*, 10–14. [CrossRef]
24. Jiang, C.; Li, B.; Guan, Z.; Yang, Z.; Zhang, L.; Zhang, L. Synthesis and recognition of novel isonucleoside triphosphates by DNA polymerases. *Bioorganic Med. Chem.* **2007**, *15*, 3019–3025. [CrossRef] [PubMed]

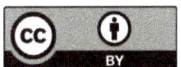 © 2019 by the authors. Licensee MDPI, Basel, Switzerland. This article is an open access article distributed under the terms and conditions of the Creative Commons Attribution (CC BY) license (http://creativecommons.org/licenses/by/4.0/).

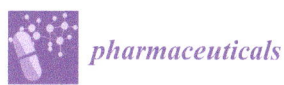

Article

Design and Synthesis of CNS-targeted Flavones and Analogues with Neuroprotective Potential Against H_2O_2- and $A\beta_{1\text{-}42}$-Induced Toxicity in SH-SY5Y Human Neuroblastoma Cells

Ana M. de Matos [1,2,3], Alice Martins [1], Teresa Man [4], David Evans [4], Magnus Walter [5], Maria Conceição Oliveira [6], Óscar López [7], José G. Fernandez-Bolaños [7], Philipp Dätwyler [8], Beat Ernst [8], M. Paula Macedo [3,9,10], Marialessandra Contino [11], Nicola A. Colabufo [11] and Amélia P. Rauter [1,2,*]

1. Center of Chemistry and Biochemistry, Faculdade de Ciências, Universidade de Lisboa, Ed. C8, Campo Grande, 1749-016 Lisboa, Portugal; amjgmatos@gmail.com (A.M.d.M); aimartins@fc.ul.pt (A.M.)
2. Centro de Química Estrutural, Faculdade de Ciências, Universidade de Lisboa, Ed. C8, Campo Grande, 1749-016 Lisboa, Portugal
3. MEDIR: Metabolic Disorders, CEDOC Chronic Diseases, Nova Medical School, Campus Sant'Ana, Rua Câmara Pestana, 6, Lab 3.8, 1150-082 Lisboa, Portugal; paula.macedo@nms.unl.pt
4. Department of Chemistry, Erl Wood Manor, Eli Lilly, Windlesham, Surrey GU20 6PH, UK; man_teresa@lilly.com (T.M.); evans_david_de@lilly.com (D.E.)
5. Abbvie Germany, Knollstr. 51, 67061 Ludwigshafen, Germany; magnus.walter@abbvie.com
6. Centro de Química Estrutural, Instiuto Superior Técnico, Ulisboa, Av. Rovisco Pais, 1049-001 Lisboa, Portugal; conceicao.oliveira@tecnico.ulisboa.pt
7. Departamento de Química Orgánica, Facultad de Química, Universidad de Sevilla, Apartado 1203, E-41071 Sevilla, Spain; osc-lopez@us.es (Ó.L.); bolanos@us.es (J.G.F.-B.)
8. Department of Pharmaceutical Sciences, University of Basel, Klingelbergstrasse 50, CH-4056 Basel, Switzerland; philipp.daetwyler@roche.com (P.D.); beat.ernst@unibas.ch (B.E.)
9. Department of Medical Sciences, IBIMED, Universidade de Aveiro, 3810-193 Aveiro, Portugal
10. APDP-ERC, APDP-Diabetes Portugal, Rua do Salitre, Nº 118-120, 1250-203 Lisboa, Portugal
11. Dipartimento di Farmacia-Scienze del Farmaco, Università degli Studi di Bari/Biofordrug, Via Edoardo Orabona, 4-70125 Bari, Italy; marialessandra.contino@uniba.it (M.C.); nicolaantonio.colabufo@uniba.it (N.A.C.)
* Correspondence: aprauter@fc.ul.pt; Tel.: +35-196-8810971

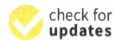

Received: 9 April 2019; Accepted: 6 June 2019; Published: 21 June 2019

Abstract: With the lack of available drugs able to prevent the progression of Alzheimer's disease (AD), the discovery of new neuroprotective treatments able to rescue neurons from cell injury is presently a matter of extreme importance and urgency. Here, we were inspired by the widely reported potential of natural flavonoids to build a library of novel flavones, chromen-4-ones and their C-glucosyl derivatives, and to explore their ability as neuroprotective agents with suitable pharmacokinetic profiles. All compounds were firstly evaluated in a parallel artificial membrane permeability assay (PAMPA) to assess their effective permeability across biological membranes, namely the blood-brain barrier (BBB). With this test, we aimed not only at assessing if our candidates would be well-distributed, but also at rationalizing the influence of the sugar moiety on the physicochemical properties. To complement our analysis, $logD_{7.4}$ was determined. From all screened compounds, the p-morpholinyl flavones stood out for their ability to fully rescue SH-SY5Y human neuroblastoma cells against both H_2O_2- and $A\beta_{1\text{-}42}$-induced cell death. Cholinesterase inhibition was also evaluated, and modest inhibitory activities were found. This work highlights the potential of C-glucosylflavones as neuroprotective agents, and presents the p-morpholinyl C-glucosylflavone **37**, which did not show any cytotoxicity towards HepG2 and Caco-2 cells at 100 μM, as a new lead structure for further development against AD.

Keywords: Alzheimer's disease; Aβ$_{1-42}$; cholinesterase inhibitors; flavones; chromen-4-ones; C-glucosyl flavonoids; PAMPA

1. Introduction

Alzheimer's disease (AD) is a chronic neurodegenerative condition currently affecting more than 40 million people worldwide [1]. Age, genetic background, and type 2 diabetes (T2D) are well-established risk factors for the development of this pathology, which leads to severe memory impairment, language problems, extreme apathy, unpremeditated aggression, and delusional symptoms [2]. The loss of independence in the performance of the simplest tasks is a major stress factor not only for AD patients, but also for relatives and caregivers. But more importantly, with no drugs being able to stop disease progression [3,4], the hope and quality of life for people living with AD is inevitably compromised unless new effective therapies are rapidly discovered.

At the molecular level, AD is a multifactorial disease [5]. Though the amyloid β (Aβ) protein is commonly placed in the center of AD aetiology, the scientific community has been conducting research to link Aβ with many other molecular players and processes known to contribute to disease development and progression, including the cellular prion protein (PrP^C) [6], tau hyperphosphorylation [7], oxidative stress, neuroinflammation [8], and insulin resistance [9], among others. Natural products, including flavonoids and their C-glucosyl derivatives, have been widely studied and found to interfere with one or more of these features [10]. Examples include chrysin (**1**) and 8-β-D-glucosylgenistein (**2**) (Figure 1). Both compounds have been studied by our group and were found to inhibit the formation of small Aβ$_{1-42}$ oligomers [11] or to interact with Aβ$_{1-42}$ peptides [12], respectively.

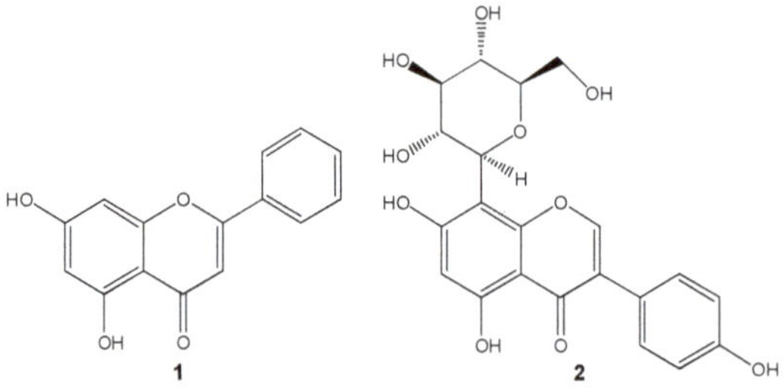

Figure 1. Chemical structure of chrysin (**1**) and 8-β-D-glucosylgenistein (**2**), two natural flavonoids with potential against Alzheimer's disease (AD). Chrysin was used as the prototype structure for chemical modification in the present work.

In this work, we were inspired by the therapeutic potential of flavonoids against AD, having chrysin (**1**) as the lead structure [11] We focused on projecting and generating a small library of flavonoids with neuroprotective potential, while displaying a suitable physicochemical profile. For that purpose, we used the 5,7-dihydroxychromen-4-one unit as the basic building block of all flavonoid structures (aglycones and C-glucosyl derivatives) for two reasons: (a) it is present in many flavonoids exhibiting neuroprotective activities, including not only chrysin [13,14], but also apigenin [15], luteolin [16], and vitexin [17,18], among others, and (b) its synthetic precursor, 2,4,6-trihydroxyacetophenone, has the ideal electron-donating capacity to act as the sugar acceptor in C-glycosylation reactions, in contrast with other polyphenols such as hydroquinone or catechol, which favor the accomplishment of highly effective synthetic routes.

In the light of our previously published data [11], we planned on executing a thorough replacement of the substituent at C-2 of the 5,7-dihydroxychromen-4-one core, with the ultimate goal of generating new compounds with potential for the establishment of interactions with Aβ$_{1-42}$. Furthermore, by synthesizing a number of flavonoids and their respective C-glucosyl derivatives, we were aiming at creating a substantial pool of data that would help us to understand the influence of the sugar moiety in their activity and/or bioavailability. Indeed, having been reported as good stabilizers of non-amyloidogenic Aβ aggregates when combined with polyphenol aglycones [19], sugars may also potentiate antioxidant and antidiabetic activities of these flavonoids [20], which is also an important feature in light of the well-established relationship between AD and type 2 diabetes (T2D) [21]. By screening our compounds against H_2O_2- and $Aβ_{1-42}$-induced cell death in SH-SY5Y human neuroblastoma cells, we have herein established a concise structure–activity relationship study on the neuroprotective effects of the molecular scaffold under investigation, focusing on the substituent at C-2 and the importance of the sugar moiety.

2. Results

Database assembly and compound selection. Following the same synthetic route developed for chrysin (**1**) in a previous study [11], we were now interested in the base-catalysed Claisen–Schmidt aldol condensation reaction for introducing structural diversity into the new flavone analogues. On the basis of the commercially available aldehydes, we then generated a database collection of 98 compounds (the aglycones), which were submitted to a selection process using the Central Nervous System (CNS)-MultiParameter Optimization (MPO) algorithm [22]. This mathematical tool enables the alignment of six key drug-like attributes: partition coefficient (ClogP), distribution coefficient (ClogD), acidity constant (pKa), molecular weight (MW), topological polar surface area (TPSA), and the number of hydrogen bond donors (HBD). Once estimated, these parameters are processed by the algorithm, which generates a desirability score in a scale from 1 to 6. This process allows the selection of compounds with chemical features that make them the most suitable to enter the central nervous system, while displaying favorable permeability, P-gp efflux, metabolic stability, and safety [22].

Using the Molecular Operating Environment (MOE) software, the required physicochemical parameters were calculated for each database compound and were subsequently processed through the CNS-MPO algorithm to generate a set of output scores. According to the creators of this tool, only molecules having a CNS-MPO desirability score above 4 are adequate for further development. Following this restriction, a diverse group of flavone analogues with different alkyl, aryl, and heteroaryl substituents at C-2 was selected (see Supplementary Materials, Table S1) and synthesized.

Synthesis. Chromones and flavones were prepared starting from MOM-diprotected acetophenone **14** (see Supplementary Materials, Scheme S1), which base-catalysed Claisen–Schmidt aldol condensation reaction with commercially available aldehydes generated chalcone and chalcone analogue intermediates in very good reaction yields (63–95%). Interestingly, the isomerization acyclic/cyclic product, resulting from chalcone/flavanone equilibrium, could be detected by liquid chromatography-mass spectrometry (LCMS) and the flavanone was the single product isolated, by reaction of the starting material with cyclobutylcarboxaldehyde (see Supplementary Materials). Subsequently, chalcones and flavanones were submitted to iodine-promoted oxidation in pyridine, followed by *p*-TsOH catalyzed deprotection to give the final products **4–12** in yields ranging from 38% to 95% (Figure 2 and Supplementary Materials).

Chrysin (**1**) and 5,7-dihydroxychromen-4-one (**13**) were also synthesized, as described in a previous study published by our group [11], with the purpose of bioactivity comparison.

For the generation of C-glucosylflavones and analogues, acetophenone C-glucosylation and selective benzylation were carried out prior to the aldol condensation step, as previously described[12] (Scheme S2, Supplementary Materials). Then, aldol condensation gave the intermediate chalcones that reacted with iodine and were debenzylated with BCl_3 at a low temperature to afford the target glucosylchromones and glucosylflavones **15–21** (see Figure 2 and Supplementary Materials for compound synthesis, and structure elucidation of intermediate compounds). Notably, some of the target glucosylflavones could not be obtained, either due to the high reactivity of the intermediates, or due to the extreme hydrophilic character of the final product, as in the case of the 2-(pyridin-4-yl)chromone, which made purification virtually unfeasible even when using reverse phase column purification techniques such as HPLC.

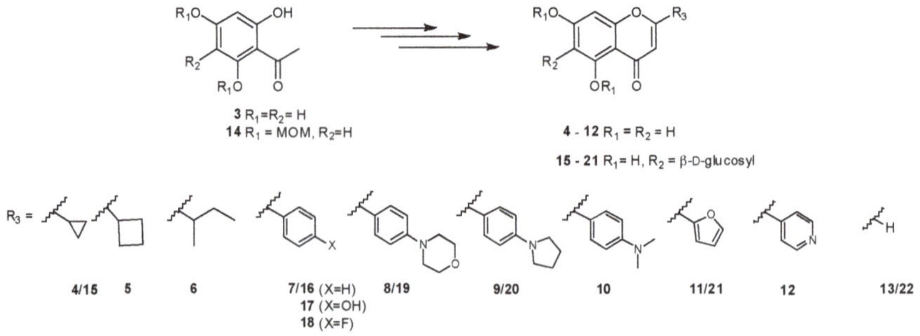

Figure 2. Structure of the new chromones, flavones and their C-glucosyl derivatives studied in this work (for the synthetic approach followed, see Supplementary Materials).

The formation of 6-glucosyl-5,7-dihydroxychromen-4-one (**22**) required a different methodology as that described for its analogues. For this task, we applied the same protocol used for generating its aglycone. Dibenzylated acetophloroglucinol derivatized with a perbenzylglucosyl group (Scheme S2B, Supplementary Materials) reacted with sodium hydride in ethyl formate at 0 °C to give an intermediate, that was subsequently dehydrated in acid medium, under reflux, affording perbenzylglucosylchromone in 84% yield. Further deprotection with BCl_3 in dichloromethane at a low temperature gave compound **22** in good yield (Scheme S2B in Supplementary Materials, that also include intermediates' synthesis and structure elucidation).

Parallel Artificial Membrane Permeability Assay (PAMPA) and log $D_{7.4}$ determination. Finding new molecules exhibiting adequate physicochemical properties for permeating the blood-brain barrier is often a challenging drawback in CNS drug discovery. Indeed, in order to fully evaluate the therapeutic potential of CNS-targeted compounds, such as those generated in the present study, the evaluation of their physicochemical and pharmacokinetic profiles is key. Hence, all synthesized compounds were tested in the parallel artificial membrane permeability assay (PAMPA) in order to measure and rationalize their potential to cross membrane barriers. Testosterone was used as the positive control in this assay. To complete our analysis, the partition coefficient at physiological pH (log$D_{7.4}$) was also determined. Ideally, log D values should be located between 1 and 4 for a good compromise between solubility and membrane permeability allowing oral availability, good cell permeation, and low metabolic susceptibility [23]. Results are presented in Table 1.

Neuroprotective activity assays against H_2O_2-induced toxicity. On the basis of previously described protocols [24–26], the flavones and analogues herein synthesized were screened for their neuroprotective effects against H_2O_2-induced oxidative stress and neuronal damage in SH-SY5Y human neuroblastoma cells by means of a thiazolyl blue tetrazolium bromide (MTT) reduction-based cell viability assay. This screening protocol aimed not only at comparing the activity of aglycones versus C-glucosyl derivatives when tested at the same concentration (50 µM), but also at distinguishing between the best candidates amongst amines, aliphatic or heteroaryl derivatives, or aromatic derivatives with electron-withdrawing substituents. In addition, all compounds were directly compared to compound **2**, a natural molecule conjectured to display neuroprotective effects [12], but with no cell-based evidence reported up to this point. Results are presented in Figure 3. All compounds were tested in the same experimental conditions without the neurotoxic agent beforehand, and none were found to significantly decrease cell viability when compared to non-treated controls (see Supplementary Materials, Table S2).

Table 1. Effective permeability (log P_e) and partition coefficient at pH 7.4 (log $D_{7.4}$) of the synthesized flavones and analogues.

Compound Nr.	Log P_e [a]	Log $D_{7.4}$ [b]
1	−4.65 ± 0.09	3.6 ± 0.4
4	−4.66 ± 0.09	2.9 ± 0.1
5	−4.51 ± 0.06	>2.5
6	−4.48 ± 0.04	>2.5
7	−4.37 ± 0.12	>2.5
8	−4.56 ± 0.04	>2.5
9	−5.31 ± 0.12	n.d.[c]
10	−4.70 ± 0.14	3.4 ± 0.2
11	−4.93 ± 0.20	>2.5
12	−4.64 ± 0.02	n.d.[c]
13	−4.76 ± 0.02	2.4 ± 0.1
15	Below detection limit	−0.6 ± 0.2
16	−8.94 ± 1.83	0.8 ± 0.3
17	−8.70 ± 1.50	0.1 ± 0.1
18	Below detection limit	−0.2 ± 0.1
19	−7.08 ± 0.91	1.2 ± 0.1
20	−6.52 ± 0.41	1.8 ± 0.2
21	−6.94 ± 0.50	−0.2 ± 0.1
22	−6.76 ± 0.11	−2.0 ± 0.2
Testosterone	−4.42 ± 0.09	-

[a]: effective permeability; [b]: partition coefficient at pH 7.4; [c]: not determined.

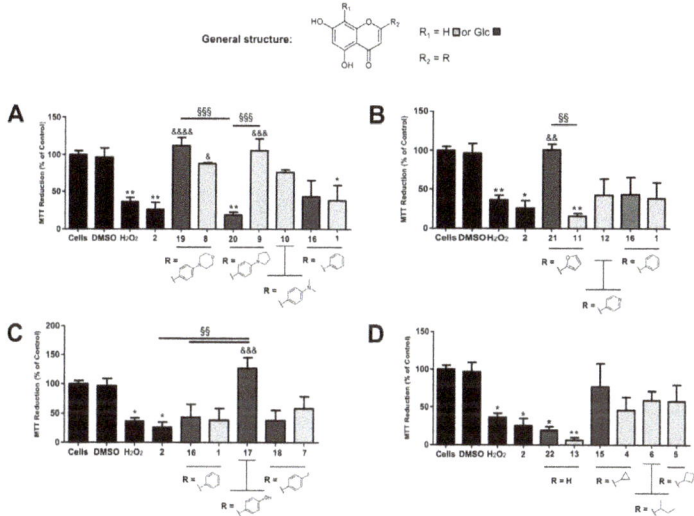

Figure 3. Neuroprotective effects of compound **2**, flavone derivatives and corresponding aglycones against H_2O_2-induced toxicity in human SH-SY5Y neuroblastoma cells via a MTT cell viability assay. (**A**) Effects caused by amine moieties in *para*-position of ring B; (**B**) effects caused by the replacement of ring B with heteroaromatic groups; (**C**) effects caused by electron withdrawing groups in *para*-position of ring B; (**D**) effects caused by the replacement of ring B with aliphatic moieties. Cells were incubated with 100 μM H_2O_2 for 24 h at 37 °C, in the presence (50 μM) or absence of each compound. The tests were performed in triplicate with a final concentration of 0.5% DMSO. Results are presented as means ± standard error. Statistical differences between groups were assessed by one-way ANOVA followed by a Tukey's post-test. * $p < 0.05$, and ** $p < 0.01$ versus cell control; & $p < 0.05$, && $p < 0.01$, &&& $p < 0.001$ and &&&& $p < 0.0001$ versus H_2O_2 control; §§ $p < 0.01$ and §§§ $p < 0.001$ versus another compound.

At 100 μM, H_2O_2 caused over 50% of cell viability loss, which is consistent with earlier published data (Figure 3) [25]. While compound **2** was not found to display neuroprotective effects against the observed H$_2$O$_2$-induced cell death in this cell line, at the tested concentration, amine derivatives were generally well-succeeded in restoring cell viability (Figure 3A). Compounds **8**, **9**, and **19** were in fact able to produce statistically significant differences when compared to H$_2$O$_2$ controls ($P < 0.5$, $P < 0.001$ and $P < 0.0001$, respectively). C-glucosides **17** and **21** were also able to rescue cells from oxidative damage caused by H$_2$O$_2$ ($P < 0.001$ and $P < 0.01$ respectively) (Figure 3B,C), while neither the remaining glycosides nor the remaining aglycones were able to lead to similar results.

Neuroprotective activity assays against Aβ$_{1-42}$-induced toxicity. From all compounds tested in the above presented assay, the pair **8** and **19** presented the strongest neuroprotective potential, with convincing proof on the importance of the aglycone for the desired neuroprotective effects against H$_2$O$_2$-induced cell injury. Both compounds were henceforth selected to be further explored, together with compound **2**, the C-analogue of chrysin (**16**), vitexin (**17**), and the pair of 4'-fluoroflavones (**7** and **18**) for comparison purposes. Here, the MTT assay was used once again to assess cell viability of SH-SY5Y cells treated with 20 µM of Aβ$_{1-42}$, in the presence of 50 µM of each compound. Similar protocols have been used to screen candidates for AD therapy [27,28]. Moreover, based on the existing evidence that *in situ* spontaneous fibrillization of Aβ$_{1-42}$ in the incubation mixture is important in the triggering of neurotoxic effects [29], we added the Aβ$_{1-42}$ peptide fragment dissolved in DMSO to the culture medium prior to incubation, together with each compound in study. Results are displayed in Figure 4. Even though there is published evidence that undifferentiated SH-SY5Y cells are not as sensitive to Aβ$_{1-42}$-induced neurite degeneration and apoptosis as differentiated ones [29], with 20 µM of Aβ$_{1-42}$ we were able to observe a significant decrease in cellular MTT reduction capacity, corresponding to roughly half of the cell viability rates observed in the non-treated control. The 4-morpholinyl derivative **19** exhibited, once more, the result with the highest significance when compared to controls. Compound **8** also displayed relevant neuroprotective effects against Aβ$_{1-42}$, contrarily to the 4'-fluoroflavone **7**.

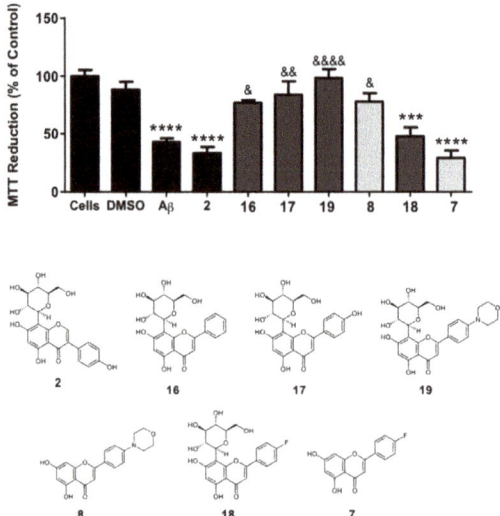

Figure 4. Neuroprotective effects of compound **2** and analogues against Aβ$_{1-42}$-induced toxicity in human SH-SY5Y neuroblastoma cells via a MTT cell viability assay. Cells were incubated with 20 µM Aβ$_{1-42}$ for 24 h at 37 °C, in the presence (50 µM) or absence of each compound. The tests were performed in triplicate with 1% DMSO (Aβ) or 1.5% DMSO (Aβ + compound – maximum DMSO percentage presented in the graph). Results are presented as means ± standard error. Statistical differences between groups were assessed by one-way ANOVA followed by a Tukey's post-test. *** $p < 0.001$ and **** $p < 0.0001$ versus cell control; & $p < 0.05$, && $p < 0.01$ and &&&& $p < 0.0001$ Aβ control.

3. Discussion

As predicted by our computational calculations, all aglycones (**1, 4–13**) presented an excellent membrane permeation capacity, as shown by the measured effective permeability for these molecules (Log P_e > −5.7). Yet, compounds **2** and **10** displayed log $D_{7.4}$ values slightly above the desired upper limit, and thus they may be associated with the risk of being retained in cell membranes and/or fat tissues. The data for C-glucosyl derivatives **15–22** exhibited much more variability. Compounds **15** and **18** displayed no detectable permeability in PAMPA. Even though compounds **16** and **17** have a slightly improved effective permeability (Log P_e ~ −9), it is still very limited to allow passive diffusion over membranes. Notably, the 4-pyrrolidinyl derivative (**38**) presented the best effective permeability from all C-glucosylflavones (log P_e = −6.520 ± 0.408) and a determined log $D_{7.4}$ (1.8 ± 0.2) within the ideal value range. Compounds **19, 21,** and **22** fell in the middle (log P_e ~ −7); however, only the 4-morpholinyl derivative **19** had a desirable log $D_{7.4}$ value (1.8 ± 0.2). Indeed, it seems that only certain aglycones are able to compensate for the hydrophilicity of the sugar moiety, either owing to their intrinsic lipophilicity, or to the resulting molecular conformation of the C-glycoside as a whole. Nevertheless, it is important to mention that, as previously described for other C-glucosyl flavonoids [30], the glucosyl moiety in these compounds might prompt their affinity towards GLUT-1 transporters in the blood-brain barrier (BBB), which may ultimately contribute to enhance their concentration near the therapeutic targets in the CNS.

The neuroprotective activity of many lead candidates, especially from natural origin, has been assessed against cellular damage induced by H_2O_2 in SH-SY5Y and other relevant neuronal cell lines over the past decades [24–26,31]. Indeed, this neurotoxic agent has been reported to cause mitochondrial and cell membrane damage, with the depletion of antioxidant enzymatic machinery leading to increased levels of reactive oxygen species (ROS) and associated neuroinflammatory processes [25]. Ultimately, H_2O_2-induced oxidative stress and inflammation trigger neuronal apoptosis through increased expression of pro-apoptotic factors such as caspase 3, and depletion of anti-apoptotic factors such as Bcl-2, which have been linked to the development and progression of AD [25,32]. As described for melittin, orientin, and bikaverin, among others, protection mechanisms offered by small molecules against H_2O_2-promoted cell damage and apoptosis may include the downregulation of pro-inflammatory transcription factors such as the nuclear factor-kappaB (NFκB), increased Bcl-2 mRNA and protein expression, inhibition of caspase expression and activity, and replenishment of neuronal pro-oxidative/antioxidant enzyme balance [24–26]. In addition, provided that Aβ oligomers have been described to enhance ROS levels and protein oxidation in neurons [33], it is important to bear in mind that other possible neuroprotective mechanisms with impacts on oxidative stress can be associated with the inhibition of Aβ oligomerization or regulation of Aβ production and/or clearance itself.

Compounds **8, 9,** and **19** were able to produce statistically significant differences when compared to H_2O_2 controls. What's more, the amine moiety was found to be critical for the neuroprotective activity, as shown by the absence of significant effects displayed by chrysin (**1**) and its C-glucosyl analogue **16**. Yet, it is herein important to distinguish between aglycones and C-glucosyl derivatives, as a consistent correlation between the presence of the sugar moiety and stimulation of cell survival could not be observed. If, on the one hand, amine aglycones **8** and **9** were able to cause significant improvements in cell viability when compared to controls, on the other hand only compound **19** produced the desired effect, with dramatic differences from that of its 4-pyrrolidinyl analogue **20**. Since both aglycones **8** and **9** are active, it is likely that the C-glucosyl moiety is detrimental in the second case. Conversely, the fact that the 4-morpholinyl group in compounds **8** and **19** induced protective effects regardless of the presence of the sugar moiety could mean that this substituent, perhaps through the presence of an endocyclic oxygen atom, is preferred for this type of activity. Interestingly, aglycone **10** was not significantly active, reinforcing that the presence of a nitrogen-containing ring in *para*-position of ring B should, indeed, be beneficial. All in all, this group of derivatives presented a major improvement when compared to compound **2**, and both unsubstituted flavones **1** and **16**, with compounds **8** and **19** as the most promising pair of flavone derivatives.

From the heteroaryl derivatives, only the C-glucosyl flavone analogue containing the 2-furanyl moiety **21** was able to produce a significant improvement in cell viability, contrarily to its aglycone **11** or the 4-pyridinyl derivative **12** (Figure 3B). Contrasting with the pair of 4-pyrrolidinyl derivatives (**9** and **20**, Figure 3A), in the case of compounds **11** and **21** it appears to be the combination of the sugar moiety with the modified aglycone that triggers the neuroprotective effect, and not the aglycone per se. Still, this combination was able to improve the activity of the C-glucosyl analogue of chrysin **16**, indicating that the replacement of ring B with a heteroaromatic ring in the presence of the sugar moiety may be advantageous. Ultimately, compound **21** succeeded at improving the activity of the lead compound **2**.

Regarding the compounds with electron-withdrawing groups in *para*-position of ring B (Figure 3C), it is interesting to note that vitexin (**17**) was able to fully recover cell viability, while compound **2** and C-glucosylchrysin (**16**) were not. These results indicate that the C-glucosylflavone scaffold may be more effective in terms of neuroprotective effects than the corresponding isoflavone, and that the hydroxy group in *para*-position of ring B is in fact beneficial for activity. What's more, from both electron withdrawing groups in *para*-position of ring B (OH- in vitexin and F- in derivatives **18** and **7**) only the hydroxy group was able to produce a relevant neuroprotective effect, which may be attributable to: (a) the formation of a phenoxyl radical stabilized by resonance due to the presence of the α,β-unsaturated ketone if the neuroprotective effect results from direct chemical ROS inactivation, or (b) the formation of hydrogen bonds with a macromolecular target, e.g., an antioxidant enzyme.

Accordingly, no significant differences between cell viability in the presence of either of the two 5,7-dihydroxychromen-4-ones (**22** and **13**) and the cell viability of H_2O_2 controls were observed in our study (Figure 3D). Even though all compounds with aliphatic substituents (**4**, **5**, and **6**) led to an increase in MTT reduction when compared to both chromen-4-ones, the increase was not significant.

From the compounds selected to be tested against $A\beta_{1-42}$-induced neurotoxicity, the 4-morpholinyl derivative **19** again presented the result with the highest significance when compared to the controls. Compound **8** also displayed relevant neuroprotective effects against $A\beta_{1-42}$ (contrarily to the 4'-fluoroflavone **7**) which once more supports the hypothesis that in this particular case, compound **8** is active per se, but its effects are maintained or potentiated by the presence of the sugar moiety. Provided that the pair of compounds **8** and **19** was active in H_2O_2-induced toxicity assay as well, whether the observed effects against $A\beta_{1-42}$ are due to a direct interaction with $A\beta$ oligomers or to the inhibition of $A\beta_{1-42}$-promoted oxidative stress (or both) remains to be clarified. Nonetheless, compound **19**, the best in the series of flavones and analogues presented in this work, also showed some inhibitory activity of acetylcholinesterase (18% at 100 µM, see Supplementary Materials, Table S3). Moreover, all compounds tested inhibited either acetylcholinesterase (AChE) and/or butyrylcholinesterase (BuChE). Chrysin was the most active butyrylcholinesterase inhibitor, while amongst the selective BuChE inhibitors, the chromen-4-one derivative **6** was indeed the most promising one. Nonetheless, compound **19** stood out as the lead molecule with potential for AD. It was tested in human epithelial colorectal adenocarcinoma (Caco-2) and liver hepatocarcinoma (HepG2) cells from concentrations ranging from 0.1 µM to 100 µM, and no significant cytotoxic effects could be observed ($IC_{50} \geq 100$ µM).

4. Materials and Methods

General Methods. HPLC grade solvents and reagents were obtained from commercial suppliers and were used without further purification. Chrysin (**1**), compound **2**, and 5,7-dihydroxychromen-4-one (**13**) were synthesized according to the methodologies previously described by us.[11,12] LCMS experiments were performed in a column XBridge C18 3.5u 2.1 × 50 mm at 1.2 mL/min and 50 °C; 10 mM ammonium bicarbonate pH 9/ACN, gradient 10 > 95% ACN in 1.5 min + 0.5 min hold. Reactions affording compounds **37** and **17** were followed by TLC, carried out on aluminum sheets (20 × 20 cm) coated with silica gel 60 F-254, 0.2 mm thick (Merck, Darmstadt, Germany) with detection by charring with 10% H_2SO_4 in ethanol. Flash column chromatography was performed using CombiFlash® Rf200 (Teledyne Isco, Lincoln, CA, USA). Preparative HPLC was performed in a Gilson apparatus using either Phenomenex Gemini NX, C18, 5 µm 30 × 100 mm or Phenomenex Gemini NX, C18, 10 µm 50 × 150 mm columns. NMR spectra for compound characterization were recorded on a Bruker AV III HD Nanobay spectrometer running at 400.13 MHz equipped with a room temperature 5 mm BBO Smartprobe. Chemical shifts are expressed in δ (ppm) and the proton coupling constants *J* in Hertz (Hz). NMR data were assigned using appropriate COSY, DEPT, HMQC, and HMBC spectra (representative examples are provided in the Supporting information appendix). Optical rotations were measured with a Perkin–Elmer 343 polarimeter. Melting points were measured using a Stuart SMP30 melting point apparatus. High-resolution mass spectra of final compounds were acquired on a Bruker Daltonics HR QqTOF Impact II mass spectrometer (Billerica, MA, USA). The nebulizer gas (N_2) pressure was set to 1.4 bar, and the drying gas (N_2) flow rate was set to 4.0 L/minute at a temperature of 200 °C. The capillary voltage was set to 4500 V and the charging voltage was set to 2000 V. Tested compounds have ≥ 95% purity as determined by LCMS. Synthesis of intermediate compounds **23–31** and **35–42** is reported in Supplementary Materials, together with their LCMS data, physical and NMR data.

General procedure for the synthesis of non-glycosylated chalcones/flavones. Each compound **23–30** was dissolved in dry pyridine (0.248 mmol in 7.33 mL). Then, catalytic amounts of I_2 (0.087 mmol, 0.35 eq.) were added and the mixture was stirred under reflux for 24 h–72 h. All reactions were followed by LCMS. Once the starting material was fully consumed, the mixture was allowed to reach room temperature and the pyridine was co-evaporated with toluene under reduced pressure. The residue was resuspended in dichloromethane, washed first with a saturated solution of sodium thiosulfate, and then with brine. The flavone was extracted with dichloromethane (3 × 30 mL), dried over $MgSO_4$, and the solution filtered and concentrated under vacuum. The residue was then resuspended in ethanol (15 mL) and *p*-TsOH (12% in AcOH, 0.1 mL) was added. The reaction was stirred under reflux for 2–24 h. After having reached completion by LCMS, the solvent was evaporated under vacuum and the residue purified using the most adequate purification method(s) to afford compounds **4–12**.

2-Cyclopropyl-5,7-dihydroxy-4H-chromen-4-one (**4**). Purified by preparative HPLC. Reaction yield over two steps: 53%; LCMS: RT = 0.52 min, *m/z* = 219.0 [M + H]$^+$ (high pH method); white solid; m.p. = 201.2–202.9 °C. ^{1}H NMR (MeOD) δ (ppm) 6.26 (d, 1H, J_{meta} = 2.1 Hz, H-8), 6.17 (d, 1H, J_{meta} = 2.1 Hz, H-6), 6.10 (s, 1H, H-3), 2.02–1.96 (m, 1H, H-1′), 1.18–1.09 (m, 4H, H-2′, H-3′). ^{13}C NMR [MeOD] δ (ppm) 181.5 (C-4), 173.5 (C-2), 166.0 (C-7), 163.4 (C-5), 159.6 (C-8a), 106.5 (C-3), 100.2 (C-6), 95.0 (C-8), 15.4 (C-1′), 9.5 (C-2′, C-3′). HRMS-ESI (*m/z*): [M + H]$^+$ calcd for $C_{12}H_{11}O_4$ 219.0652, found 219.0642.

2-Cyclobutyl-5,7-dihydroxy-4H-chromen-4-one (**5**). Purified by preparative HPLC. Reaction yield over two steps: 85%; LCMS: RT = 0.72 min, *m/z* = 233.0 [M + H]$^+$ (high pH method); white solid; m.p. = 200.3–201.5 °C. ^{1}H NMR (MeOD) δ (ppm) 6.34 (d, 1H, J_{meta} = 2.1 Hz, H-8), 6.18 (d, 1H, J_{meta} = 2.1 Hz, H-6), 6.03 (s, 1H, H-3), 3.53 (td, 1H, *J* = 8.0 Hz, H-1′), 2.37–2.31 (m, 4H, H-2′, H-4′), 2.17–2.06 (m, 1H, H-3′a), 1.99–1.91 (m, 1H, H-3′). ^{13}C NMR [(CD$_3$)OD] δ (ppm) 183.4 (C-4), 174.1 (C-2), 166.0 (C-7), 163.3 (C-5), 159.9 (C-8a), 106.5 (C-3), 100.0 (C-6), 94.9 (C-8), 39.5 (C-1′), 27.5 (C-2′, C-4′), 19.0 (C-3′). HRMS-ESI (*m/z*): [M + H]$^+$ calcd for $C_{13}H_{13}NO_4$ 233.0808, found 233.0804.

5,7-Dihydroxy-2-(1-methylpropyl)-4H-chromen-4-one (**6**). Purified by preparative HPLC. Reaction yield over three steps: 67%; LCMS: RT = 1.10 min, *m/z* = 235.0 [M + H]$^+$ (low pH method); brown solid; m.p. = 192.5–193.8 °C. ^{1}H NMR (MeOD) δ (ppm) 6.33 (d, 1H, J_{meta} = 2.2 Hz, H-8), 6.20 (d, 1H, J_{meta} = 2.2 Hz, H-6), 6.05 (s, 1H, H-3), 2.65 (sextet, 1H, $J_{1′-1″~1′-2′}$ = 7.4 Hz, H-1′), 1.80–1.59 (m, 2H, H-2′), 1.30 (d, 3H, $J_{1″-1′}$ = 7.4 Hz, H-1″), 0.95 (t, 3H, $J_{3′-2′}$ = 7.4 Hz, H-3′). ^{13}C NMR [MeOD] δ (ppm) 184.1 (C-4), 175.8 (C-2), 166.0 (C-7), 163.5 (C-5), 159.9 (C-8a), 107.6 (C-3), 105.4 (C-4a), 100.0 (C-6), 94.8 (C-8), 41.7 (C-1′), 28.6 (C-2′), 18.2 (C-1″), 11.9 (C-3′). HRMS-ESI (*m/z*): [M + H]$^+$ calcd for $C_{13}H_{15}O_4$ 235.0965, found 235.0962.

4′-Fluoro-5,7-dihydroxyflavone (**7**). Purified by preparative HPLC. Reaction yield over two steps: 38%; LCMS: RT = 1.10 min, *m/z* = 273.0 [M + H]$^+$ (low pH method); white solid; m.p. = 264.8–265.5 °C. ^{1}H NMR [MeOD] δ (ppm) 8.05 (dd, 2H, *J*$_{ortho}$ = 8.9 Hz, *J*$_{2′-F=6′-F}$ = 5.2 Hz, H-2′, H-6′), 7.31 (t, 2H, *J*$_{ortho}$~*J*$_{3′-F=5′-F}$ = 8.7 Hz, H-3′, H-5′), 6.73 (s, 1H, H-3), 6.50 (d, 1H, *J*$_{meta}$ = 2.2 Hz, 1H, H-8), 6.24 (d, 1H, *J*$_{meta}$ = 2.2 Hz, H-6). ^{13}C NMR [MeOD] δ (ppm) 183.8 (C-4), 166.3 (C-7), 164.7 (C-5), 163.3 (d, *J*$_{C-F}$ = 259.3 Hz, C-4′), 159.5 (C-8a), 130.1 (d, *J*$_{C-F}$ = 9.0 Hz, C-2′, C-6′), 127.6 (C-1′), 117.3 (d, *J*$_{C-F}$ = 22.5 Hz, C-3′, C-5′), 106.0 (C-3, C-4a), 100.3 (C-6), 95.2 (C-8). HRMS-ESI (*m/z*): [M + H]$^+$ calcd for C$_{15}$H$_{10}$FO$_4$ 273.0558, found 273.0554.

5,7-Dihydroxy-4′-(morpholin-4-yl)flavone (**8**). Purified by preparative HPLC. Reaction yield over two steps: 68%; LCMS: RT = 1.07 min, *m/z* = 340.0 [M + H]$^+$ (low pH method); orange solid; m.p. = 234.0–235.6 °C. ^{1}H NMR (MeOD) δ (ppm) 7.87 (d, 2H, *J*$_{ortho}$ = 9.0 Hz, H-2′ and H-6′), 7.06 (d, 2H, H-3′ and H-5′), 6.58 (s, 1H, H-3), 6.45 (d, 1H, *J*$_{meta}$ = 2.2 Hz, H-8), 6.21 (d, 1H, *J*$_{meta}$ = 2.1 Hz, H-6), 3.86–3.83 (m, 4H, NCH$_2$CH$_2$O), 3.34 (NCH$_2$CH$_2$O, overlapped with methanol-*d*$_4$ peak). ^{13}C NMR (MeOD) δ (ppm) 183.8 (C-4), 165.9 (C-2), 163.7 (C-7 and C-5), 159.4.0 (C-8a), 155.3 (C-4′), 128.9 (C-2′, C-6′), 121.8 (C-1′), 115.4 (C-3′, C-5′), 105.3 (C-4a), 103.3 (C-3), 100.1 (C-6), 95.0 (C-8), 67.7 (NCH$_2$CH$_2$O), 48.1 (NCH$_2$CH$_2$O). HRMS-ESI (*m/z*): [M + H]$^+$ calcd for C$_{19}$H$_{18}$NO$_5$ 340.1179, found 340.1175.

5,7-Dihydroxy-4′-(pyrrolidin-1-yl)flavone (**9**). Purified by preparative HPLC. Reaction yield over two steps: 95%; LCMS: RT = 1.08 min, *m/z* = 324.0 [M + H]$^+$ (high pH method); orange solid; m.p. = 282.4–283.6 °C. ^{1}H NMR [(CD$_3$)$_2$CO] δ (ppm) 7.89 (d, 2H, *J*$_{ortho}$ = 9.0 Hz, H-2′ and H-6′), 6.70 (s, 1H, H-3), 6.65 (d, 2H, H-3′ and H-5′), 6.46 (d, 1H, *J*$_{meta}$ = 2.2 Hz, H-8), 6.16 (d, 1H, *J*$_{meta}$ = 2.2 Hz, H-6), 3.35–3.33 (m, NCH$_2$CH$_2$), 2.00–1.97 (m, 4H, NCH$_2$CH$_2$). ^{13}C NMR [(CD$_3$)$_2$CO] δ (ppm) 181.5 (C-4), 164.6 (C-2), 163.9 (C-7), 161.5 (C-5), 157.2 (C-8a), 150.1 (C-4′), 128.0 (C-2′, C-6′), 116.0 (C-1′), 111.7 (C-3′, C-5′), 103.6 (C-4a), 100.9 (C-3), 98.7 (C-6), 93.9 (C-8), 47.4 (NCH$_2$CH$_2$), 25.0 (NCH$_2$CH$_2$). HRMS-ESI (*m/z*): [M + H]$^+$ calcd for C$_{19}$H$_{18}$NO$_4$ 324.1230, found 324.1225.

4′-Dimethylamino-5,7-dihydroxyflavone (**10**). Purified by preparative HPLC. Reaction yield over two steps: 54%; LCMS: RT = 1.12 min, *m/z* = 298.0 [M + H]$^+$ (low pH method); orange solid; m.p. = 291.3–292.7 °C. ^{1}H NMR [(CD$_3$)$_2$SO] δ (ppm) 13.11 (s, 1H, OH-5), 7.88 (d, 2H, *J*$_{ortho}$ = 9.0 Hz, H-2′ and H-6′), 6.80 (d, 2H, H-3′ and H-5′), 6.71 (s, 1H, H-3), 6.46 (d, 1H, *J*$_{meta}$ = 2.1 Hz, H-8), 6.17 (d, 1H, *J*$_{meta}$ = 2.1 Hz, H-6), 3.03 [s, 6H, N(CH$_3$)$_2$]. ^{13}C NMR [(CD$_3$)$_2$SO] δ (ppm) 181.5 (C-4), 164.3 (C-2), 163.8 (C-7), 161.4 (C-5), 157.2 (C-8a), 152.6 (C-4′), 127.8 (C-2′, C-6′), 116.5 (C-1′), 111.6 (C-3′, C-5′), 103.6 (C-4a), 101.2 (C-3), 98.6 (C-6), 93.8 (C-8), 39.6 [N(CH$_3$)$_2$]. HRMS-ESI (*m/z*): [M + H]$^+$ calcd for C$_{17}$H$_{16}$NO$_4$ 298.1074, found 298.101.

2-(Furan-2-yl)-5,7-dihydroxy-4H-chromen-4-one (**11**). Purified by preparative HPLC. Reaction yield over two steps: 59%; LCMS: RT. = 0.99 min, *m/z* = 298.0 [M + H]$^+$ (low pH method); white solid; m.p. = 239.3–240.8 °C. ^{1}H NMR [(CD$_3$)$_2$CO] δ (ppm) 12.87 (s, 1H, OH-5), 7.92 (d, 1H, *J*$_{5′-4′}$ = 1.6 Hz, H-5′), 7.34 (d, 1H, *J*$_{4′-3′}$ = 3.5 Hz, H-3′), 6.77 (dd, 1H, *J*$_{5′-4′}$ = 3.5 Hz, *J*$_{3′-4′}$ = 1.8 Hz, H-4′), 6.49–6.48 (m, 2H, H-3, H-8), 6.27 (d, 1H, *J*$_{meta}$ = 1.8 Hz, H-6). ^{13}C NMR [(CD$_3$)$_2$CO] δ (ppm) 182.7 (C-4), 164.9 (C-2), 156.3 (C-7)*, 163.1 (C-5), 158.0 (C-8a)*, 147.8 (C-5′), 146.9 (C-2′), 114.8 (C-3′), 113.9 (C-4′), 104.0 (C-4a), 103.9 (C-3), 100.1 (C-6), 95.0 (C-8). HRMS-ESI (*m/z*): [M + H]$^+$ calcd for C$_{13}$H$_{19}$O$_5$ 245.0444, found 245.0438. *Permutable signals.

5,7-Dihydroxy-2-(pyridin-4-yl)-4H-chromen-4-one (**12**). Purified by preparative HPLC. Reaction yield over three steps: 87%; LCMS: RT = 0.43 min, *m/z* = 256.0 [M + H]$^+$ (low pH method);: orange oil. ^{1}H NMR (MeOD) δ (ppm) 8.79 (d, 2H, H-3′, H-5′), 8.37 (d, 2H, *J*$_{ortho}$ = 6.6 Hz, H-2′, H-6′), 6.74 (s, 1H, H-3), 6.30 (d, 1H, *J*$_{meta}$ = 1.8 Hz, H-8), 6.10 (d, 1H, *J*$_{meta}$ = 1.8 Hz, H-6). ^{13}C NMR (MeOD) δ (ppm) 180.7 (C-4), 171.1 (C-2), 169.8 (C-7), 161.0 (C-5), 155.6 (C-8a), 151.6 (C-1′), 143.3 (C-3′, C-5′), 128.1 (C-2′,

C-6′), 103.4 (C-3), 103.2 (C-4a), 99.6 (C-6), 92.7 (C-8). HRMS-ESI (*m/z*): [M + H]$^+$ calcd for $C_{14}H_{10}NO_4$ 256.0604, found 256.0600.

General procedure for the synthesis of C-glucosylflavones. Each C-glucosylchalcone **35–41** was dissolved in dry pyridine (0.172 mmol in 5.11 mL). Then, catalytic amounts of I_2 (0.060 mmol, 0.35 eq.) were added and the mixture was stirred under reflux for 48–72 h. All reactions were followed by LCMS. Once the starting material was fully consumed, the mixture was allowed to reach room temperature and the pyridine was co-evaporated with toluene under reduced pressure. The residue was resuspended in dichloromethane, washed first with a saturated solution of sodium thiosulfate, and then with brine. The flavone was extracted with dichloromethane (3 × 30 mL), dried over $MgSO_4$, and the solution filtered and concentrated under vacuum. The residue was then resuspended in extra dry dichloromethane (7.10 mL) and stirred at −78 °C under N_2 saturated atmosphere. A 1 M solution of BBr_3 in dichloromethane (1.72 mL, 1.72 mmol, 10 eq.) was added in a dropwise manner over 5 min, and the reaction stirred for 2–4 h. After having reached completion by LCMS, the reaction was quenched with a 1:1 mixture of dichloromethane/methanol (ca. 15 mL) and the reaction was stirred for approximately 20 min at room temperature. The solvent was evaporated under vacuum and the residue purified using the most adequate purification method(s) to afford compounds **15–21**.

2-Cyclopropyl-8-(β-D-glucopyranosyl)-5,7-dihydroxy-4-chromen-4-one (**15**). Purified by preparative HPLC. Reaction yield over two steps: 37%; LCMS: RT = 0.51 min, *m/z* = 381.0 [M + H]$^+$ (low pH method); yellowish oil. ^{1}H NMR (MeOD) δ (ppm) 6.23 (s, 1H, H-6), 6.20 (s, 1H, H-3), 4.86 (H-1″, overlapped with the methanol-d_6 water peak), 3.92–3.87 (m, 2H, H-2″, H-6″a), 3.75–3.64 (m, 1H, H-6″b), 3.47–3.42 (m, 3H, H-3″, H-4″, H-5″), 2.06–2.00 (m, 1H, H-1′), 1.46–1.43 (m, 1H, H-2′a)*, 1.28–1.22 (m, 1H, H-3′a)*, 1.18–1.09 (m, 2H, H-2′b, H-3′b). ^{13}C NMR (MeOD) δ (ppm) 183.6 (C-4), 173.3 (C-2), 164.4 (C-7), 162.7 (C-5), 160.4 (C-8a), 106.8 (C-8), 105.5 (C-3), 104.9 (C-4a), 99.3 (C-6), 82.8 (C-5″), 80.1 (C-3″), 74.9 (C-1″), 73.3 (C-2″), 72.6 (C-4″), 63.4 (C-6″), 15.7 (C-1′), 10.0, 9.6 (C-2′, C-3′). *Permutable signals. HRMS-ESI (*m/z*): [M + H]$^+$ calcd for $C_{18}H_{21}O_9$ 381.1180, found 381.1176.

8-(β-D-Glucopyranosyl)-5,7-dihydroxyflavone (**16**). Purified by preparative HPLC, followed by Isolute SCX-2 column chromatography (Biotage). Reaction yield over two steps: 88%; LCMS: RT = 0.49 min, *m/z* = 414.80 [M − H]$^-$ (high pH method); yellow solid; m.p. = 188.1–189.2 °C. ^{1}H NMR (MeOD) δ (ppm) 8.13, 8.03 (d, 2H, J_{ortho} = 7.1 Hz, H-2′ and H-6′)*, 7.58–7.54 (m, 3H, H-3′, H-4′ and H-5′), 6.75 (s, 1H, H-3), 6.30 (s, 1H, H-6), 5.00 (d, 1H, $J_{1″-2″}$ = 9.9 Hz, H-1″)*, 4.11 (t, 1H, $J_{2″-1″}$~$_{2″-3″}$ = 9.3 Hz, H-2″), 3.97 (br d, 1H, $J_{6″a-6″b}$ = 12.1 Hz, H-6″a)*, 3.81 (dd, 1H, $J_{6″b-6″a}$ = 12.1 Hz, $J_{6″b-5″}$ = 5.3 Hz, H-6″a), 3.68 (t, 1H, $J_{4″-3″~4″-5″}$ = 9.2 Hz, H-4″), 3.55–3.48 (m, 2H, H-3″ and H-5″). ^{13}C NMR (MeOD) δ (ppm) 184.2 (C-4), 166.0 (C-2), 164.8 (C-7), 162.8 (C-5), 158.2 (C-8a), 133.1 (C-3′ and C-5′), 132.8 (C-1′), 130.2 (C-4′), 128.1, 127.8 (C-2′ and C-6′)*, 105.8 (C-3), 105.1 (C-8), 104.6 (C-4a), 99.6 (C-6), 82.9 (C-5″), 80.2 (C-3″), 75.3 (C-1″), 72.8 (C-2″), 72.3, 71.5 (C-4″)*, 63.1, 62.7 (C-6″)*. *Two peaks were observed due to the presence of rotamers. HRMS-ESI (*m/z*): [M + H]$^+$ calcd for $C_{21}H_{21}O_9$ 417.1180, found 417.1174.

8-(β-D-Glucopyranosyl)-5,7,4′-trihydroxyflavone (**17**). Purified by column chromatography (DCM/MeOH 1:0 to 5:1). Isolated yield over two steps: 7%; R_f = 0.43 (EtOAc/EtOH 6:1). ^{1}H NMR (MeOD) δ (ppm) 7.93 (d, 2H, J_{ortho} = 8.6 Hz, H-2′, H-6′), 6.91 (d, 2H, J_{ortho} = 8.8 Hz, H-3′, H-5′), 6.49 (s, 1H, H-3), 6.14 (s, 1H, H-6), 5.05 (d, 1H, $J_{1″-2″}$ = 9.7 Hz, H-1″), 4.17–4.10 (m, 1H, H-2″), 3.94 (d, 1H, $J_{6″a-6″b}$ = 12.0 Hz, H-6″a), 3.79 (dd, 1H, $J_{6″b-6″a}$ = 12.1 Hz, $J_{6″b-5″}$ = 5.5 Hz, H-6″b), 3.65 (t, 1H, $J_{4″-3″}$ = $J_{4″-5″}$ = 9.2 Hz, H-4″), 3.56–3.48 (m, 2H, H-3″, H-5″). ^{13}C NMR (MeOD) δ (ppm) 182.1 (C-4), 168.2 (C-4′), 164.4 (C-7), 163.3 (C-2), 161.2 (C-5), 160.8 (C-8a), 129.8 (C-2′, C-6′), 124.6 (C-1′), 117.3 (C-3′, C-5′), 106.2 (C-4a), 104.5 (C-8), 102.8 (C-3), 99.3 (C-6), 82.8 (C-2″), 80.7 (C-5″), 78.5 (C-3″), 74.4 (C-1″), 72.5 (C-4″), 61.4 (C-6″). HRMS-ESI (*m/z*): [M + H]$^+$ calcd for $C_{21}H_{21}O_{10}$ 433.1129, found 433.1120.

4′-Fluoro-8-(β-D-glucopyranosyl)-5,7-dihydroxyflavone (**18**). Purified by preparative HPLC. Reaction yield over two steps: 45%; LCMS: RT= 0.71 min, m/z = 433.00 [M - H]$^-$ (low pH method); colorless oil. ^{1}H NMR (MeOD) δ (ppm) 8.12 (dd, 2H, J_{ortho} = 8.20 Hz, J_{H-F} = 5.9 Hz, H-2′, H-6′), 7.27 (t, 2H, $J_{ortho-H-F}$ = 8.7 Hz, H-3′, H-5′), 6.52 (s, 1H, H-3), 6.02 (s, 1H, H-6), 5.04 (d, 1H, $J_{1''-2''}$ = 9.3 Hz, H-1″), 4.11 (t, 1H, $J_{2''-1''}$ = $J_{2''-3''}$ = 9.2 Hz, H-2″), 3.89 (dd, 1H, $J_{6''a-6''b}$ = 12.3 Hz, $J_{6''a-5''}$ = 1.8 Hz, H-6″a), 3.80 (dd, 1H, $J_{6''b-6''a}$ = 12.1 Hz, $J_{6''b-5''}$ = 4.8 Hz, H-6″b), 3.65 (t, 1H, $J_{4''-3''}$ = $J_{4''-5''}$ = 9.3 Hz, H-4″), 3.51 (t, 1H, $J_{3''-2''}$ = $J_{3''-4''}$ = 9.0 Hz, H-3″), 3.48–3.44 (m, 1H, H-5″). ^{13}C NMR (MeOD) δ (ppm) 182.5 (C-4), 167.5 (C-2), 166.0 (d, J_{C-F} = 251.2 Hz, C-4′), 163.3 (C-7), 161.9 (C-5), 159.1 (C-8a), 130.3 (d, J_{C-F} = 8.8 Hz, C-2′, C-6′), 129.9 (d, J_{C-F} = 3.2 Hz, C-1′), 117.0 (d, J_{C-F} = 22.5 Hz, C-3′, C-5′), 105.6 (C-4a), 104.8 (C-3), 104.4 (C-6), 104.1 (C-8), 82.6 (C-5″), 80.9 (C-3″), 76.0 (C-1″), 73.8 (C-2″), 72.1 (C-4″), 62.8 (C-6″). HRMS-ESI (m/z): [M + H]$^+$ calcd for $C_{21}H_{20}FO_9$ 435.1086, found 435.1083.

8-(β-D-Glucopyranosyl)-5,7-dihydroxy-4′-(morpholin-4-yl)flavone (**19**). Purified by preparative HPLC. Reaction yield over two steps: 74%; LCMS: RT = 0.57 min, m/z = 500.0 [M − H]$^-$ (high pH method); orange solid; m.p. = 210.5–211.4 °C; $[\alpha]_D^{20}$ = + 10 (c 0.5 MeOH); ^{1}H NMR (MeOD) δ (ppm) 7.94, 7.84 (d, 2H, J_{ortho} = 8.3 Hz, H-2′ and H-6′)*, 7.01 (d, 2H, J_{ortho} = 8.6 Hz, H-3′ and H-5′), 6.52 (s, 1H, H-3), 6.26 (s, 1H, H-6), 5.05, 4.99 (d, 1H, $J_{1''-2''}$ = 9.9 Hz, H-1″)*, 4.14 (t, 1H, $J_{2''-1''}$ = $J_{2''-3''}$ = 9.5 Hz, H-2″), 3.98–3.79 (m, 6H, H-6″a, H-6″b and NCH$_2$CH$_2$O), 3.70 (t, 1H, $J_{4''-3''}$ = $J_{4''-5''}$ = 9.6 Hz, H-4″), 3.57–3.53 (m, 1H, H-3″), 3.49–3.46 (m, 1H, H-5″), 3.32–3.20 (NCH$_2$CH$_2$O, superimposed with the MeOD peak). ^{13}C NMR (MeOD) δ (ppm) 184.0 (C-4), 166.5 (C-2), 164.4 (C-7), 162.6 (C-5), 158.0 (C-8a), 155.1 (C-4′), 129.5, 129.1 (C-2′ and C-6′)*, 122.0 (C-1′), 115.3 (C-3′ and C-5′), 105.8 (C-4a), 105.2 (C-8), 103.0 (C-3), 99.4 (C-6), 82.8 (C-5″), 80.3 (C-3″), 75.3 (C-1″), 72.9 (C-2″), 72.3 (C-4″), 67.7 (NCH$_2$CH$_2$O), 63.1 (C-6″), 40.4 (NCH$_2$CH$_2$O). *Peaks were observed due to the presence of rotamers. HRMS-ESI (m/z): [M + H]$^+$ calcd for $C_{25}H_{28}NO_{10}$ 502.1708, found 502.1695.

8-(β-D-Glucopyranosyl)-5,7-dihydroxy-4′-(pyrrolidin-1-yl)flavone (**20**). Purified by preparative HPLC. Reaction yield over two steps: 80%; LCMS: RT = 0.86 min, m/z = 486.00 [M + H]$^+$ (low pH method); orange oil. ^{1}H NMR (MeOD) δ (ppm) 7.93 (d, 2H, J_{ortho} = 8.2 Hz, H-2′ and H-6′)*, 6.67 (d, 2H, J_{ortho} = 8.3 Hz, H-3′ and H-5′), 6.50 (s, 1H, H-3), 6.25 (s, 1H, H-6), 4.99 (d, 1H, $J_{1''-2''}$ = 9.9 Hz, H-1″)*, 4.16 (t, 1H, $J_{2''-1''}$ = $J_{2''-3''}$ = 9.4 Hz, H-2″), 3.98 (d, 1H, $J_{6-a''-6-b''}$ = 11.8 Hz, H-6″a)*, 3.80 (dd, 1H, $J_{6-b''-6-a''}$ = 11.9 Hz, $J_{6-b'',5''}$ = 5.8 Hz, H-6″b), 3.70 (t, 1H, $J_{4''-3''}$ = $J_{4''-5''}$ = 9.2 Hz, H-4″), 3.56–3.46 (m, 2H, H-3″, H-5″), 3.38–3.35 (m, 4H, NCH$_2$CH$_2$), 2.07 (s, 4H, NCH$_2$CH$_2$). ^{13}C NMR (MeOD) δ (ppm) 181.6 (C-4), 167.6 (C-2), 165.5 (C-7), 162.6 (C-5), 160.4 (C-8a), 156.4 (C-4′), 129.7 (C-2′ and C-6′), 121.7 (C-1′), 112.8 (C-3′ and C-5′), 105.0 (C-4a), 104.5 (C-8), 101.5 (C-3), 97.9 (C-6), 82.9 (C-5″), 80.3 (C-3″), 75.3 (C-1″), 72.9 (C-2″), 72.4 (C-4″), 63.2 (C-6″), 49.1 (NCH$_2$CH$_2$, overlapped with the MeOD peak), 26.4 (NCH$_2$CH$_2$). *Peaks were observed due to the presence of rotamers. HRMS-ESI (m/z): [M + H]$^+$ calcd for $C_{25}H_{28}NO_9$ 486.1759, found 486.1743.

2-(Furan-2-yl)-8-(β-D-glucopyranosyl)-5,7-dihydroxy-4H-chromen-4-one (**21**). Purified by preparative HPLC. Reaction yield over two steps: 56%; LCMS: RT = 0.62 min, m/z = 404.80 [M − H]$^-$ (low pH method); yellowish oil. ^{1}H NMR (MeOD) δ (ppm) 7.82 (d, 1H, $J_{2'-3'}$ = 3.5 Hz, H-2′), 7.33 (br s, 1H, H-4′), 6.72 (dd, 1H, $J_{3'-4'}$ = 1.8 Hz, H-3′), 6.53 (s, 1H, H-3), 6.28 (s, 1H, H-6), 4.96 (d, 1H, $J_{1''-2''}$ = 9.4 Hz, H-1″), 4.16 (t, 1H, $J_{2''-1''}$ = $J_{2''-3''}$ = 9.4 Hz, H-2″), 3.89 (d, 1H, $J_{6-a'',6-b''}$ = 11.6 Hz, H-6″a), 3.73 (dd, 1H, $J_{6-b''}$ = $J_{5''}$ = 5.1 Hz, H-6″b), 3.64 (t, 1H, $J_{4''-3''}$ = $J_{4''-5''}$ = 9.4 Hz, H-4″), 3.53 (t, 1H, $J_{4''-3''\sim 4''-5''}$ = 9.2 Hz, H-3″), 3.46–3.41 (m, 1H, H-5″). ^{13}C NMR (MeOD) δ (ppm) 183.7 (C-4), 167.2 (C-2), 164.9 (C-7), 162.9 (C-5), 157.3 (C-8a), 148.0 (C-2′), 147.3 (C-1′), 115.6 (C-4′), 113.9 (C-3′), 107.2 (C-4a), 106.0 (C-8), 103.5 (C-3), 99.6 (C-6), 82.6 (C-5″), 80.1 (C-3″), 75.0 (C-1″), 72.9 (C-2″), 72.3 (C-4″), 63.0 (C-6″). HRMS-ESI (m/z): [M + H]$^+$ calcd for $C_{19}H_{19}NO_{10}$ 407.0973, found 407.0965.

8-(β-D-Glucopyranosyl)-5,7-dihydroxy-4H-chromen-4-one (**22**). Compound **42** (0.195 g, 0.221 mmol, 1 eq.) was dissolved in anhydrous DCM (5 mL). The mixture was stirred at −78 °C, and BCl$_3$ (1M solution in DCM, 2.21 mL, 2.21 mmol, 10 eq.) was added in a dropwise manner over 5 min. The reaction was complete after 1 h, as detected by LCMS, and was quenched with a 1:1 mixture of DCM/MeOH (40 mL). The mixture was stirred for approximately 20 min at room temperature. The solvent was evaporated under vacuum and the residue purified by column chromatography (DCM-MeOH 1:0 to 4:1). Compound **22** was obtained as a white solid; m.p. = 192.5–193.0 °C; $[\alpha]_D^{20}$ = + 16 ° (c 0.5 MeOH). Reaction yield: 45%; LCMS: RT = 0.41 min, m/z = 338.80 [M - H]$^-$ (low pH method). ^{1}H NMR (MeOD) δ (ppm) 8.04 (d, 1H, J_{cis} = 5.8 Hz, H-2), 6.28 (s, 1H, H-6), 6.24 (d, 1H, J_{cis} = 5.9 Hz, H-3), 4.91 (d, 1H, $J_{1''-2''}$ = 9.9 Hz, H-1''), 4.07 (t, 1H, $J_{2''-1''-2''-3''}$ = 9.3 Hz, H-2''), 3.88 (dd, 1H, $J_{6-a''-6-b''}$ = 12.1 Hz, $J_{6-a''-5''}$ = 2.1 Hz, H-6''a), 3.71 (dd, 1H, $J_{6-b''-6-a''}$ = 12.0 Hz, $J_{6-b''-5''}$ = 5.4 Hz, H-6''b), 3.50–3.41 (m, 3H, H-3'', H-4'', H-5''). ^{13}C NMR (MeOD) δ 183.7 (C-4), 165.0 (C-7), 163.0 (C-5), 158.0 (C-8a and C-2), 111.5 (C-3), 106.8 (C-4a), 104.9 (C-8), 100.5 (C-6), 82.6 (C-5''), 80.1 (C-3''), 75.4 (C-1''), 72.8 (C-2''), 71.8 (C-4''), 62.9 (C-6''). HRMS-ESI (m/z): [M + H]$^+$ calcd for $C_{15}H_{17}NO_9$ 341.0867, found 341.0865.

Log $D_{7.4}$ determination. The in-silico prediction tool ALOGPS [4] was used to estimate the octanol-water partition coefficients (log P) of the compounds. Depending on these values, the compounds were classified either as hydrophilic (log P below zero), moderately lipophilic (log P between zero and one), or lipophilic (log P above one) compounds. For each category, two different ratios (volume of octan-1-ol to volume of buffer) were defined as experimental parameters (Table 2).

Table 2. Compound classification based on estimated log P values.

Compound Category	log P	Ratios (Octan-1-ol:Buffer)
hydrophilic	<0	30:140, 40:130
moderately lipophilic	0–1	70:110, 110:70
lipophilic	>1	3:180, 4:180

Equal amounts of phosphate buffer (0.1 M, pH 7.4) and octan-1-ol were mixed and shaken vigorously for 5 min to saturate the phases. The mixture was left until separation of the two phases, and the buffer was retrieved. Stock solutions of the test compounds were diluted with buffer to a concentration of 1 µM. For each compound, three determinations per octan-1-ol:buffer ratio were performed in different wells of a 96-well plate. The respective volumes of buffer-containing analyte (1 µM) were pipetted to the wells and covered by saturated octan-1-ol according to the chosen volume ratio. The plate was sealed with aluminum foil, shaken (1350 rpm, 25 °C, 2 h) on a Heidolph Titramax 1,000 plate-shaker (Heidolph Instruments GmbH & Co. KG, Schwabach, Germany) and centrifuged (2,000 rpm, 25 °C, 5 min, 5804 R Eppendorf centrifuge, Hamburg, Germany). The aqueous phase was transferred to a 96-well plate for analysis by liquid chromatography-mass spectrometry (LCMS, see below). Log P coefficients were calculated from the octan-1-ol:buffer ratio (o:b), the initial concentration of the analyte in buffer (1 µM), and the concentration of the analyte in buffer (cB) according to the following equation:

$$\log P = \log\left(\frac{1\ \mu M - c_B}{c_B} \times \frac{1}{o:b}\right) \tag{1}$$

Results are presented as the mean ± SD of three independent experiments. If the mean of two independent experiments obtained for a given compound did not differ by more than 0.1 units, the results were accepted.

Parallel artificial membrane permeability assay (PAMPA). Effective permeability (log P_e) was determined in a 96-well format with PAMPA [34]. For each compound, measurements were performed at pH 7.4 in quadruplicates. Four wells of a deep well-plate were filled with 650 µL of PRISMA HT universal buffer, adjusted to pH 7.4 by adding the requested amount of NaOH (0.5 M). Samples (150 µL) were withdrawn from each well to determine the blank spectra by UV/Vis-spectroscopy (190 to 500 nm, SpectraMax 190, Molecular Devices, Silicon Valley, CA, USA). Then the analyte, dissolved in DMSO

(10 mM), was added to the remaining buffer to yield 50 µM solutions. To exclude precipitation, the optical density (OD) was measured at 650 nm, and solutions exceeding OD 0.01 were filtrated. Afterwards, samples (150 µL) were withdrawn to determine the reference spectra. Further 200 µL were transferred to each well of the donor plate of the PAMPA sandwich (pIon, P/N 110 163). The filter membranes at the bottom of the acceptor plate were infused with 5 µL of GIT-0 Lipid Solution and 200 µL of Acceptor Sink Buffer were filled into each acceptor well. The sandwich was assembled, placed in the GutBox™, and left undisturbed for 16 h. Then, it was disassembled and samples (150 µL) were transferred from each donor and acceptor well to UV-plates for determination of the UV/Vis spectra. Effective permeability (log Pe) was calculated from the compound flux deduced from the spectra, the filter area, and the initial sample concentration in the donor well with the aid of the PAMPA Explorer Software (pIon, version 3.5).

LC-MS measurements. Analyses were performed using a 1100/1200 Series HPLC System coupled to a 6410 Triple Quadrupole mass detector (Agilent Technologies, Inc., Santa Clara, CA, USA) equipped with electrospray ionization. The system was controlled with the Agilent MassHunter Workstation Data Acquisition software (version B.01.04). The column used was an AtlantisR T3 C18 column (2.1 × 50 mm) with a 3 µm-particle size (Waters Corp., Milford, MA, USA). The mobile phase consisted of eluent A: 10 mM ammonium acetate, pH 5.0 in 95:5, H_2O:MeCN; and eluent B: MeCN containing 0.1% formic acid. The flow rate was maintained at 0.6 mL/min. The gradient was ramped from 95% A/5% B to 5% A/95% B over 1 min, and then held at 5% A/95% B for 0.1 min. The system was then brought back to 95% A/5% B, resulting in a total duration of 4 min. MS parameters such as fragmentor voltage, collision energy, and polarity were optimized individually for each drug, and the molecular ion was followed for each compound in the multiple reaction monitoring mode. The concentrations of the analytes were quantified by the Agilent Mass Hunter Quantitative Analysis software (version B.01.04).

Neuroprotective assays in human neuroblastoma (SH-SY5Y) cells. SH-SY5Y cells were grown in Dulbecco's Modified Eagle Medium (DMEM, Gibco, Life Technologies) supplemented with 10% fetal bovine serum (FBS, Biochrom GmbH) and 1% Penicillin-Streptomycin (Gibco, Life Technologies) in a humidified incubator at 37 °C, 5% CO_2. For the neuroprotective activity assay, undifferentiated SGSY-5Y cells were plated onto 96-well flat-bottomed microtiter plates at a density of 1×10^4 cells/well in DMEM supplemented with 2% FBS and preincubated for 24 h at 37 °C, 5% CO_2. Compounds (stored as 10 mM solutions in DMSO at −20 °C) were then added to achieve a final concentration of 50 µM and, after 30 min, cells were incubated in the presence or absence of 20 µM Aβ protein fragment 1-42 (Sigma-Aldrich, dissolved in DMSO and stored in 2 mM aliquots at −20 °C) or 100 µM of H_2O_2 (Sigma-Aldrich, dissolved to 10 mM in 0.9% NaCl aqueous solution immediately prior to the assay) overnight at 37 °C, 5% CO_2. The final DMSO percentage was 0.5% for compounds in the presence of H_2O_2, 1% for cells incubated only with Aβ, or 1.5% for cells incubated with compounds and Aβ, thus, controls for each DMSO percentage were also run. The following morning, 20 µL of a 5 mg/mL solution of 3-(4,5-dimethylthiazol-2-yl)-2,5-diphenyltetrazolium bromide (MTT, Sigma-Aldrich) in PBS (Gibco, Life Technologies) was added to each well and the plates were further incubated for 4 h at 37 °C, followed by the addition of DMSO (200 µL) to each well in order to dissolve the resulting formazan crystals. After 2 h incubating at 37 °C, the optical density (OD) at 540 nm (with a 620 nm reference filter) was measured in an Amersham Biosciences Biotrak II Plate Reader. The percentage of MTT reduction was determined according to Equation (1). All experiments were performed in triplicate and results are presented as means ± standard error. Differences between experimental conditions were compared for statistical significance by one-way ANOVA followed by a Tukey's post-test, an analysis carried out using GraphPad Prism Software (LA Jolla, CA, USA). Differences were considered significant when $P < 0.05$. In order to exclude direct MTT reduction, compounds were also tested in (a) the absence of cells and (b) in the absence of both cells and culture medium, using the same experimental conditions described above.

$$\text{MTT Reduction (\% of Control)} = \left[\frac{OD_{sample} - OD_{medium}}{OD_{cell\ control} - OD_{medium}}\right] \times 100 \qquad (2)$$

Cell viability assay in human epithelial colorectal adenocarcinoma (Caco-2) and human liver hepatocellular (HepG2) cells. Caco-2 and HepG2 Cells were cultured in DMEM-Dulbecco's modified Eagle's medium (Sigma-Aldrich) supplemented with 10% (*v*/*v*) inactivated fetal bovine serum (PAA Laboratories GmbH), 2 mM L-glutamine (Sigma-Aldrich), 100 U/mL penicillin and 100 µg/mL streptomycin (Sigma-Aldrich), in a humidified incubator at 37 °C with a 5% CO_2 atmosphere. Cells (3×10^4 cells/well) were seeded into 96-well plates and incubated at 37 °C in 5% CO_2 atmosphere. After 24 h, compounds were added at different concentrations (0.1–100 µM) and incubated in the same conditions. DMSO controls were performed to evaluate a possible solvent cytotoxicity, while pure DMSO was used as a cytotoxic drug. After the established incubation time with compounds, MTT (5 mg/mL) in PBS (Sigma-Aldrich) was added (10 µL) to each well. After 3 h incubation at 37 °C, in 5% CO_2, the supernatant was removed. The formazan crystals were solubilized using ethanol/DMSO (1:1) (100 µL), and the absorbance values were determined at 570 nm on the microplate reader Victor3 from PerkinElmer Life Sciences.

5. Conclusions

In the present work, we have generated a library of chemically diverse flavone analogues and their C-glucosyl derivatives, and explored the structural requirements for neuroprotective activity and therapeutic potential against AD.

With imposed physicochemical properties upon their design as CNS-targeted agents, all synthesized aglycones were found to have good effective permeability and adequate $logD_{7.4}$ values, indicating that, as expected, they have adequate pharmacokinetic and safety profiles for administration, with the ability to cross cell membrane barriers, including gastrointestinal epithelia and the BBB. Even though not all C-glucosyl derivatives were able to achieve the same outcomes due to the presence of the polar sugar moiety, some of them presented a promising compromise between effective permeability and lipophilicity. From these compounds, the *p*-morpholinyl derivative **37** stood out for having fully rescued SH-SY5Y human neuroblastoma cells from H_2O_2- and $A\beta_{1-42}$-induced toxicity in a screening MTT assay. Importantly, it was the only compound in which the aglycone (**8**) was also active, pointing towards aglycone specificity for the desired activity. The ability of the sugar moiety to maintain or even potentiate the activity in this compound (**8/19**) definitely comes across as a benefit, since according to previously published indications, the sugar may enhance the antioxidant properties of the compound as a whole, while helping to maintain $A\beta_{1-42}$ peptides in their disaggregated state [19,20]. Furthermore, our results support the use of C-glucosylflavones for neuroprotective applications in detriment of the corresponding isoflavones by providing a direct comparison between two scaffolds from natural origin—compound **2** and vitexin **17**—in more than one cell-based assay. Compound **19** also exhibits a modest acetylcholinesterase inhibitory activity, thus coming across as a new multitarget lead compound for AD. This promising and non-toxic morpholinyl flavone derivative ultimately offers a relevant improvement when compared to the natural products chrysin (**1**) and **2**, which served as the inspiration for our work owing to their reported neuroprotective potential.

Supplementary Materials: The following are available online at http://www.mdpi.com/1424-8247/12/2/98/s1, Table S1: Structure, physicochemical properties and CNS-MPO score of the flavone analogues selected for synthesis. All physicochemical properties were calculated using MOE software; Table S2: Cytotoxic activity of each compound assessed in SH-SY5Y neuroblastoma cells via an MTT cell viability assay; Experimental procedures for cholinesterase inhibition assays; Table S3: Acetylcholinesterase (AChE) and butyrylcholinesterase (BuChE) inhibitory efficacy of chrysin (**1**), 8-glucosylgenistein (**2**) and some of the synthesized flavone analogues at 100 µM; Synthetic approaches for chromones, flavones and the corresponding C-glucosyl derivatives; Scheme S1: Synthesis of selected flavones and analogues (A) via chalcone formation and (B) via flavanone formation; Scheme S2: Synthesis of (A) C-glucosyl flavones and analogues and (B) the 6-glucosyl-5,7-dihydroxychromen-4-one (**41**); Preparation procedures, physical and LCMS data, and NMR spectra of intermediate compounds.

Author Contributions: Compound design, synthesis and characterization were carried out by A.M.d.M., under the supervision of M.W., T.M., D.E. (Eli Lilly) and A.P.R. PAMPA and logD determinations were conducted by

A.M.d.M. and P.D. under the supervision of B.E. Neuroprotective activity assays were performed by A.M.d.M. under the supervision of M.P.d.M. Cholinesterase inhibition assays were conducted by Ó.L. and J.G.F.-B. HRMS of final compounds was accomplished by M.C.O. Cytotoxicity assays were conducted by A.M. under the supervision of M.C. and N.A.C. This paper was written by A.M.d.M., revised by D.E., M.P.M., and B.E., revised and modified by A.P.

Funding: This research was funded by the FP7—Seventh framework programme of the European Community, FP7-PEOPLE-2013-IAPP, grant number 612347, and by Fundação para a Ciência e a Tecnologia, project UID/Multi/0612/2019 and grant number SFRH/BD/93170/2013.

Acknowledgments: The authors thank Fundação para a Ciência e a Tecnologia for financial support through the project UID/Multi/0612/2019 and for the PhD grant attributed to Ana Marta de Matos (SFRH/BD/93170/2013). The European Union is also gratefully acknowledged for the support of the project entitled "Diagnostic and Drug Discovery Initiative for Alzheimer's Disease" (D3i4AD), FP7-PEOPLE-2013-IAPP, GA 612347.

Conflicts of Interest: There are no conflicts of interest to declare.

References

1. World Health Organization. *Dementia Fact Sheet*; World Health Organization: Geneva, Switzerland, 2017.
2. Förstl, H.; Kurz, A. Clinical features of Alzheimer's disease. *Eur. Arch. Psychiatry Clin. Neurosci.* **1999**, *249*, 288–290. [CrossRef]
3. Yiannopoulou, K.G.; Papageorgiou, S.G. Current and future treatments for Alzheimer's disease. *Ther. Adv. Neurol. Disord.* **2013**, *6*, 19–33. [CrossRef]
4. Frozza, R.L.; Lourenco, M.V.; De Felice, F.G. Challenges for Alzheimer's Disease Therapy: Insights from Novel Mechanisms Beyond Memory Defects. *Front. Neurosci.* **2018**, *12*, 37. [CrossRef]
5. Alkadhi, K.; Eriksen, J. The Complex and Multifactorial Nature of Alzheimer's Disease. *Curr. Neuropharmacol.* **2011**, *9*, 586. [CrossRef] [PubMed]
6. Zhou, J.; Liu, B. Alzheimer's Disease and Prion Protein. *Intractable Rare Dis. Res.* **2013**, *2*, 35–44. [CrossRef] [PubMed]
7. Chong, F.P.; Ng, K.Y.; Koh, R.Y.; Chye, S.M. Tau Proteins and Tauopathies in Alzheimer's Disease. *Cell. Mol. Neurobiol.* **2018**, *38*, 965–980. [CrossRef] [PubMed]
8. Dyall, S.C. Amyloid-Beta Peptide, Oxidative Stress and Inflammation in Alzheimer's Disease: Potential Neuroprotective Effects of Omega-3 Polyunsaturated Fatty Acids. *Int. J. Alzheimer's Dis.* **2010**, *2010*, 274128. [CrossRef]
9. Neth, B.J.; Craft, S. Insulin Resistance and Alzheimer's Disease: Bioenergetic Linkages. *Front. Aging Neurosci.* **2017**, *9*, 345. [CrossRef]
10. Baptista, F.I.; Henriques, A.G.; Silva, A.M.; Wiltfang, J.; da Cruz e Silva, O.A. Flavonoids as Therapeutic Compounds Targeting Key Proteins Involved in Alzheimer's Disease. *ACS Chem. Neurosci.* **2014**, *5*, 83–92. [CrossRef]
11. Matos, A.M.; Cristóvão, J.S.; Yashunsky, D.V.; Nifantiev, N.E.; Viana, A.S.; Gomes, C.M.; Rauter, A.P. Synthesis and effects of flavonoid structure variation on amyloid-beta aggregation. *Pure Appl. Chem.* **2017**, *89*, 1305–1320. [CrossRef]
12. Jesus, A.R.; Dias, C.; Matos, A.M.; De Almeida, R.F.M.; Viana, A.S.; Marcelo, F.; Ribeiro, R.T.; Macedo, M.P.; Airoldi, C.; Nicotra, F.; et al. Exploiting the therapeutic potential of 8-β-D-glucopyranosylgenistein: Synthesis, antidiabetic activity, and molecular interaction with islet amyloid polypeptide and amyloid β-peptide (1-42). *J. Med. Chem.* **2014**, *57*, 9463–9472. [CrossRef]
13. Nabavi, S.F.; Braidy, N.; Habtemariam, S.; Orhan, I.E.; Daglia, M.; Manayi, A.; Gortzi, O.; Nabavi, S.M. Neuroprotective effects of chrysin: From chemistry to medicine. *Neurochem. Int.* **2015**, *90*, 224–231. [CrossRef] [PubMed]
14. Vedagiri, A.; Thangarajan, S. Mitigating effect of chrysin loaded solid lipid nanoparticles against Amyloid β25-35 induced oxidative stress in rat hippocampal region: An efficient formulation approach for Alzheimer's disease. *Neuropeptides* **2016**, *58*, 111–125. [CrossRef] [PubMed]
15. Balez, R.; Steiner, N.; Engel, M.; Muñoz, S.S.; Lum, J.S.; Wu, Y.; Wang, D.; Vallotton, P.; Sachdev, P.; O'Connor, M.; et al. Neuroprotective effects of apigenin against inflammation, neuronal excitability and apoptosis in an induced pluripotent stem cell model of Alzheimer's disease. *Sci. Rep.* **2016**, *6*, 31450. [CrossRef]
16. Lin, P.; Tian, X.H.; Yi, Y.S.; Jiang, W.S.; Zhou, Y.J.; Cheng, W.J. Luteolin-induced protection of H_2O_2-induced apoptosis in PC12 cells and the associated pathway. *Mol. Med. Rep.* **2015**, *12*, 7699–7704. [CrossRef] [PubMed]

17. Shan, S.; Chen, L.; Zhang, B.; Zhao, X. Neuroprotective effects of vitexin AGAINST isoflurane-induced neurotoxicity by targeting the TRPV1 and NR2B signaling pathways. *Mol. Med. Rep.* **2016**, *14*, 5607–5613.
18. Malar, D.S.; Suryanarayanan, V.; Prasanth, M.I.; Singh, S.K.; Balamurugan, K.; Devi, K.P. Vitexin inhibits Aβ$_{25-35}$ induced toxicity in Neuro-2a cells by augmenting Nrf-2/HO-1 dependent antioxidant pathway and regulating lipid homeostasis by the activation of LXR-α. *Toxicol. In Vitro* **2018**, *50*, 160–171. [CrossRef] [PubMed]
19. Ladiwala, A.R.A.; Mora-Pale, M.; Lin, J.C.; Bale, S.S.; Fishman, Z.S.; Dordick, J.S.; Tessier, P.M. Polyphenolic glycosides and aglycones utilize opposing pathways to selectively remodel and inactivate toxic oligomers of amyloid β. *ChemBioChem* **2011**, *12*, 1749–1758. [CrossRef] [PubMed]
20. Xiao, J. Dietary Flavonoid Aglycones and Their Glycosides: Which Show Better Biological Significance? *Crit. Rev. Food Sci. Nutr.* **2017**, *57*, 1874–1905. [CrossRef] [PubMed]
21. de Matos, A.M.; de Macedo, M.P.; Rauter, A.P. Bridging Type 2 Diabetes and Alzheimer's Disease: Assembling the Puzzle Pieces in the Quest for the Molecules with Therapeutic and Preventive Potential. *Med. Res. Rev.* **2018**, *38*, 261–324. [CrossRef] [PubMed]
22. Wager, T.T.; Hou, X.; Verhoest, P.R.; Villalobos, A. Moving beyond rules: The development of a central nervous system multiparameter optimization (CNS MPO) approach to enable alignment of drug-like properties. *ACS Chem. Neurosci.* **2010**, *1*, 435–449. [CrossRef] [PubMed]
23. Di, L.; Kerns, E.H. Profiling drug-like properties in discovery research. *Curr. Opin. Chem. Boil.* **2003**, *7*, 402–408. [CrossRef]
24. Law, B.N.T.; Ling, A.P.K.; Koh, R.Y.; Chye, S.M.; Wong, Y.P. Neuroprotective effects of orientin on hydrogen peroxide-induced apoptosis in SH-SY5Y cells. *Mol. Med. Rep.* **2014**, *9*, 947–954. [CrossRef] [PubMed]
25. NirmalaDevi, D.; Venkataramana, M.; Chandranayaka, S.; Ramesha, A.; Jameel, N.M.; Srinivas, C. Neuroprotective effects of bikaverin on H_2O_2-induced oxidative stress mediated neuronal damage in SH-SY5Y cell line. *Cell. Mol. Neurobiol.* **2014**, *34*, 973–985. [CrossRef] [PubMed]
26. Han, S.M.; Kim, J.M.; Park, K.K.; Chang, Y.C.; Pak, S.C. Neuroprotective effects of melittin on hydrogen peroxide-induced apoptotic cell death in neuroblastoma SH-SY5Y cells. *BMC Complement. Altern. Med.* **2014**, *14*, 286. [CrossRef] [PubMed]
27. Zhao, J.; Liu, F.; Huang, C.; Shentu, J.; Wang, M.; Sun, C.; Chen, L.; Yan, S.; Fang, F.; Wang, Y.; et al. 5-Hydroxycyclopenicillone Inhibits β-Amyloid Oligomerization and Produces Anti-β-Amyloid Neuroprotective Effects In Vitro. *Molecules* **2017**, *22*, 1651. [CrossRef] [PubMed]
28. Oguchi, T.; Ono, R.; Tsuji, M.; Shozawa, H.; Somei, M.; Inagaki, M.; Mori, Y.; Yasumoto, T.; Ono, K.; Kiuchi, Y. Cilostazol Suppresses Aβ-induced Neurotoxicity in SH-SY5Y Cells through Inhibition of Oxidative Stress and MAPK Signaling Pathway. *Front. Aging Neurosci.* **2017**, *9*, 337. [CrossRef]
29. Krishtal, J.; Bragina, O.; Metsla, K.; Palumaa, P.; Tõugu, V. In situ fibrillizing amyloid-beta 1-42 induces neurite degeneration and apoptosis of differentiated SH-SY5Y cells. *PLoS ONE* **2017**, *12*, e0186636. [CrossRef]
30. Zhang, Y.; Zhang, T.; Wang, F.; Xie, J. Brain tissue distribution of spinosin in rats determined by a new high-performance liquid chromatography-electrospray ionization-mass/mass spectrometry method. *J. Chromatogr. Sci.* **2015**, *53*, 97–103. [CrossRef]
31. Zhong, L.; Zhou, J.; Chen, X.; Lou, Y.; Liu, D.; Zou, X.; Yang, B.; Yin, Y.; Pan, Y. Quantitative proteomics study of the neuroprotective effects of B12 on hydrogen peroxide-induced apoptosis in SH-SY5Y cells. *Sci. Rep.* **2016**, *6*, 22635. [CrossRef]
32. Rohn, T.T.; Head, E. Caspases as Therapeutic Targets in Alzheimer's Disease: Is It Time to "Cut" to the Chase? *Int. J. Clin. Exp. Pathol.* **2009**, *2*, 108–118. [PubMed]
33. Butterfield, D.A.; Boyd-Kimball, D. Oxidative Stress, Amyloid-β Peptide, and Altered Key Molecular Pathways in the Pathogenesis and Progression of Alzheimer's Disease. *J. Alzheimer's Dis.* **2018**, *62*, 1345–1367. [CrossRef] [PubMed]
34. Kansy, M.; Senner, F.; Gubernator, K. Physicochemical high throughput screening: Parallel artificial membrane permeation assay in the description of passive absorption processes. *J. Med. Chem.* **1998**, *41*, 1007–1010. [CrossRef] [PubMed]

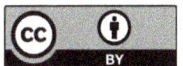

© 2019 by the authors. Licensee MDPI, Basel, Switzerland. This article is an open access article distributed under the terms and conditions of the Creative Commons Attribution (CC BY) license (http://creativecommons.org/licenses/by/4.0/).

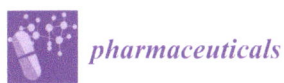

Article

Chain-Branched Polyhydroxylated Octahydro-*1H*-Indoles as Potential Leads against Lysosomal Storage Diseases

Juan C. Estévez [1,2], Marcos A. González [1,2], M. Carmen Villaverde [2], Yuki Hirokami [3], Atsushi Kato [3], Fredy Sussman [1], David Reza [1,2] and Ramón J. Estévez [1,2,*]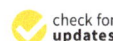

[1] Centro Singular de Investigación en Química Biolóxica e Materiais Moleculares, Universidade de Santiago de Compostela, 15782 Santiago de Compostela, Spain; juancarlos.estevez@usc.es (J.C.E.); mar.gonzalez.castro@gmail.com (M.A.G.); fredy.sussman@usc.es (F.S.); david.reza@gmail.com (D.R.)
[2] Departamento de Química Orgánica, Universidade de Santiago de Compostela, 15782 Santiago de Compostela, Spain; mc.villaverde@usc.es
[3] Department of Hospital Pharmacy, University of Toyama, Toyama 930-0194, Japan; yuhi@saitama-med.ac.jp (Y.H.); kato@med.u-toyama.ac.jp (A.K.)
* Correspondence: ramon.estevez@usc.es; Tel.: +34-881815731

Received: 13 February 2019; Accepted: 19 March 2019; Published: 29 March 2019

Abstract: Here, the synthesis and glycosidase inhibition properties of the two first known 3-ethyloctahydro-1*H*-indole-4,5,6-triols are reported. This study shows the transformation of D-glucose into polyhydroxylated 1-(2-nitrocyclohexane) acetaldehydes, followed by a protocol involving the formation of the azacyclopentane ring. Results of inhibitory potency assays and docking calculations show that at least one of them could be a lead for optimization in the search for compounds that behave like folding chaperones in lysosomal storage diseases.

Keywords: sugars; iminosugars; glycosidase inhibition

---

1. Introduction

Iminosugars [1–4] and aminocarbasugars [5–7] are sugar mimics that inhibit a variety of enzymes of therapeutic interest, including glycosidases and glycosyltransferases. They have been shown to be lead molecules for the treatment of diseases such as diabetes, viral infections, or lysosomal storage disorders. Some representative examples are included in Figure 1. Thus, the *N*-alkylated 1-deoxynojirimycin miglitol (**II**) (Glyset®) [8,9] and the aminocarbasugar voglibose (**IV**) [10,11] have been approved for the treatment of type II diabetes [12,13], and miglustat (**III**) (Zavesca®) is prescribed for the treatment of Gaucher disease [14,15]. The bicyclic iminosugar castanospermine (**V**) [16,17] is a polyhydroxylated indolizidine alkaloid [3,18] that can be considered as a conformational restricted analogue of miglitol. This compound and its derivatives have received considerable attention as potential antineoplastic and immunosuppressive agents, but, unfortunately, they have shown toxicity to human cells [19–22]. This led to the study of analogues of these leads aimed at altering their activity and toxicity profile. Specifically, the polyhydroxylated octahydroindole (**VI**) and its *N*-hydroxyalkyl derivatives were studied as castanospermine analogues where the position of the *N*-atom was changed, allowing them to be considered as conformational restricted carbasugars [23,24].

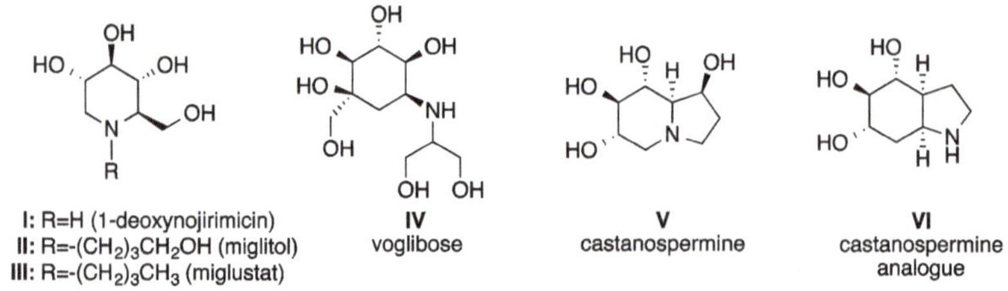

Figure 1. Selection of iminosugars and aminocarbasugars.

As a contribution to the search for new castanospermine analogues, and as a part of ongoing project on synthetic application of nitro sugars and related compounds [25], we report herein the synthesis and biological evaluation of compounds **10** and **13** as novel polyhydroxylated octahydroindoles bearing an alkyl substituent at the C-3 position. Results of the inhibitory potency assays and docking calculations have shown that at least one of them could be a lead for optimization in the search for compounds that behave like folding chaperones, useful as drugs against lysosomal storage diseases like G_{M1} gangliosidosis and Morquio B disease [26].

2. Results

2.1. Chemical Synthesis

Michael addition of carbonyl synthetic equivalents to electron-deficient nitro alkenes has proven to be a promising method for the enantioselective synthesis of γ−nitro acids [27,28]. In this regard, carbasugar nitro olefins are suitable scaffolds for this and other synthetic purposes [29], although they are practically unexplored. They include in their structure a preformed carbocyclic ring bearing several hydroxy substituents in a well-defined spatial orientation and a nitroethylene subunit suitable for Michael addition of nucleophiles.

In order to apply this methodology, the key six-membered nitroolefin **4b** was obtained from the known nitro sugar **1** [30], according to a protocol developed by us for the synthesis of the first polyhydroxylated 1-nitrocyclohexane [31].

Removal of the isopropylidene protecting group of **1** under acidic conditions [trifluoracetic acid (TFA)/H_2O] was followed by a potassium carbonate-promoted intramolecular Henry reaction of the resulting ε-nitro aldehyde **3** (the open form of the tricomponent mixture **2** + **3**), which was directly reacted with potassium carbonate in methanol followed by acetic anhydride and a catalytic amount of dimethoxyaminopyridine (DMAP) in order to promote its dehydration aimed at obtaining the cyclic nitroolefin **4b**, via **4a** (Scheme 1).

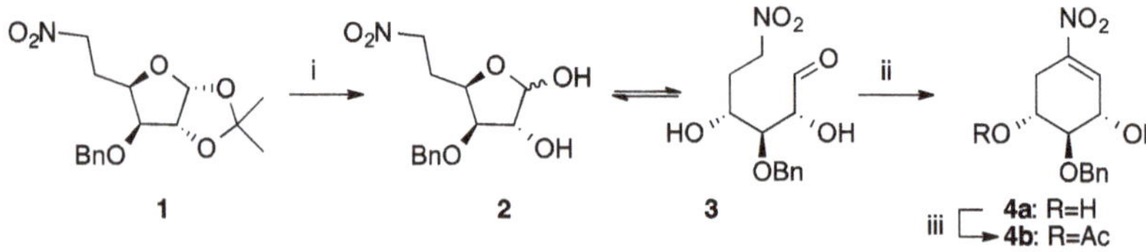

Scheme 1. Conditions: (i) TFA/H_2O, rt, 5 h. (ii) 2% K_2CO_3/MeOH, rt, 4 h. (iii) Ac_2O, DMAP (cat), Et_2O, rt, 6 h (77%, three steps).

Michael addition of butyraldehyde to **4b**, catalyzed by pyrrolidine, resulted in an epimeric mixture of γ-nitro aldehydes **5** and **6**, which were isolated by column chromatography (Scheme 2). The stereochemical outcome of this reaction, which is controlled by the substrate, can be rationalized on the basis of the Felkin–Ahn rule.

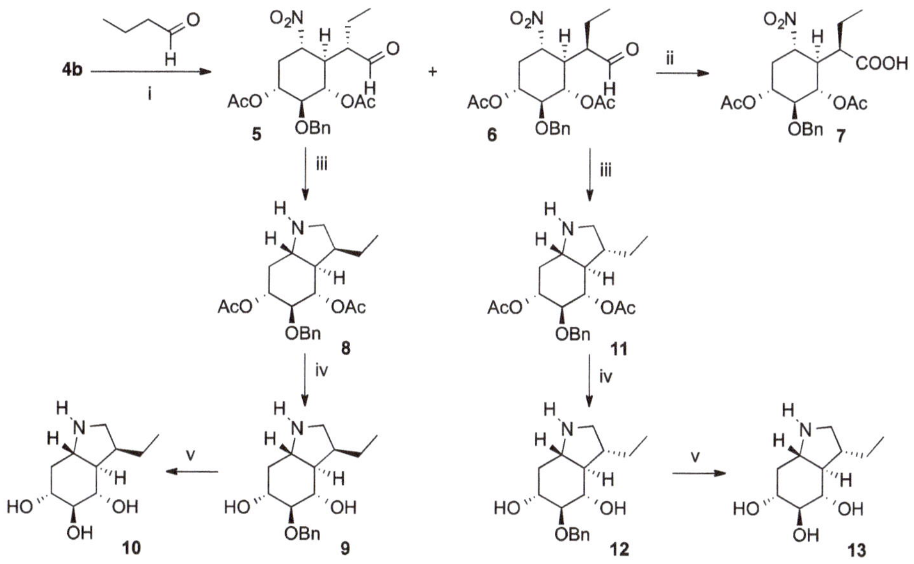

Scheme 2. Conditions: (i) pyrrolidine, CH$_2$Cl$_2$, rt, 3 h (50% for **5**, 21% for **6**); (ii) NaClO$_2$/NaH$_2$PO$_4$, 2-methyl-2-butene, *t*-BuOH/H$_2$O (3:1), rt, 2 h, 88%; (iii) Zn dust, MeOH/AcOH (1:1), 0 °C, 14 h (90% for **8**, 85% for **11**); (iv) 1 M NaOH/MeOH, rt, 4 h /69% for **9** and for **12**); (v) 10% Pd/C, MeOH, H$_2$ (1 atm) (87% for **10**, 88% for **13**).

The structure of compounds **5** and **6** were unambiguously identified by X-ray experiments (Figure 2). In the latter case this was corroborated by the X-ray structure of the corresponding carboxylic acid **7**, which was obtained by (2,2,6,6-tetramethylpiperidin-1-yl)oxyl (TEMPO) oxidation of **6**.

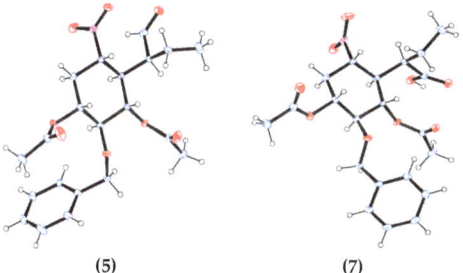

Figure 2. X-ray structures of compounds **5** and **7**.

Finally, γ−nitroaldehydes **5** and **6** were satisfactorily converted into the corresponding octahydroindoles **10** and **13** (Scheme 2). Reaction of compound **5** with Zn dust in an acidic media for 14 h directly provided the corresponding octahydroindole **8**, by the reduction of the nitro group to amino, followed by a spontaneous reductive amination of the resulting γ−amino aldehyde. Basic hydrolysis of **8** with NaOH resulted in a selective hydrolysis of its acetate subunits to give derivative **9**. Catalytic hydrogenation of **9** gave the trihydroxylated octahydroindole **10**. On the other hand, the epimeric octahydroindole **13** was similarly obtained from γ−nitro aldehyde **6** via compounds **11** and **12**.

2.2. Glycosidase Inhibition Assays

Table 1 displays results of the inhibition of a variety of glycosidases by iminosugars **10** and **13**, as the inhibition percentage at 1000 µM. As seen from this table, these compounds display by far the highest inhibition activity against bovine β-galactosidase (amongst all enzymes assayed), albeit at levels under 50%.

Table 1. Data on inhibition of various glycosidases by compounds **10** and **13**.

Enzyme	Compound 10	Compound 13	Miglitol (IC$_{50}$)
α-Glucosidase			
Yeast	16% [a]	19.5% [a]	70 µM
Rice	0% [a]	0% [a]	0.17 µM
Rat intestinal maltase	4.1% [a]	0% [a]	>1000 µM
β-Glucosidase			
Almond	12% [a]	5% [a]	>1000 µM
Bovine liver	0% [a]	21.7% [a]	>1000 µM
α-Galactosidase			
Coffee beans	15.9% [a]	0% [a]	>1000 µM
	0% [a]	21.7% [a]	
β-Galactosidase			
Bovine liver	45.6% [a]	35.8% [a]	>1000 µM
Lactase	0.6% [a]	7.4% [a]	>1000 µM
α-Mannosidase			
Jack bean	0% [a]	0% [a]	
β-Mannosidase			
Snail	0% [a]	2.3% [a]	>1000 µM
α-L-Fucosidase			
Bovine kidney	7.5% [a]	12.9% [a]	>1000 µM
α-L-Rhamnosidase			
Penicillium decumbens	0% [a]	0% [a]	803
β-Glucronidase			
E.coli	18.1% [a]	12.3% [a]	>1000 µM
α,α-Trehalase			
Porcine kidney	0% [a]	0% [a]	131
Amyloglucosidase			
Aspergillus niger	0% [a]	0% [a]	>1000 µM

[a] inhibition % at 1000 µM.

2.3. Docking Studies

To further shed some light on the differences between the inhibition activities of these compounds for lysosomal β-galactosidase (β-Gal), we performed docking simulations that included the above mentioned compounds **10** and **13**, as well as galactose, a catalytic product of this enzyme. We included this latter compound as a point of reference, since the structure of its complex with human β-galactosidase (with whom the bovine variant shares a highly conserved binding domain) is known.

The docking results for these compounds are summarized in Table 2. This table lists the scoring value for the top-scoring poses obtained in three docking calculations that differ in the options used in this work, which include "early termination search", "diverse solutions", and docking runs that allow for active site side chain flexibility (see methods section for details). The table also includes the hydrogen bond pattern between the ligands and some residues of the protein.

Table 2. Results of the docking simulations and score values for the top pose of each run.

Ligand	Protein Residue HB	Fitness & Search Options [a]									
		Early Termination			Diverse Solutions			Side Flexible Search			
		CHEM	GOLD	PLP	CHEM	GOLD	PLP	CHEM	GOLD	PLP	PDB
Galactose	Galactose score	21.88	54.49	55.63	18.57	50.17	52.84	12.57	53.60	42.29	-
	Tyr83(OH)	3-OH	3-OH	3-OH		3-OH	3-OH		3-OH	3-OH	3-OH
	Ala128(N)		3-OH				3-OH	3-OH	3-OH	3-OH	3-OH
	Glu129(OE1)	6-OH	6-OH	4,6-OH	6-OH	4-OH	4,6-OH	4,6-OH	4-OH	4-OH	6-OH
	Glu129(OE2)	4-OH	4-OH	4-OH	4-OH	4-OH	4-OH		6-OH	6-OH	4-OH
	Asn187(ND2)	2-OH	2-OH	2-OH	2-OH	2-OH	2-OH		2-OH		2-OH
	Asn187(OD)							2-OH			
	Glu188(OE1)	1-OH	1-OH	1-OH	1-OH	1-OH	1-OH		1-OH	1-OH	1-OH
	Glu188(OE2)		1-OH				1-OH	1-OH		1,2-OH	1-OH
	Glu268(OE1)	2-OH	2-OH				2-OH		2-OH	2-OH	2-OH
	Glu268(OE2)	2-OH	2-OH	2-OH	2-OH	2-OH	2-OH		2-OH		2-OH
	Tyr333(OH)	6-OH	6-OH	6-OH	6-OH	6-OH	6-OH		6-OH	6-OH	6-OH
10	10 score	27.58	44.31	49.82	27.19	44.25	45.78	20.47	52.90	38.17	
	Tyr83(OH)	6-OH	6-OH	6-OH	6-OH	5-OH	6-OH	6-OH	5-OH	6-OH	
	Ile126(O)	6-OH		6-OH			6-OH		5-OH	6-OH	
	Ala128(N)	6-OH		6-OH					5-OH	6-OH	
	Glu129(OE1)	N	N	N	N	6-OH	N			N	
	Glu129(OE2)							N	6-OH	N	
	Asn187(ND2)	5-OH	5,6-OH	5-OH	5-OH		5,6-OH		4-OH		
	Asn187(OD)							5,6-OH	4-OH	5,6-OH	
	Glu188(OE1)	4,5-OH	4,5-OH	4,5-OH	4,5-OH		4,5-OH	4,5-OH		4,5-OH	
	Glu188(OE2)			4-OH					4-OH		
	Glu268(OE1)			4-OH		4-OH			4-OH		
	Glu268(OE2)		6-OH		6-OH		6-OH				
	Tyr333(OH)				N		N				
13	13 score	25.37	46.53	43.62	25.53	45.76	43.10	17.65	56.23	39.34	
	Tyr83(OH)		5-OH		5,6-OH	5-OH		6-OH		6-OH	
	Ile126(O)										
	Ala128(N)		5-OH					6-OH			
	Glu129(OE1)	6-OH		6-OH		6-OH	6-OH	4-OH		N	
	Glu129(OE2)				N			5-OH			
	Asn187(ND2)				5 OH				6-OH	5-OH	
	Asn187(OD)								6-OH	5-OH	
	Glu188(OE1)		4-OH		4-OH			N			
	Glu188(OE2)			4-OH	4-OH	4-OH			5-OH	4-OH	
	Glu268(OE1)	4,5-OH	4-OH	4,5-OH	4-OH	4,5-OH	4,5-OH		6-OH	5-OH	
	Glu268(OE2)		4-OH		5-OH	4,5-OH					
	Tyr333(OH)	6-OH		6-OH			6-OH				

[a] The color codes in this table are used to indicate the number of runs that share the same top exit pose. See text below for further explanation.

In this table we have used a color code for every scoring value as well as the hydrogen bond pattern. It is used to identify common poses obtained across different docking simulations. Compounds whose poses share the same color in different docking runs have a similar top exit pose. For instance, most of the scoring values in the docking results for galactose are colored with a single color (green), to indicate that there seems to be a consensus on the pose reached by these compounds, which reproduces the one found in the crystal structure of the β-galactosidase-galactose complex found in Protein Data Bank (PDB) entry 3HTC (see Figure 3). This outcome serves to validate the docking protocol used for these calculations. Docking of ligand **10** produces a similar pose in most of the cases (see Figure 4), colored cyan in Table 2. Compound **13** displays a larger number of different poses than compound **10**, indicating this latter ligand fits better in the binding site, a result that may underlie its higher inhibitory activity (see Table 1). Figure 5 shows the poses that result for compound **13** using all the three scoring functions. Most of the poses obtained for this ligand are un-colored, in order to point out that these are single binding conformations which do not display comparable poses amongst the different docking runs. The only pose that is reproduced in more than one run (for this compound) was obtained with GoldScore and has the largest number of hydrogen bonds.

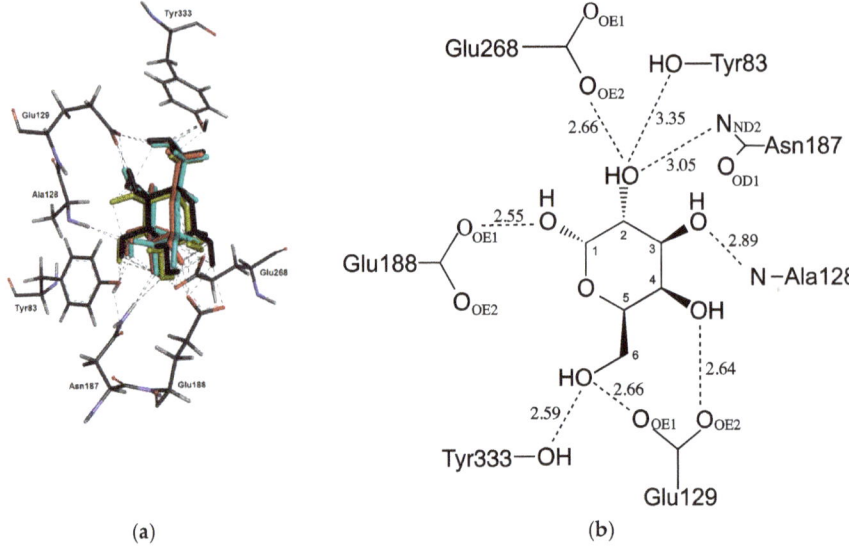

Figure 3. (**a**) Top galactose poses obtained in early termination runs with the various scoring functions used, superimposed on the one observed in the crystal structure, drawn in yellow. The ChemScore structure is drawn in red, while the GoldScore and ChemPLP are drawn in black and cyan, respectively. (**b**) Hydrogen bond interactions between the ligand and the protein residues, resulting from the GoldScore scoring protocol run, observed as well in PDB entry 3THC [32].

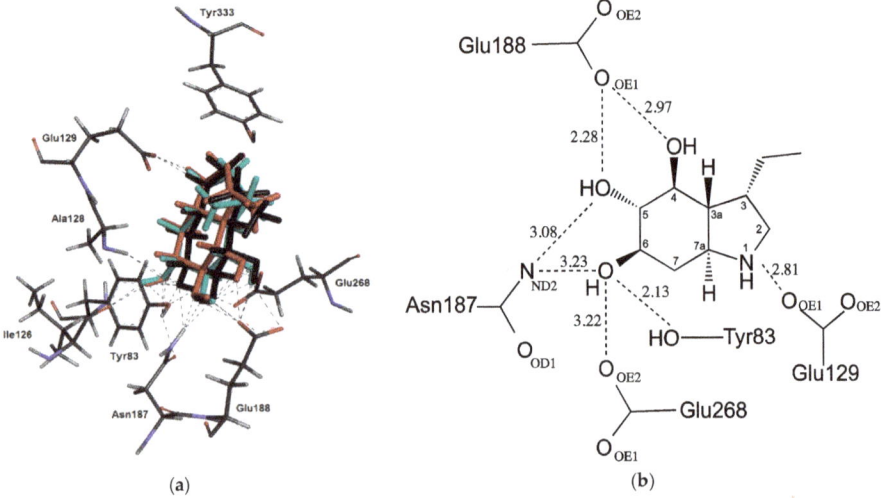

Figure 4. (**a**) Top poses obtained for compound **10** in early termination runs with the various scoring functions used. The ChemScore structure is drawn in red, while the GoldScore and ChemPLP are drawn in black and cyan, respectively. (**b**) Hydrogen bond interactions between the ligand and the protein residues, resulting from the GoldScore scoring protocol run.

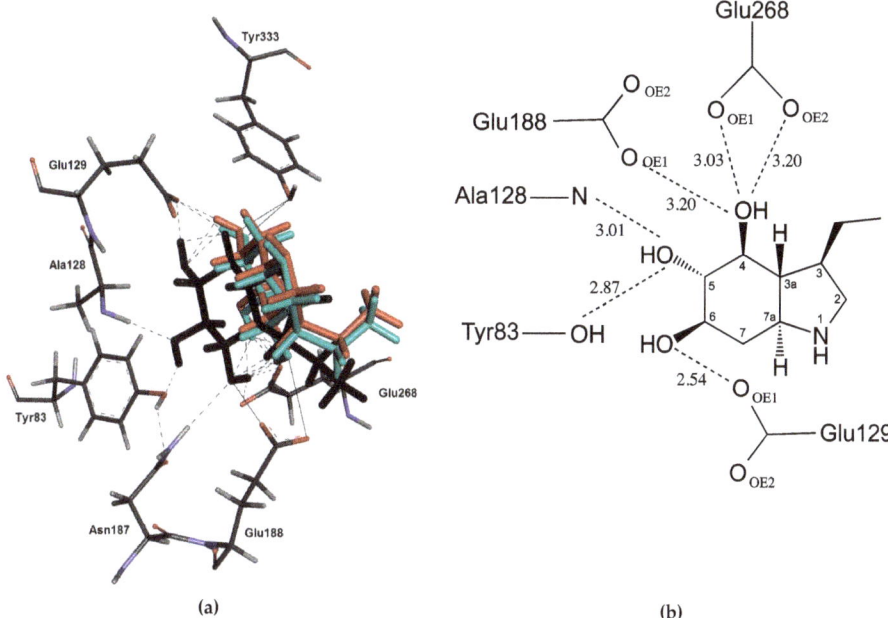

Figure 5. (a) Top poses obtained for compound **13** in early termination runs with the various scoring functions used. The ChemScore structure is drawn in red, while the GoldScore and ChemPLP are drawn in black and cyan, respectively. (b) Hydrogen bond interactions between the ligand and the protein residues, resulting from the GoldScore scoring protocol run.

To further asses the uniqueness of the binding poses for the three ligands used in our studies we have reviewed the "early termination" protocol results. In this protocol the best pose search is terminated as soon as a specified number of runs have a similar solution, within a given Root Mean Square Deviation (RMSD) of each other (see methods section). The results show that the number of runs increases for the weaker binder (compound **13**) as compared to compound **10**, indicating a lack of consensus for the best pose for the former. For instance, compound **13** does not find a consensus solution with the ChemPLP scoring function in the early termination run. Finally, cluster analysis results indicate that the latter compound present fewer clusters at the RMSD cut-off used in this study (results not shown), an outcome that further validates the hypothesis behind the difference in affinity.

3. Discussion

This work presents new synthetic routes to polyhydroxylated octahydroindoles with pharmacological chaperone (PC) therapeutic potential aimed at autosomal recessive diseases like G_{M1} gangliosidosis and Morquio B, a group of lysosomal storage disorders resulting from the abnormal metabolism of macro-substances such as glycosphingolipids, glycogen, mucopolysaccharides, and glycoproteins [33]. This abnormal metabolism may result in neurodegenerative disorders as well as dwarfism and skeletal abnormalities [34].

These diseases are caused by mutations in the lysosomal β-galactosidase (β-Gal), which are frequently related to misfolding and subsequent endoplasmic reticulum-associated degradation [26]. PC therapy is a novel approach that uses small molecule ligands of the mutant enzyme to promote the correct folding and prevent endoplasmic reticulum-associated degradation while promoting trafficking to the lysosome [33]. The affinity of the leads for the enzyme should not be high since it is desirable that the activity of the enzyme should be preserved. The range of affinities for these compounds usually span from the milli- to the micro-molar level. Some of the efficacious leads are galactose analogues. In this family of ligands the hydroxyl groups serve to maintain the structural binding specificity. The compounds studied here (**10** and **13**) are polyhydroxylated octahydroindoles and hence represent a departure from the galactose analogue paradigm. The results indicate that these compounds display inhibitory potency only for β-Gal at a milli-molar level, making them a good starting point for further development as PCs. The docking calculations performed herein for these compounds have allowed us to rationalize the small difference in binding between these compounds. As seen above, compound **10** displays a single well defined binding pose, while its epimer **13** loses this pose specificity, an outcome that may explain the observed binding affinity order.

The β-galactosidase mutations that originate the four phenotypes of the G_{M1} gangliosidosis and Morquio B diseases have been identified and have been mapped into the crystallographic structure of this molecule. Most mutations fall outside the active site and hence will not disturb the ligand–protein interactions. Actually, one of the phenotypes of this disease does not present any mutations in the active site. The other three phenotypes each present a single mutation that could affect the hydrogen bond pattern described above or ligand–protein van der Waals contacts [34]. As a conclusion, the present work opens new venues for PC therapies other than galactose analogs. It will be desirable in the future to carry out the binding kinetics and docking studies of our compounds with the few known β-galactosidase active site mutants in order to advance in the lead compound generation.

4. Materials and Methods

4.1. Methods for the Glycosidase Inhibition Studies

The enzymes α-glucosidase (from yeast, rice), β-glucosidase (from almonds, bovine liver), α-galactosidase (from coffee beans), β-galactosidase (from bovine liver), α-mannosidase (from jack beans), β-mannosidase (from snails), α-L-fucosidase (from bovine kidney), α-L-rhamnosidase (from *Penicillium decumbens*), β-glucuronidases (from *Escherichia coli*), α,α-trehalase (from porcine kidney), amyloglucosidase (from *Aspergillus niger*), *p*-nitrophenyl glycosides, and various disaccharides were purchased from Sigma-Aldrich Co. Brush border membranes were prepared from the rat small intestine according to the method of Kessler et al. [35], and were assayed at pH 6.8 for rat intestinal maltase using maltose. For rat intestinal glucosidases and porcine kidney trehalase activities, the reaction mixture (0.2 mL) contained 25 mM substrate and the appropriate amount of enzyme, and the incubations were performed for 10 min at 37 °C. The reaction was stopped by heating at 100 °C for 3 min. After centrifugation (600 g; 10 min), 0.035 mL of the resulting reaction mixture were added to 2.1 mL of the Glucose CII-test Wako (Wako Pure Chemical Ind., Osaka, Japan). The absorbance at 505 nm was measured to determine the amount of the released D-glucose. Other glycosidase activities were determined using an appropriate *p*-nitrophenyl glycoside as substrate at the optimum pH of each enzyme. The reaction mixture (0.2 mL) contained 2 mM of the substrate and the appropriate amount of enzyme. The reaction was stopped by adding 0.4 mL of 400 mM Na_2CO_3. The released *p*-nitrophenol was measured spectrometrically at 400 nm.

4.2. Docking Protocol

We carried out the docking simulations with the suite of modules resident in the program GOLD [36]. We scored the poses with three of the scoring resident functions (i.e., GoldScore [37,38], ChemScore [39–41], and ChemPLP [42]).

For the docking predictions to our target we used the X-ray structure of human β-galactosidase (hβ-Gal) bound to galactose (PDB entry 3THC) [34]. As a first step we selected the catalytic domain (residues 29 to 360) and we cleaned up the target structure discarding alternative conformations and adding hydrogen atoms, using the Discovery Studio (DS) modules [43]. We defined the binding site as including all the β-Gal catalytic domain atom residues that lay at 6 Å from the ligand (i.e., β-galactose). We performed the docking simulations using three different approaches in the GOLD "Fitness Search

Options" running setup: in the first one we used the "allow early termination" option, which instructs GOLD to terminate docking of a ligand as soon as a specified number of runs have a similar solution, within a given RMSD of each other. In the second one we used the "generate diverse solutions" option in which diversity is reinforced during the ligand mapping stage. This aim is reached by comparing the RMSD of the current solution against those that have already been generated. If the RMSD is below the diversity threshold or the maximum of solutions per cluster has been reached, the mapping is rejected and the process repeated until an acceptable solution is generated. In the last one we used the "allow early termination" option but leaving flexibility of the side chains of the active site residues Tyr83, Glu129, Asn187, Glu188, Glu268, and Tyr333. In all cases the docking conformations generated by the genetic algorithm were evaluated by the all three scoring functions mentioned above. In the case of galactose, we validated our methodology by searching for poses similar to the crystallographic one. In the case of ligands **10** and **13** we performed an additional analysis, searching (across all docking options) for hydrogen bond interactions similar to the ones observed in the galactose complex.

4.3. Chemical Synthesis Methods

Melting points were determined using a Kofler Thermogerate apparatus and are uncorrected. Specific rotations were recorded on a JASCO DIP-370 optical polarimeter, infrared spectra on a MIDAC FTIR spectrophotometer, and nuclear magnetic resonance spectra on a Bruker WM-250 or a Varian Mercury 300 apparatus. Mass spectra were obtained on a Kratos MS 50 TC mass spectrometer. Elemental analyses were obtained from the Elemental Analysis Service at the University of Santiago de Compostela. Thin layer chromatography (tlc) was performed using Merck GF-254 type 60 silica gel and ethyl acetate/hexane mixtures as eluents; the tlc spots were visualized with Hanessian mixture. Column chromatography was carried out using Merck type 9385 silica gel. Solvents were purified as in reference [44].

*4.3.1. (1R,2S,3S)-2-(Benzyloxy)-5-nitrocyclohex-4-ene-1,3-diyl diacetate (**4b**)*

A 2:1 TFA/H$_2$O mixture (90 mL) was added to compound **1** (285 mg, 0.88 mmol) and the resulting mixture was stirred at room temperature for 5 h. The solvents were evaporated under vacuum and co-evaporated with toluene (3 × 10 mL). The crude was solved in methanol (20 mL), 2% aq. K$_2$CO$_3$ (9 mL) were added, and the mixture was stirred at room temperature for 4 h. The reaction was then neutralized with DOWEX 50WX4-50 (previously acidified at pH = 1), filtered and concentrated to dryness, to provide **4a**.

Ac$_2$O (1.8 mL, 19.4 mmol) and a catalytic amount of DMAP (30 mg) were added to a solution of crude **4a** in Et$_2$O (60 mL) and the resulting solution was stirred at room temperature for 12 h. The reaction was then concentrated to dryness and the residue was solved in CH$_2$Cl$_2$ (30 mL) and washed with H$_2$O (3 × 15 mL). The organic layer was dried (anhydrous Na$_2$SO$_4$), filtered and concentrated to dryness. The residue was purified by flash column chromatography (AcOEt/Hex 1:3) to give compound **4b** (237 mg, 77% yield), as an amorphous white solid. $[\alpha]_D^{20}$: +69.5 (c 2.2, CHCl$_3$). ^{1}H-RMN (Cl$_3$CD, 250 MHz, ppm): 1.96 (s, 3H, CH$_3$); 1.98 (s, 3H, CH$_3$); 2.66–2.77 (m, 1H, H-6); 2.99–3.10 (m, 1H, H-6′); 3.81 (dd, J = 6.9 Hz, J = 4.3 Hz, 1H); 4.64 (s, 2H, CH$_2$Ph); 5.15 (dt, J = 7.0, J = 5.3 Hz, 1H, H-1); 5.51 (tt, J = 4.1 Hz, J = 1.9 Hz, 1H, H-3); 6.99 (d, J = 3.4 Hz, 1H, H-4); 7.17–7.32 (m, 5H, 5xH-Ar). ^{13}C-RMN (Cl$_3$CD, 62.5 MHz, ppm): 20.8 (CH$_3$); 20.9 (CH$_3$); 27.4 (CH$_2$); 67.9 (CH); 68.7 (CH); 73.7 (CH$_2$); 75.1 (CH); 127.7 (CH); 127.8 (2xCHAr); 128.2 (CHAr); 128.6 (2xCHAr); 137.4 (C); 148.2 (C); 169.7 (CO); 170.0 (CO). IR (ν, cm^{-1}): 1747 (s, C=O); 1528 (m, NO$_2$); 1340 (m, NO$_2$). HRMS (ESI$^+$): calculated for C$_{17}$H$_{19}$NNaO$_7$ [M + Na]$^+$: 372.1054. Found: 372.1061.

*4.3.2. (1R,2S,3S,4R,5S)-2-(Benzyloxy)-5-nitro-4-((S)-1-oxobutan-2-yl)cyclohexane-1,3-diyl diacetate (**5**) and (1R,2S,3S,4R,5S)-2-(benzyloxy)-5-nitro-4-((R)-1-oxobutan-2-yl)cyclohexane-1,3-diyl diacetate (**6**)*

n-Butanal (211 µL, 2.34 mmol) and pyrrolidine (99 µL, 1.21 mmol) were added to a solution of nitroolefin **4b** (157 mg, 0.45 mmol) in CH$_2$Cl$_2$ (4 mL). The resulting solution was stirred at room temperature for 3 h and then was concentrated to dryness. Flash column chromatography of the residue (EtOAc/hexane 1:4) provided compound **5** (98 mg, 50% yield, white solid) and its epimer **6** (21% yield, clear gum).

Compound **5**. m.p.: 112.5–114.0 °C (EtOAc/Hex). $[\alpha]_D^{20}$ = −17.3° (c 1.5, CHCl$_3$). ^{1}H–RMN (Cl$_3$CD, 250 MHz, ppm): 0.88 (t, J = 7.3 Hz, 3H, CH$_2$CH$_3$); 1.13–1.33 (m, 2H, CH$_2$CH$_3$); 1.74 (s, 3H, CH$_3$); 1.92 (s, 3H, CH$_3$); 1.75–2.13 (m, 2H, H-6+H-6′); 2.63 (dt, J = 4.2 Hz; J = 12.2 Hz, 1H, H-4); 2.92 (td, J = 1.9 Hz; J = 11.5 Hz, 1H, H-2a); 3.54 (t, J = 9.4 Hz, 1H, H-2); 4.54 (ABq, J = 11.4 Hz, 2H, CH$_2$Ph); 4.61–4.93 (m, 3H, H-1 + H-3 + H-5); 7.12–7.28 (m, 5H, 5xAr-H); 9.44 (d, J = 1.1 Hz, 1H, H-C=O). ^{13}C-RMN (Cl$_3$CD, 62.5 MHz, ppm): 13.5 (CH$_3$); 16.0 (CH$_2$); 20.6 (CH$_3$); 20.9 (CH$_3$); 33.8 (CH$_2$); 44.0 (CH); 52.3 (CH); 69.1 (CH); 70.3 (CH); 75.1 (CH$_2$); 81.5 (CH); 82.2 (CH); 127.7 (2xCH-Ar); 128.0 (CH-Ar); 128.6 (2xCH-Ar); 137.6 (C); 169.1 (CO); 169.8 (CO); 200.1 (CO). IR (ν, cm^{-1}): 1745 (s, C=O); 1556 (s, NO$_2$), 1369 (s, NO$_2$). MS-ESI$^+$ (m/z, %): 444.1 (100, [M + Na]$^+$). EA: Calculated for C$_{21}$H$_{27}$NO$_8$: C, 59.85; H, 6.46; N, 3.32. Found: C, 59.84; H, 6.54; N, 3.16.

Compound **6**. $[\alpha]_D^{20}$ = −1.9° (c 1.0, CHCl$_3$). ^{1}H-RMN (Cl$_3$CD, 250 MHz, ppm): 0.89 (t, J = 7.1 Hz, 3H, -CH$_2$CH$_3$); 1.15–1.52 (m, 2H, -CH$_2$CH$_3$); 1.90 (s, 3H, CH$_3$); 1.91 (s, 3H, CH$_3$); 1.74–2.07 (m, 2H, H-6 + H-6′); 2.51 (dt, J = 12.1 Hz, J = 4.41 Hz,1H, H-4); 2.75–2.85 (m, 1H, H-2a); 3.58 (t, J = 9.2 Hz, 1H, H-2); 4.52-4.67 (m, 3H, CH$_2$Ph + H-5); 4.81 (ddd, J = 4.6 Hz; J = 9.5 Hz; J = 11.6 Hz, 1H, H-1); 5.01 (dd, $J_{3,2}$ = 9.2 Hz; $J_{3,4}$ = 11.1 Hz, 1H, H-3); 7.14–7.30 (m, 5H, 5xAr-H); 9.44 (s, 1H, H-C=O). ^{13}C-RMN (Cl$_3$CD, 62.5 MHz, ppm): 13.2 (CH$_3$); 17.4 (CH$_2$); 20.9 (CH$_3$); 21.0 (CH$_3$); 33.9 (CH$_2$); 43.5 (CH); 51.5 (CH); 70.2 (CH); 70.5 (CH); 75.2 (CH$_2$); 80.6 (CH); 81.9 (CH); 127.6 (2xCH-Ar); 128.0 (CH-Ar); 128.6 (2xCH-Ar); 137.8 (C); 169.8 (2xCO); 201.3 (CO). IR (ν, cm^{-1}): 1752 (s, C=O); 1718 (s, C=O), 1555 (s, NO$_2$), 1372 (s, NO$_2$). HRMS (ESI$^+$): Calculated for C$_{21}$H$_{27}$NNaO$_8$ [M + Na]$^+$: 444.1629. Found: 444.1623.

4.3.3. (R)-2-((1R,2S,3S,4R,6S)-2,4-Diacetoxy-3-(benzyloxy)-6-nitrocyclohexyl)butanoic acid (**7**)

2-Methyl-2-butene (115 μL, 1.09 mmol), NaH$_2$PO$_4$.2H$_2$O (50 mg, 0.32 mmol) and NaClO$_2$ (13.5 mg, 0.15 mmol) were added to a 0 °C cooled solution of aldehyde **6** (115 mg, 0.27 mmol) in a 5:2 ^{t}BuOH/H$_2$O mixture (7 mL). The reaction was then stirred at room temperature for 2 h, the ^{t}BuOH was removed under vacuum, and the resulting mixture was extracted with EtOAc (3 × 10 mL). The organic layers were dried (anhydrous Na$_2$SO$_4$), filtered, and the solvents were removed under vacuum. The residue was submitted to flash column chomathography (EtOAc/Hexane 1:2) to give compound **7** (105 mg, 88% yield), as a solid mp: 146.8-148.1 °C (EtOAc/Hexane). $[\alpha]_D^{20}$ = +10.8° (c 1.4, CHCl$_3$). ^{1}H-RMN (Cl$_3$CD, 250 MHz, ppm): 0.92 (t, J = 7.2 Hz, 3H, CH$_2$CH$_3$); 1.38–2.10 (m, 2H, CH$_2$CH$_3$); 1.94 (s, 3H, CH$_3$); 1.98 (s, 3H, CH$_3$); 2.18–2.24 (m, 2H, H-5 + H-5′); 2.59 (dt, J = 4.6 Hz; J = 12.3 Hz, 1H, H-1); 2.80 (td, J = 1.9 Hz; J = 11.2 Hz, 1H, H-2a); 3.61 (t, J = 9.1 Hz, 1H, H-3); 4.57–4.70 (m, 3H, CH$_2$Ph + H-6); 4.92 (tdd, J = 11.5 Hz, J = 8.8 Hz, J = 5.1 Hz, 1H, H-2); 5.15 (dd, J = 9.0 Hz; J = 11.2 Hz, 1H, H-4); 7.20–7.36 (m, 5H, 5xAr-H); 9.24 (sa, 1H CO$_2$H). ^{13}C-RMN (Cl$_3$CD, 62.5 MHz, ppm): 13.0 (CH$_3$); 21.0 (2xCH$_3$); 21.5 (CH$_2$); 34.3 (CH$_2$); 45.2 (CH); 45.6 (CH); 70.3 (CH); 70.6 (CH); 74.9 (CH$_2$); 82.0 (CH); 82.2 (CH); 127.8 (2xCH-Ar); 127.9 (CH-Ar); 128.6 (2xCH-Ar); 137.9 (C); 169.8 (CO); 169.9 (CO); 177.5 (CO). IR (ν, cm^{-1}): 1746 (s, C=O); 1711 (s, C=O), 1557 (s, NO$_2$); 1370 (s, NO$_2$). HRMS (ESI$^+$): Calculated for C$_{21}$H$_{27}$NNaO$_9$ [M + Na]$^+$: 460.1578. Found: 460.1555.

4.3.4. (3S,3aR,4S,5S,6R,7aS)-5-(Benzyloxy)-3-ethyloctahydro-1H-indole-4,6-diyl diacetate (**8**)

Zinc dust (969 mg, 14.82 mmol) was added to a 0 °C cooled solution of aldehyde **5** (250 mg, 0.59 mmol) in a 1:1 MeOH/AcOH mixture (15 mL) and the resulting suspension was stirred at 0 °C for 14 h. The reaction was filtered through a celite pad, which was eluted with methanol, and the filtrate was concentrated to dryness. The residue was disolved in Cl$_2$CH$_2$ (15 mL) and was washed with saturated aq. NaHCO$_3$ (2x10 mL). The organic layer was dried (anhydrous Na$_2$SO$_4$), filtered, and concentrated to dryness under vacuum. Flash column chromatography of the resulting oil (CH$_2$Cl$_2$/MeOH 9:1) provided compound **8** (206 mg, 90% yield,), as a white amorphous solid. $[\alpha]_D^{20}$ = −10.8 (c 1.8, CHCl$_3$).

¹H-RMN (Cl₃CD, 250 MHz, ppm): 0.77 (t, *J* = 7.4 Hz, 3H, CH₂CH₃); 1.09–1.49 (m, 5H, H-3 + H-7 + H-7' + CH₂-CH₃); 1.90 (s, 3H, CH₃); 1.91 (s, 3H, CH₃); 2.06 (bs, 1H, NH); 2.27 (ddd, *J* = 3.4 Hz, *J* = 5.1 Hz, *J* = 11.7 Hz, 1H, H-3a); 2.65–2.74 (m, 2H, H-2 + H-2'); 3.21 (t, *J* = 10.0 Hz, 1H, H-7a); 3.53 (t, *J* = 9.3 Hz, 1H, H-5); 4.58 (ABq, *J* = 11.6 Hz, 2H, CH₂Ph); 4.89 (ddd, *J* = 5.1 Hz, *J* = 9.5 Hz, *J* = 11.3 Hz, 1H, H-6); 4.99 (dd, *J* = 9.1 Hz, *J* = 11.1 Hz, 1H, H-4); 7.16–7.28 (m, 5H, 5x-Ar-H). ¹³C-RMN (Cl₃CD, 62.5 MHz, ppm): 12.0 (CH₃); 21.0 (2xCH₃); 21.9 (CH₂); 35.3 (CH₂); 39.7 (CH); 51.4 (CH₂); 52.0 (CH); 54.5 (CH); 71.1 (CH); 73.5 (CH); 74.7 (CH₂); 84.8 (CH); 127.4 (2xCH-Ar); 127.5 (CH-Ar); 128.3 (2xCH-Ar); 138.3 (C); 169.8 (CO); 169.9 (CO). IR (ν, cm⁻¹): 3205 (b, NH), 1740 (s, C=O). HRMS (ESI⁺): Calculated for C₂₁H₃₀NO₅ [M + H]⁺: 376.2118. Found: 376.2122.

4.3.5. (3S,3aR,4S,5S,6R,7aS)-5-(Benzyloxy)-3-ethyloctahydro-1H-indole-4,6-diol (**9**)

A 1 M NaOH methanolic solution (1 mL, 1 mmol) was added to a solution of amine **8** (30 mg, 0.08 mmol) in methanol (2 mL) and the resulting solution was stirred at room temperature for 4 h. Half of the methanol was then evaporated, and the reaction was neutralized with saturated NH₄Cl solution and extracted with ethyl acetate (3 × 10 mL). The joined organic layers were dried (anhydrous Na₂SO₄), filtered, and concentrated to dryness under vacuum. Purification of the resulting oil by flash column chromathography (CH₂Cl₂/MeOH 7:1) gave compound **9** (16 mg, 69% yield), as a clear gum. [α]$_D^{20}$ = +3.0 (c 1.0, CH₃OH) ¹H-RMN (CD₃OD, 250 MHz, ppm): 0.88 (t, *J* = 7.3 Hz, 3H, CH₂-CH₃); 1.19–1.58 (m, 4H); 1.92–2.07 (m, 2H); 2.18 (ddd. *J* = 3.4 Hz, *J* = 5.0 Hz, *J* = 11.7 Hz, 1H, H-3a); 2.68–2.88 (m, 2H, H-2' + H-7a); 3.15 (t, *J* = 8.8 Hz, 1H); 3.31–3.46 (m, 1H); 3.54–3.64 (m, 1H, H-6); 4.83 (s, 2H, CH₂Ph); 7.18–7.31 (m, 3H, 3xAr-H); 7.37–7.42 (m, 2H, 2xAr-H). ¹³C-RMN (CD₃OD, 62.5 MHz, ppm): 12.7 (CH₃); 28.1 (CH₂); 36.7 (CH₂); 45.3 (CH); 52.3 (CH₂); 54.8 (CH); 59.4 (CH); 72.7 (CH); 75.8 (CH); 76.6 (CH); 90.4 (CH); 128.5 (CH-Ar); 129.2 (4xCH-Ar); 140.5 (C). IR (ν, cm⁻¹): 3371 (b, NH + OH). HRMS (ESI⁺): Calculated for C₁₇H₂₆NO₃, [M + H]⁺: 292.1907. Found: 292.1902

4.3.6. (3S,3aR,4S,5S,6R,7aS)-3-Ethyloctahydro-1H-indole-4,5,6-triol (**10**)

Pd/C 10% (15 mg) was added to a deoxygenated solution of amine **9** (15 mg, 0.05 mmol) in methanol (2 mL) and the resulting suspension was stirred at room temperature for 6 h, under a hydrogen atmosphere (P = 1 atm). The reaction was then filtered through a celite pad, eluted with methanol, and the filtrate concentrated to dryness. Flash column chromatography of the residue (CH₂Cl₂/MeOH 5:1) allowed isolation of compound **10** (9 mg, 87% yield) as a yellow oil. [α]$_D^{20}$ = +16.4 (c 0.9, MeOH). ¹H-RMN (CD₃OD, 250 MHz, ppm): 0.91 (t, *J* = 7.4 Hz, 3H, CH₂CH₃); 1.22–1.39 (m, 1H); 1.49–1.69 (m, 2H); 1.91–2.20 (m, 2H), 2.28 (dt, 1H, *J* = 11.5 Hz, *J* = 4.2 Hz, 1H); 2.99–3.19 (m, 3H), 3.40–3.64 (m, 3H). ¹³C-RMN (CD₃OD, 62,5 MHz, ppm): 12.5 (CH₃); 28.0 (CH₂); 33.5 (CH₂); 39.2 (CH); 42.6 (CH); 62.7 (CH₂); 66.9 (CH); 72.0 (CH); 75.4 (CH); 81.2 (CH). IR (ν, cm⁻¹): 3405 (b, NH + OH). HRMS (ESI+): Calculated for C₁₀H₂₀NO₃ [M + H]⁺: 202.1438. Found: 202.1438.

4.3.7. (3R,3aR,4S,5S,6R,7aS)-5-(Benzyloxy)-3-ethyloctahydro-1H-indole-4,6-diyl diacetate (**11**)

Starting from aldehyde **6** (100 mg, 0.24 mmol) and following the same procedure as for compound **8**, compound **11** was obtained (76 mg, 85% yield), as a white amorphous solid. [α]$_D^{20}$ = +9.3 (c 1.8, CHCl₃). ¹H-RMN (Cl₃CD, 250 MHz, ppm): 0.79–0.93 (m, 4H), 0.97–1.12 (m, 1H), 1.18–1.51 (m, 4 H), 1.76–1.83 (m, 1H), 1,93 (s, 3H, CH₃), 1,96 (s, 3H, CH₃), 2.35 (ddd, *J* = 11.6 Hz, *J* = 5.0 Hz, *J* = 3.7 Hz, 1H), 2.80 (td, *J* = 11.2 Hz, *J* = 3.3 Hz, 1H), 3.18–3.24 (m, 1H), 3.53–3.59 (m, 1H), 4.62 (ABq, *J* = 11.6 Hz, 2H, CH₂Ph), 4.93 (ddd, *J* = 11.4 Hz, *J* = 9.6 Hz, *J* = 4.9 Hz, 1H), 5.13 (dd, *J* = 11.6 Hz, *J* = 8.7 Hz, 1H), 7.21–7.33 (m, 5H, 5xAr-H). ¹³C-RMN (Cl₃CD, 62.5 MHz, ppm): 12.1 (CH₃); 21.1 (CH₃); 21.2 (CH₃); 22.1 (CH₂); 35.4 (CH₂); 39.9 (CH); 51.5 (CH₃); 52.1 (CH); 54.6 (CH); 71.3 (CH); 73.7 (CH); 74.9 (CH₂); 85.0 (CH); 127.6 (2xCH); 127.7 (2xCH); 128.5 (CH); 138.4 (C); 170.0 (CO); 170.1 (CO). IR (ν, cm⁻¹): 3220 (b, NH); 1741 (s, C=O). HRMS (ESI⁺): Calculated for C₂₁H₃₀NO₅ [M + H]⁺: 376.2118. Found: 376.2122.

4.3.8. (3R,3aR,4S,5S,6R,7aS)-5-(Benzyloxy)-3-ethyloctahydro-1H-indole-4,6-diol (12)

Reaction of amine **11** (54 mg, 0.14 mmol) under the same conditions as for the preparation of amine **9** gave compound **12** (29 mg, 69% yield), as a clear gum. $[\alpha]_D^{20}$ = +18.2 (c 2.1, CH$_3$OH). ^{1}H-RMN (CD$_3$OD, 250 MHz, ppm): 0.92 (t, J = 7.3 Hz, 3H, CH$_2$CH$_3$); 1.13 (tq, J = 13.4 Hz, J = 7.0 Hz, 1H, H-CHCH$_3$); 1.27–1.48 (m, 1H, H-CHCH$_3$); 1.61 (td, J = 11.4 Hz, J = 7.6 Hz, 1H, H-7); 1.76 (dtd, J = 14.9 Hz, J = 7.5 Hz, J = 3.3 Hz,1H, H-7′); 2.11–2.25 (m, 2H, H-3 + H-3a); 2.61 (td, J = 11.6 Hz, J = 3.5 Hz, 1H, H-7a + H-2); 2.77 (dd, J = 11.5 Hz, J = 3.2 Hz, 1H); 3.19–3.27 (m, 2H, H-2 + H-5); 3.52–3.65 (m, 2H); 4.87–4.91 (m, 2H, CH$_2$Ph); 7.22–7.37 (m, 3H, 3xAr-H), 7.46–7.49 (m, 2H, 2xAr-H). ^{13}C-RMN (CD$_3$OD, 62.5 MHz, ppm): 12.4 (CH$_3$); 23.1 (CH$_2$); 38.7 (CH$_2$); 41.1 (CH); 52.1 (CH$_2$); 55.2 (CH); 56.0 (CH); 71.8 (CH); 73.1 (CH); 76.5 (CH); 91.1 (CH$_2$); 128.5 (2xCH); 129.2 (3xCH); 140.6 (C). IR (ν, cm^{-1}): 3371 (b, NH + OH). HRMS (ESI+): Calculated for C$_{17}$H$_{26}$NO$_3$ [M + H]$^+$: 292.1907. Found: 292.1909.

4.3.9. (3R,3aR,4S,5S,6R,7aS)-3-ethyloctahydro-1H-indole-4,5,6-triol (13)

Following the same procedure as for amine **9**, amine **12** (18 mg, 0.06 mmol) gave compound **13** (11 mg, 88% yield), as a yellow solid. $[\alpha]_D^{20}$ = +36.4 (c 1.1, CH$_3$OH). ^{1}H-RMN (CD$_3$OD, 250 MHz, ppm): 0.90 (t, 3H, J = 7.3 Hz, CH$_2$CH$_3$); 1.10–1.43 (m, 3H); 1.81–1.96 (m, 2H); 2.11–2.46 (m, 4H); 3.13–3.67 (m, 3H). ^{13}C-RMN (CD$_3$OD, 62.5 MHz, ppm): 12.1 (CH$_3$); 24.1 (CH$_2$); 35.2 (CH); 38.3 (CH$_2$); 52.5 (CH); 63.6 (CH$_2$); 63.7 (CH); 71.5 (CH); 72.2 (CH); 82.3 (CH). IR (ν, cm^{-1}): 3408 (b, NH + OH). HRMS (ESI$^+$): Calculated for C$_{10}$H$_{20}$NO$_3$ [M + H]$^+$: 202.1438. Found: 202.1438.

X-ray crystal structure for compound **5**, X-ray crystal structure for compound **7**, ^{1}H NMR and ^{13}C NMR spectra for compounds **4b**, **5**, **6**, **7**, **8**, **9**, **10**, **11**, **12**, and **13** are in Supplementary Materials.

Supplementary Materials: The following are available online at http://www.mdpi.com/1424-8247/12/2/47/s1.

Author Contributions: R.J.E., M.C.V. and A.K. conceived the original concept; R.J.E. and J.C.E. developed the synthetic methodology; M.C.V. and F.S. performed the docking studies; R.J.E., A.K., F.S., and M.C.V. interpreted the resulting data; J.C.E., M.G., and Y.H. performed experimental work; R.J.E., A.K., F.S. and M.C.V. performed writing—original draft preparation; R.J.E., A.K., F.S., and M.C.V. performed writing—reviewing and editing; R.J.E. and A.K. were responsible for supervision, project administration, and funding acquisition.

Funding: This work has received financial support from the Spanish Ministry of Science and Innovation (CTQ2009-08490), the Xunta de Galicia (Centro Singular de Investigación de Galicia, accreditation 2016–2019, ED431B 2018/13; Project CN2011/037 and Project GRC2014/040), and the European Union (European Regional Development Fund-ERDF). It has also received a Grant-in-Aid for Scientific Research (C) from the Japanese Society for the Promotion of Science (JSPS KAKENHI Grant Number JP17K08362) (AK).

Conflicts of Interest: The authors declare no conflict of interest.

References

1. Compain, P.; Martin, O.R. (Eds.) *Iminosugars: From Synthesis to Therapeutic Applications*; Wiley: Hoboken, NJ, USA, 2007; ISBN 978-0-470-03391-3.
2. Horne, G.; Wilson, F.X.; Tinsley, J.; Williams, D.H.; Storer, R. Iminosugars past, present and future: Medicines for tomorrow. *Drug Discov. Today* **2011**, *16*, 107–118. [CrossRef]
3. Stütz, A.E. (Ed.) *Iminosugars as Glycosidase Inhibitors: Nojirimycin and Beyond*; Wiley-VCH: New York, NY, USA, 1999; ISBN 9783527295449.
4. Harit, V.K.; Ramesh, N.G. Amino-functionalized iminocyclitols: Synthetic glycomimetics of medicinal interest. *RSC Adv.* **2016**, *6*, 109528–109607. [CrossRef]
5. Arjona, O.; Gómez, A.M.; López, J.C.; Plumet, J. Synthesis and conformational and biological aspects of carbasugars. *Chem. Rev.* **2007**, *107*, 1919–2036. [CrossRef]
6. Chen, X.; Fan, Y.; Zheng, Y.; Shen, Y. Properties and production of valienamine and its related analogues. *Chem. Rev.* **2003**, *103*, 1955–1977. [CrossRef] [PubMed]
7. Trapero, A.; Egido-Gabás, M.; Bujons, J.; Llebaria, A. Synthesis and evaluation of hydroxymethylaminocyclitols as glycosidase inhibitors. *J. Org. Chem.* **2015**, *80*, 3512–3529. [CrossRef]

8. Johnston, P.S.; Coniff, R.F.; Hoogwerf, B.J.; Santiago, J.V.; Pi-Sunyer, F.X.; Krol, A. Effects of the carbohydrase inhibitor miglitol in sulfonylurea-treated NIDDM patients. *Diabetes Care* **1994**, *17*, 20–29. [CrossRef] [PubMed]
9. Campbell, L.K.; Baker, D.E.; Campbell, R.K. Miglitol: Assessment of its role in the treatment of patients with diabetes mellitus. *Ann. Pharmacother.* **2000**, *34*, 1291–1301. [CrossRef] [PubMed]
10. Horii, S.; Fukase, H.; Matsuo, T.; Kameda, Y.; Asano, N.; Matsui, K. Synthesis and α-D-glucosidase inhibitory activity of *N*-substituted valiolamine derivatives as potential oral antidiabetic agents. *J. Med. Chem.* **1986**, *29*, 1038–1046. [CrossRef] [PubMed]
11. Matsumoto, K.; Yano, M.; Miyake, S.; Ueki, Y.; Yamaguchi, Y.; Akazawa, S.; Tominaga, Y. Effects of voglibose on glycemic excursions, insulin secretion, and insulin sensitivity in non-insulin-ireated NIDDM patients. *Diabetes Care* **1998**, *21*, 256–260. [CrossRef] [PubMed]
12. Krentz, A.J.; Bailey, C.J. Oral antidiabetic agents: Current role in type 2 diabetes mellitus. *Drugs* **2005**, *65*, 385–411. [CrossRef]
13. Joubert, P.H.; Venter, H.L.; Foukaridis, G.N. The effect of miglitol and acarbose after an oral glucose load: A novel hypoglycaemic mechanism? *Br. J. Clin. Pharmacol.* **1990**, *30*, 391–396. [CrossRef] [PubMed]
14. Ficicioglu, C. Review of miglustat for clinical management in Gaucher disease type I. *Ther. Clin. Risk Manag.* **2008**, *4*, 425–431. [CrossRef] [PubMed]
15. Elstein, D.; Hollak, C.; Aerts, J.M.F.G.; van Weely, S.; Maas, M.; Cox, T.M.; Lachmann, R.H.; Hrebicek, M.; Platt, F.M.; Butters, T.D.; et al. Sustained therapeutic effects of oral miglustat (Zavesca, *N*-butyldeoxynojirimycin, OGT 918) in type I Gaucher disease. *J. Inherit. Metab. Dis.* **2004**, *27*, 757–766. [CrossRef]
16. Molyneux, R.J.; Roitman, J.N.; Dunnheim, G.; Szumilo, T.; Elbein, A.D. 6-Epicastanospermine, a novel indolizidine alkaloid that inhibits α-glucosidase. *Arch. Biochem. Biophys.* **1986**, *251*, 450–457. [CrossRef]
17. Kang, M.S.; Liu, P.S.; Bernotas, R.C.; Harry, B.S.; Sunkara, P.S. Castanospermine analogues: Their inhibition of glycoprotein processing α-glucosidases from porcine kidney and B16F10 cells. *Glycobiology* **1995**, *5*, 147–152. [CrossRef] [PubMed]
18. Michael, J.P. Indolizidine and quinolizidine alkaloids. *Nat. Prod. Rep.* **1999**, *16*, 675–696. [CrossRef]
19. Goss, P.E.; Baker, M.A.; Carver, J.P.; Dennis, J.W. Inhibitors of carbohydrate processing: A new class of anticancer agents. *Clin. Cancer Res.* **1995**, *1*, 935–944.
20. Molyneux, R.J.; Pan, Y.T.; Tropea, J.E.; Benson, M.; Kaushal, G.P.; Elbein, A.D. 6,7-Di*epi*castanospermine, a tetrahydroxyindolizidine alkaloid inhibitor of amyloglucosidase. *Biochemistry* **1991**, *30*, 9981–9987. [CrossRef]
21. Pastuszak, I.; Molyneux, R.J.; James, L.F.; Elbein, A.D. Lentiginosine, a dihydroxyindolizidine alkaloid that inhibits amyloglucosidase. *Biochemistry* **1990**, *29*, 1886–1891. [CrossRef]
22. Michalik, A.; Hollinshead, J.; Jones, L.; Fleet, G.W.J.; Yu, C.-Y.; Hu, X.-G.; van Well, R.; Horne, G.; Wilson, F.X.; Kato, A.; et al. Steviamine, a new indolizidine alkaloid from *Stevia rebaudiana*. *Phytochem. Lett.* **2010**, *3*, 136–138. [CrossRef]
23. Gravier-Pelletier, C.; Maton, W.; Le Merrer, Y. A straightforward route to indolizidine and quinolizidine analogs as new potential antidiabetics. *Synlett* **2003**, 333–336.
24. Gravier-Pelletier, C.; Maton, W.; Bertho, G.; Le Merrer, Y. Synthesis and glycosidase inhibitory activity of enantiopure polyhydroxylated octahydroindoles and decahydroquinolines, analogs to castanospermine. *Tetrahedron* **2003**, *59*, 8721–8730. [CrossRef]
25. González, M.A.; Estévez, A.M.; Campos, M.; Estévez, J.C.; Estévez, R.J. Protocol for the incorporation of γ-amino acids into peptides: Application to (−)-shikimic acid based 2-aminomethyl- cyclohexanecarboxylic acids. *J. Org. Chem.* **2018**, *83*, 1543–1550. [CrossRef]
26. Suzuki, H.; Ohto, U.; Higaki, K.; Mena-Barragán, T.; Aguilar-Moncayo, M.; Ortiz Mellet, C.; Nanba, E.; Garcia-Fernandez, J.M.; Suzuki, Y.; Shimizu, T. Structural basis of pharmacological chaperoning for human β-Galactosidase. *J. Biol. Chem.* **2014**, *289*, 14560–14568. [CrossRef] [PubMed]
27. Ono, N. *The Nitro Group in Organic Synthesi*; Wiley-VCH: Weinheim, Germany, 2001; ISBN 0-471-22448-0.
28. Guo, L.; Chi, Y.; Almeida, A.M.; Guzei, I.A.; Parker, B.K.; Gellman, S.H. Stereospecific synthesis of conformationally constrained γ-amino acids: New foldamer building blocks that support helical secondary structure. *J. Am. Chem. Soc.* **2009**, *131*, 16018–16020. [CrossRef]

29. Bhorkade, S.B.; Gavhane, K.B. Multigram synthesis of an advanced nitroalkene intermediate: Application in synthesis of octahydroindol-2-one derivative featuring diastereoselective Michael addition of diethylmalonate. *Tetrahedron Lett.* **2016**, *57*, 2575–2578. [CrossRef]
30. Ballini, R.; Palestini, C. A new, highly efficient synthesis of conjugated nitrocycloalkenes. *Tetrahedron Lett.* **1994**, *35*, 5731–5734. [CrossRef]
31. Otero, J.M.; Barcia, J.C.; Salas, C.O.; Thomas, P.; Estévez, J.C.; Estévez, R.J. Studies on the Michael addition of naphthoquinones to sugar nitro olefins: First synthesis of polyhydroxylated hexahydro-*11H*-benzo[a]carbazole-5,6-diones and hexahydro-11*bH*-benzo[b]carbazole-6,11-diones. *Tetrahedron* **2012**, *68*, 1612–1621. [CrossRef]
32. Laskowski, R.A.; Jablonska, J.; Pravda, L.; Varekova, R.S.; Thornton, J.M. PDBsum: Structural summaries of PDB entries. *Protein Sci.* **2018**, *27*, 129–134. [CrossRef]
33. Fan, J.-Q. A counterintuitive approach to treat enzyme deficiencies: Use of enzyme inhibitors for restoring mutant enzyme activity. *Biol. Chem.* **2008**, *389*, 1–11. [CrossRef]
34. Ohto, U.; Usui, K.; Ochi, T.; Yuki, K.; Satow, Y.; Shimizu, T. Crystal structure of human β-galactosidase. Structural basis of G_{M1} gangliosidosis and Morquio B diseases. *J. Biol. Chem.* **2012**, *287*, 1801–1812. [CrossRef] [PubMed]
35. Kessler, M.; Acuto, O.; Storelli, C.; Murer, H.; Müller, M.; Semenza, G. A modified procedure for the rapid preparation of efficiently transporting vesicles from small intestinal brush border membranes. Their use in investigating some properties of D-glucose and choline transport systems. *Biochim. Biophys. Acta* **1978**, *506*, 136–154. [CrossRef]
36. *GOLD.*; Version 5.1; Cambridge Crystallographic Data Centre: Cambridge, UK, 2011.
37. Jones, G.; Willett, P.; Glen, R.C. Molecular recognition of receptor sites using a genetic algorithm with a description of desolvation. *J. Mol. Biol.* **1995**, *245*, 43–53. [CrossRef]
38. Jones, G.; Willett, P.; Glen, R.C.; Leach, A.R.; Taylor, R. Development and validation of a genetic algorithm for flexible docking. *J. Mol. Biol.* **1997**, *267*, 727–748. [CrossRef] [PubMed]
39. Baxter, C.A.; Murray, C.W.; Clark, D.E.; Westhead, D.R.; Eldridge, M.D. Flexible docking using Tabu search and an empirical estimate of binding affinity. *Proteins* **1998**, *33*, 367–382. [CrossRef]
40. Eldridge, M.D.; Murray, C.W.; Auton, T.R.; Paolini, G.V.; Mee, R.P. Empirical scoring functions: I. The development of a fast empirical scoring function to estimate the binding affinity of ligands in receptor complexes. *J. Comput. Aided Mol. Des.* **1997**, *11*, 425–445. [CrossRef] [PubMed]
41. Verdonk, M.L.; Cole, J.C.; Hartshorn, M.J.; Murray, C.W.; Taylor, R.D. Improved protein-ligand docking using GOLD. *Proteins* **2003**, *52*, 609–623. [CrossRef]
42. Korb, O.; Stützle, T.; Exner, T.E. Empirical scoring functions for advanced protein-ligand docking with PLANTS. *J. Chem. Inf. Model.* **2009**, *49*, 84–96. [CrossRef]
43. *Discovery Studio, Versions 2.1 and 2.5*; Acceelrys Inc.: San Diego, CA, USA, 2009.
44. Perrin, D.D.; Armarego, W.L.F. *Purification of Laboratory Chemicals*; Pergamon: New York, NY, USA, 1988.

Sample Availability: Samples of the compounds **10** and **13** are available from the authors.

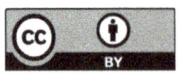

© 2019 by the authors. Licensee MDPI, Basel, Switzerland. This article is an open access article distributed under the terms and conditions of the Creative Commons Attribution (CC BY) license (http://creativecommons.org/licenses/by/4.0/).

Communication

Development of a Microwave-assisted Chemoselective Synthesis of Oxime-linked Sugar Linkers and Trivalent Glycoclusters

Katherine McReynolds *[,](image) **Dustin Dimas** [†], **Grace Floyd** [‡] **and Kara Zeman**

Department of Chemistry, California State University, Sacramento, 6000 J Street, Sacramento, CA 95819-6057, USA; Dustin.Dimas-1@ou.edu (D.D.); gracepfloyd@gmail.com (G.F.); karazeman@csus.edu (K.Z.)
* Correspondence: kdmcr@csus.edu; Tel.: +01-916-278-6551
† Current address: Department of Chemistry and Biochemistry, The University of Oklahoma, 101 Stephenson Parkway, SLSRC, Room 1000, Norman, OK 73019-5251, USA.
‡ Current address: Biocare Medical, 60 Berry Dr., Pacheco, CA 94553, USA.

Received: 19 February 2019; Accepted: 8 March 2019; Published: 14 March 2019

Abstract: A rapid, high-yielding microwave-mediated synthetic procedure was developed and optimized using a model system of monovalent sugar linkers, with the ultimate goal of using this method for the synthesis of multivalent glycoclusters. The reaction occurs between the aldehyde/ketone on the sugars and an aminooxy moiety on the linker/trivalent core molecules used in this study, yielding acid-stable oxime linkages in the products and was carried out using equimolar quantities of reactants under mild aqueous conditions. Because the reaction is chemoselective, sugars can be incorporated without the use of protecting groups and the reactions can be completed in as little as 30 min in the microwave. As an added advantage, in the synthesis of the trivalent glycoclusters, the fully substituted trivalent molecules were the major products produced in excellent yields. These results illustrate the potential of this rapid oxime-forming microwave-mediated reaction in the synthesis of larger, more complex glycoconjugates and glycoclusters for use in a wide variety of biomedical applications.

Keywords: Microwave reactions; chemoselective; oxime; aminooxy; glycoclusters; multivalent

---

1. Introduction

Multivalent glycoconjugates such as glycoclusters, glycodendrimers, glyconanoparticles and glycan microarrays have found a wide range of applications in biochemistry and medicine from studying protein-carbohydrate interactions to developing potential therapeutic agents [1–4]. It has long been recognized in nature that proteins and their binding partners are often displayed in a multivalent fashion. It is also well known for carbohydrate-containing molecules that their binding interactions with their biological partners are much stronger when present in multiple copies rather than in a 1:1 ratio. This is known as the multivalent or cluster glycoside effect [2,3,5,6].

Given the complexity and size of multivalent glycoconjugates, as well as the requirement for multiple simultaneous reactions to append the sugars, it is critical that a synthetic strategy be developed to create these molecules in an efficient and fully functionalized manner. Commonly, carbohydrate chemistry requires multiple protection/deprotection steps due to the similar reactivity of the hydroxyl groups present. This can lead to time-consuming reaction pathways with low yielding final products. Some studies have sought to simplify the attachment of the carbohydrates to the multivalent scaffold. We previously showed that we could use amide coupling between the carboxylic acid-containing unprotected sugar, sialic acid and a poly(amidoamine) (PAMAM) dendrimer core to create a fully substituted 2nd generation 16-mer glycodendrimer that showed μM activity against

HIV-1 [7]. However, this strategy is only applicable to sugars with either an existing amine or carboxylic acid group or would require the introduction of these groups, leading to further steps. Another approach uses click chemistry, however, this still requires functionalization of the carbohydrate moiety with either an alkyne or an azide group, requiring a multi-step synthetic process involving protecting group chemistry to install those groups [2,8–10].

As an alternative strategy to either amide or click chemistry, we sought a streamlined synthetic process that would allow us to use unprotected carbohydrates in the coupling step to a multivalent scaffold molecule to create the desired fully substituted glycoclusters. This involved a two-part simplification strategy. First, a chemoselective oxime-forming reaction was selected [11,12]. Oxime linkages are known to be both acid- and glycosidase-stable, making them more robust than glycosidic linkages for biological applications [13–15]. The oximation reaction occurs under mild, aqueous conditions between an aminooxy-containing molecule, here a monovalent linker or a multivalent core [16] and an unprotected reducing aldose (hemiacetal) or ketose (hemiketal) sugar [17,18]. Oxime linkages in sugars can exist in an equilibrium mixture containing two forms in protic solutions, the ring opened oxime, with E/Z isomers (major products) and the ring-closed glycoside, comprised of the α- and β-anomers (minor products, Figure 1) [11,19]. The second simplification to the synthetic process involved the use of a microwave-mediated reaction for the formation of the oxime linkage. This was done for multiple reasons. First, to shorten the reaction times from several hours down to minutes in duration [20]. Next, to synthesize the desired glycoconjugates in good yields and for the multivalent glycoclusters, to ensure that simultaneous reactions of each sugar with the complementary aminooxy group on the linker/core molecule could be achieved. Finally, to simplify the process and ensure reproducibility of the reaction through the use of programmed methods. These characteristics of microwave-mediated reactions make them particularly attractive for the synthesis of carbohydrate-containing molecules, which can be sensitive to long and harsh reaction conditions [21]. Additionally, there are only a few reports of microwave-assisted reactions for the purpose of synthesizing multivalent glycoconjugates [22–30]. Most of these reports focus on the use of microwave irradiation to mediate click chemistry reactions. There is only one reported use of alternate microwave-mediated reactions to form multivalent oxime-linked glycopeptoids [30]. In this paper, Carrasco and coworkers reported the microscale microwave-assisted synthesis of a glycopeptoid using a 50 to 100-fold excess of sugar.

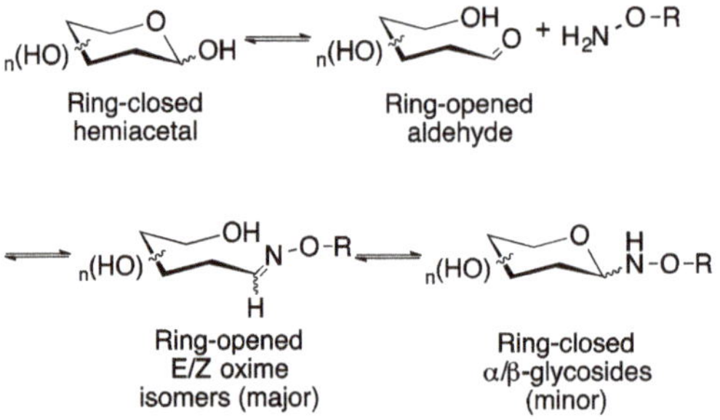

Figure 1. Reaction of a typical reducing aldose sugar with an aminooxy-containing compound in a protic solvent such as water results in the initial formation of the ring-opened E/Z oximes, which over time in aqueous solution, will equilibrate with the ring closed glycosides.

Other traditional, non-microwave-mediated studies similarly show the use of multiple equivalents of sugar relative to oxime forming partners. For simple monovalent systems, 2–3 equivalents of aldose sugar were reacted with aminooxy-containing linkers/peptides, both in the presence/absence of aniline for 1–48 h at 25 °C or 60 °C [31]. Here, Jensen and coworkers reported yields for the GlcNAc oxime linker as 7 and 72% for a 1-h reaction conducted at 25 or 60 °C., respectively, for the non-aniline catalyzed reaction, illustrating that elevated temperatures alone improved reaction rates. For the same GlcNAc reaction conducted with 0.1 M aniline included, the yields were 20 and 80% for a 1 or 6 h reaction time at 25 °C, respectively [31]. For the ketose sialic acid sugars, Szabo and coworkers reported the synthesis of sialic acid and tetrasialic acid conjugated to one side of a di-aminooxy linker [32]. The reactions were carried out at 37 °C for 22 h using 19 equivalents of the linker to the sugar to avoid crosslinking. These reactions resulted in yields of 33 and 50%, respectively, for sialic acid and tetrasialic acid-linked monovalent conjugates. Finally, for an example of a traditional multivalent oxime-forming reaction, Renaudet et al. reported yields of 66, 65 and 74% for the syntheses of tetravalent oxime-linked glycopeptoids using the anomeric aminooxy-sugars α-Fuc, β-Fuc and β-Gal and a tetra-aldehyde-bearing cyclic peptide. The reactions were conducted at 37 °C for 2 h and utilized 2 equivalents of sugar per reactive site [33].

Here we report the development of an efficient microwave-mediated method used to synthesize both mono- and multivalent oxime-linked linkers and glycoclusters, respectively. Our method uses *equimolar* ratios of sugar:aminooxy-linker/core and can be completed in as little as 30 min of total reaction time, such that many reactions can be completed in the space of a day and precious/rare glycans used sparingly. This microwave procedure is also simple to set up and operate, making it possible for the rapid production of a wide variety of glycoconjugates by junior researchers/technicians in the lab. Reaction condition uniformity can also be maintained through the use of a programmed method, thereby increasing method consistency and minimizing trial-to-trial variation. Through our microwave-mediated procedure, we have been able to demonstrate both the preparative production of sugar-linkers in a single step, such that they can be isolated and utilized in further synthetic transformations or the facile synthesis of novel glycoclusters in excellent yields that can then be readily incorporated into biological studies. Finally, we have also illustrated that we can create large quantities of the sugar-linker conjugates using our microwave-mediated conditions in good yields without the addition of the common catalyst, aniline [31,34]. Removal of the aniline catalyst and using the microwave to shorten the reaction time both lend themselves to making the reaction greener overall.

2. Results

In this paper we outline the successful combination of chemoselectivity with a microwave-mediated reaction for purposes of synthesizing a series of oxime-linked monovalent sugar-linker molecules and three trivalent glycoclusters. We first evaluated seven common aldose mono-, di- and tri-saccharides (*N*-acetyl glucosamine, cellobiose, gentiobiose, lactose, maltose, maltotriose and melibiose, **1–7**, Scheme 1) for the preparation of the monovalent sugar linkers. This chemistry was undertaken to determine the optimum microwave reaction conditions necessary for the reaction in equimolar quantities of sugar to aminooxy-linker. The study had a goal of minimizing the use of excess reactants, particularly if expensive/difficult to create sugars were to be used, which would also serve to simplify the purification process. Traditionally, aniline is used as a catalyst in oxime-forming reactions because it yields significant increases to the reaction rate [31,34]. Therefore, in our development of the microwave-mediated method, we evaluated whether or not aniline was required to improve the yields for oxime formation or whether it could be omitted to make the reaction greener and easier to purify, without significantly sacrificing the reaction yield. The resultant sugar-linker molecules are useful intermediates in the development of multivalent glycoconjugates. The trivalent glycoclusters synthesized in this study provide proof of concept for the synthesis of higher order glycoclusters efficiently and excellent isolated yields via a chemoselective microwave synthesis.

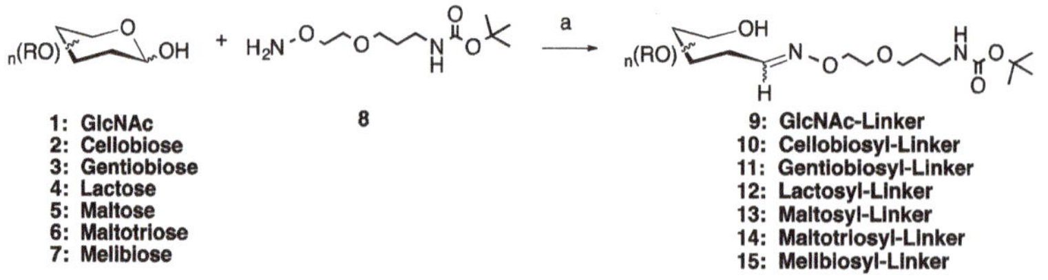

Scheme 1. Microwave synthesis of sugar linker conjugates **9–15**. (a) 0.1 M NH$_4$OAc, pH 4.5, 25% of 400 W, 50 °C, 30 min. Optional: 0.1.

1: GlcNAc
2: Cellobiose
3: Gentiobiose
4: Lactose
5: Maltose
6: Maltotriose
7: Melibiose

9: GlcNAc-Linker
10: Cellobiosyl-Linker
11: Gentiobiosyl-Linker
12: Lactosyl-Linker
13: Maltosyl-Linker
14: Maltotriosyl-Linker
15: Meliblosyl-Linker

For the trivalent glycocluster synthesis, we employed both an aldose reducing disaccharide, cellobiose (**2**, Scheme 2) and two ketose sugars, sialic acid (N-acetyl neuraminic acid, Neu5Ac, **18**, Scheme 3) and the α-2→8-linked dimer of sialic acid (disialic acid) (**19**, Scheme 3) [35]. These sugars were chosen to illustrate that the microwave reaction worked efficiently for both types of sugars and that the glycosidic bonds present in **2** and **19** would be stable to the microwave heating conditions at a pH of 4.5. Sialic acid-containing glycans are widely found in nature and are important markers in disease states such as cancer, influenza and meningococcal meningitis [36,37]. The produced glycoclusters contain the acid/glycosidase stable oxime linkage, which can help ensure the integrity of the molecules if they are ultimately used in biological applications [13–15]. It is also worth noting that longer oligosaccharides may be necessary given that the reducing end sugar will exist as a mixture of the native closed ring conformation and the open ring oxime, which may impact the resultant biological activity.

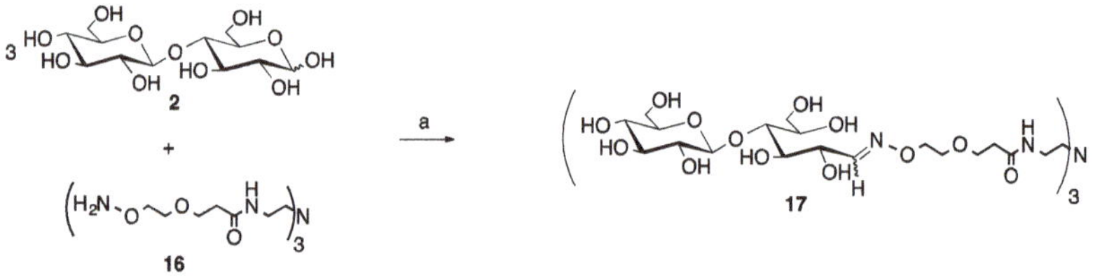

Scheme 2. Microwave synthesis of trivalent cellobiose glycocluster (**17**, 94% yield). (a) 0.1 M NH$_4$OAc, pH 4.5, 0.1 M aniline, 25% of 400 W, 30 min.

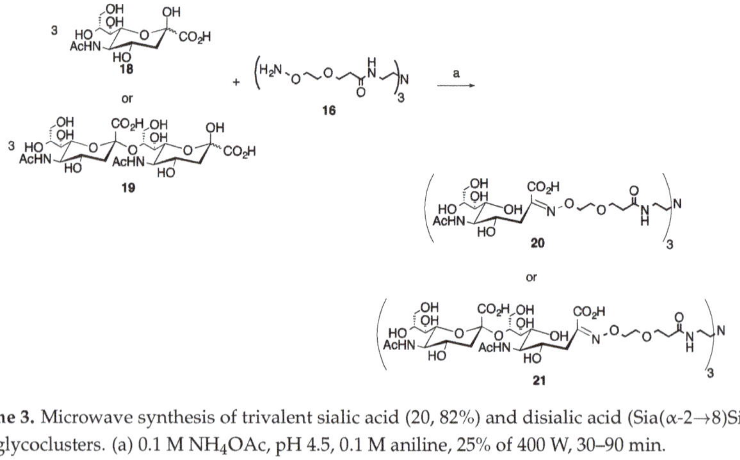

Scheme 3. Microwave synthesis of trivalent sialic acid (**20**, 82%) and disialic acid (Sia(α-2→8)Sia, **21**, 88%) glycoclusters. (a) 0.1 M NH$_4$OAc, pH 4.5, 0.1 M aniline, 25% of 400 W, 30–90 min.

2.1. Medium Scale Microwave-mediated Synthesis of Monovalent Sugar-Linkers

To begin the medium scale (≤0.250 mmol) synthesis of the monovalent sugar linker molecules, a bifunctional, hydrophilic aminooxy-Boc-protected amine linker was used (**8**, Scheme 1) [16]. This was combined 1:1 with any of the seven off-the-shelf aldose mono-, di- and tri-saccharides (**1–7**) in 0.1 M ammonium acetate, pH 4.5, in the presence or absence of 0.1 M aniline. The reactions were carried out in a CEM MARS 5 laboratory-grade microwave. Many different combinations of power level and time were attempted, with the optimum combination found to be 30 min at 25% of 400 W, with a 50 °C maximum temperature. Upon completion of the reaction, the solution was freeze dried then purified by flash chromatography on silica gel in a 6:4:0.5 mixture of chloroform:methanol:water. Examination of the pooled fractions by ^{1}H NMR showed no evidence of degradation of either the products or unreacted starting materials (See Supplementary Materials for details). This initial set of reactions, using the aniline catalyst, gave rise to 73–93% yields of the Boc-protected sugar linker products (**9–15**, Table 1), while the same reactions conducted without the aniline catalyst resulted in yields ranging from 60–68%, a decrease of 9–28%, depending on the sugar used.

Table 1. Summary of sugar-linker 50 °C traditional and microwave syntheses. Medium scale (≤0.250 mmol) reactions were run in the presence or absence of 0.1 M aniline (final concentration), while the large scale (≥0.800 mmol) reactions were all run in the presence of 0.1 M aniline as a catalyst. The Δ% yield column compares the yields of the medium scale aniline catalyzed reaction with the uncatalyzed reaction of the same scale. For the large-scale reactions, the comparison is between the medium and large-scale aniline-catalyzed reactions.

Sugar	Additive	% Yield	% Yield
Medium Scale (≤0.250 mmol)			
Non-Microwave Conditions:			
Cellobiose	0.1 M Aniline	65	
	N/A	56	−9
Microwave-Mediated Conditions:			
GlcNAc	0.1 M Aniline	78	
	N/A	68	−10
Cellobiose	0.1 M Aniline	76	
	N/A	63	−13
Gentiobiose	0.1 M Aniline	73	
	N/A	60	−13
Lactose	0.1 M Aniline	93	
	N/A	65	−28
Maltose	0.1 M Aniline	74	
	N/A	65	−9
Maltotriose	0.1 M Aniline	92	
	N/A	68	−24
Melibiose	0.1 M Aniline	80	
	N/A	68	−12
Large Scale (≥0.800 mmol)			
GlcNAc	0.1 M Aniline	79	1
Cellobiose	0.1 M Aniline	75	−1
Gentiobiose	0.1 M Aniline	65	−8
Lactose	0.1 M Aniline	63	−30
Maltose	0.1 M Aniline	62	−12
Maltotriose	0.1 M Aniline	64	−28
Melibiose	0.1 M Aniline	60	−20

For further comparison, two traditional, non-microwave-mediated reactions to yield the Boc-protected cellobiosyl-linker (**10**) were carried out at 50 °C for 30 min in the presence or absence of the aniline catalyst. Cellobiose was chosen for the sugar, as it represents a typical aldose disaccharide. For the aniline-catalyzed reaction, a 65% yield of **10** resulted, while for the non-catalyzed reaction a yield of 56% of **10** was observed (Table 1). Comparing these results against **10** synthesized in the microwave, modest yield improvements were noted in the microwave mediated reactions. The microwave aniline-catalyzed reaction gave rise to an 11% higher yield and the non-aniline catalyzed microwave reaction resulted in a 7% higher yield. Overall the average % yield increase for all 7 aldoses for the microwave versus traditional reactions in the presence of aniline was 16% and 9% for the non-aniline catalyzed reactions. Interestingly, the average magnitude of the difference between aniline versus non-aniline catalyzed reactions was greater (~15%) for the microwave-mediated reactions than for the traditional heated reactions (9%). These results indicate that modest improvements of yield can be gained by using microwave-mediated conditions, using equimolar quantities of sugar and linker. In addition, if desired, it was found that the aniline catalyst could be left out of the reaction mixture to simplify product purification and make the reaction greener, all without unreasonable yield losses.

2.2. Large Scale Microwave-mediated Synthesis of Monovalent Sugar-Linkers

To further evaluate reaction scalability, the microwave reaction was then carried out on the same seven aldose sugars at higher quantities ($\geq$0.800 mmol) using identical microwave reaction conditions as described above. All of the reactions included the 0.1 M aniline catalyst to maximize the yields. Here it was found that the isolated yields in the large-scale reactions ranged from 60–79%, a decrease of 1–30% compared to the medium scale aniline-catalyzed reactions, again depending on the sugar incorporated (Table 1). We noted that the decreases in the yields for the medium scale reactions in the absence of aniline were similar to the decreases seen in the larger scale microwave-mediated reactions in the presence of the aniline catalyst. This means that while the microwave can be an excellent tool for shortening the reaction times for these reactions, a balance must be struck between reaction scale and reaction time savings. For our purposes, it made sense to significantly scale up the reactions, given that the sugars used were all commercially available and the linker could be produced efficiently in large quantities as well [16]. These new monovalent sugar-linker molecules are useful intermediates that can be utilized in the synthesis of further glycoconjugates. Once the Boc group is removed, the resultant amine can be used in amide coupling reactions to attach the sugar linker to whatever carboxyl-containing scaffold/surface is desired.

2.3. Multivalent Glycocluster Microwave-mediated Synthesis

Based on the results for the model monovalent sugar linkers, we moved into the microwave-mediated synthesis of multivalent glycoclusters. With multivalent scaffolds, in addition to the desired fully functionalized product (here the trisubstituted glycocluster), under-substituted products are possible (un-, mono- and disubstituted glycoclusters). It was hypothesized that by utilizing our best reaction conditions developed for the equimolar system described above (25% of 400 W power, 30 min, 0.1 M aniline), that the production of under-substituted products would be limited. The synthesis of three novel trivalent glycoclusters was undertaken beginning with the optimized conditions and included one aldose disaccharide, cellobiose (**2**, Scheme 2), as well as a ketose monosaccharide sialic acid (**18**, Scheme 3) and a ketose disaccharide, α-2$\rightarrow$8-disialic acid (**19**, Scheme 3), with a previously synthesized trivalent aminooxy-terminated hydrophilic core (**16**) [16]. Here, cellobiose was chosen as a representative aldose disaccharide and both sialic acid and α-2$\rightarrow$8-disialic acid [35] were chosen to represent more hindered, less reactive ketose substrates to show the utility of this method for these interesting, biologically important sugars.

Beginning with a 3:1 ratio of cellobiose to the trivalent core (**2** and **16**, respectively), the 30-min reaction time was sufficient to produce only the desired trivalent product, **17**, in 94% yield following purification via size exclusion chromatography (SEC, Scheme 2). This reaction was carried out on a 10-fold lower scale than the monovalent, aniline-catalyzed reaction, which is one possible reason why the yields were higher. No under-substituted products (un-, mono- or disubstituted), sugar degradation or unreacted starting materials were observed for this reaction by ^{1}H NMR upon purification.

For the ketoses, the sialic acid (**18**) reaction with the trivalent core (**16**, Scheme 3), a 3:1 ratio of sugar to core was utilized. The reaction was carried out as described above for 30 min and after purification by SEC, an 82% yield of the desired trivalent product (**20**) was achieved. However, unlike the reaction to produce **17**, where no under-substituted products were produced, the disubstituted byproduct was isolated from a separate peak from the SEC purification and identified by ^{1}H NMR. Carrying this method forward, the disaccharide ketose, disialic acid, **19**, was reacted in a 3:1 sugar to core (**16**) ratio under the same conditions as used for sialic acid. However, it was noted that 30 min was not sufficient to achieve a good yield for the desired trivalent product, **21**. This is likely due to steric issues, so two additional 30-min cycles were carried out under the same conditions for a total of 90 min of microwave reaction time. After purification by SEC, an 88% yield of the desired trivalent product (**21**) was achieved. Similar to the sialic acid reaction, the disubstituted byproduct was isolated from a separate peak after SEC purification and was identified by ^{1}H NMR. No other under-substituted products or other byproducts were noted from the pooled column fractions for any of the observed peaks, showing again that the microwave-mediated reaction conditions are mild enough to use for these more expensive sugars.

3. Discussion

In conclusion, the development of an efficient microwave-mediated oxime forming reaction between equimolar quantities of unprotected aldose or ketose sugars and either a monovalent or trivalent aminooxy-containing linker or core was undertaken with the aims to create a facile and reproducible method that resulted in decreased reaction times, minimization of the amounts of sugars/catalysts used to reduce costs and make the reactions greener, while still creating the desired glycoconjugates efficiently and in good to excellent yields. We began our studies with the formation of model monovalent oxime-linked sugar linker molecules at two different preparative reaction scales (medium and large). This was done to determine the optimum microwave-mediated conditions necessary to achieve the best yields in the smallest amount of time without requiring an excess of either the sugar or linker molecules. Once this was accomplished, the microwave reaction conditions were then applied to more complex multivalent systems, such that biologically relevant glycoclusters could be prepared in their desired fully substituted forms in a matter of minutes in a single chemoselective step.

To begin with the monovalent oxime-linked sugar linkers, first a medium scale reaction ($\leq$0.250 mmol) was tested both in the presence and absence of 0.1 M aniline as a catalyst and equimolar quantities of sugar and linker. The aniline-based reaction conditions were superior to the reactions without aniline, which was not unexpected, however, if greener reaction conditions are sought or simplified purification procedures are desired, the reactions still work well without the catalyst when the reaction is carried out using microwave conditions. When the reaction was scaled up to a more preparative scale ($\geq$0.800 mmol) in the presence of 0.1 M aniline, slightly lower yields were obtained, however, the yields were considered to be acceptable, given the ease of setup and the short reaction time needed to produce larger quantities of simple glycoconjugates.

The real advantage of using a microwave-mediated reaction in the formation of oxime-linked glycoconjugates was realized when the method was applied to one disaccharide aldose and two ketose sugars in a multivalent reaction. The complete substitution of multivalent glycoclusters can be difficult to achieve, as multiple, simultaneous reactions are required between the individual sugars and the reactive moieties on the multivalent scaffold. However, in this study using our optimized microwave-mediated reaction conditions developed with the monovalent sugar linkers, it was found that the tri-cellobiosyl product (**17**) was synthesized in a 94% yield, with no under-substitution products observed, while the tri-sialic acid (**20**) and trivalent di-sialic acid (**21**) were the predominant products formed in 82 and 88% yields, respectively. For the latter two reactions, the only other observed minor product in each case was the disubstituted glycocluster.

This newly developed microwave method allows for the efficient production of monovalent or multivalent glycoconjugates. It offers ease of set-up, consistent trial-to-trial reaction control through the use of programmable methods, short reaction times and good yields of the desired products, all while utilizing equimolar quantities of the reactant oxime-forming partners. This method, when applied to larger, more complex/hindered oligosaccharides gives rise to primarily the desired fully substituted products, with minimal to no production of undesired under-substituted products. This is valuable, particularly when one is working with sugars that are rare or expensive to produce/purchase.

4. Materials and Methods

4.1. General Methods

Unless otherwise noted all chemicals were purchased from commercial sources and used without further purification/treatment. All microwave reactions were carried out in a CEM MARS 5 microwave. All reaction solutions were freeze dried upon reaction completion prior to purification. Size exclusion chromatography (SEC) separations were conducted on either a BioRad BioLogic DuoFlow 10 system or a Pharmacia LC 500 system, using a BioRad 2.5 × 120 cm column packed with BioGel P-10 in 0.03 M NH_4HCO_3. 3.5 mL fractions were collected, and the absorbance measured at 214 nm and 225 nm. ^1H and ^{13}C spectra (internal methanol standard) in D_2O were collected on a Bruker Avance III 500 MHz spectrometer. ^1H NMR integration data for **17**, **20** and **21** were normalized to 1/3 of the total molecule. Mass spectrometry data were obtained at the Campus Chemical Instrument Center (CCIC) Mass Spectrometry and Proteomics Facility at The Ohio State University (OSU).

4.2. Synthesis of Monovalent Sugar-Linkers

4.2.1. General Procedure for the Medium-Scale (0.187–0.250 mmol) Synthesis of Sugar-Linkers

Without Aniline-microwave or Traditional Heating

Compounds 9–15 were synthesized using 1 equivalent of the aminooxy linker (**Compound 8**) [16], prepared as a 100 mg/mL solution in methanol. The appropriate volume of this solution was transferred to a flask and evaporated under reduced pressure, then freeze-dried to get an accurate mass of the oil. Next, 1 equivalent of: *N*-acetylglucosamine, cellobiose, gentiobiose, lactose, maltose, maltotriose or melibiose was separately added to each flask containing **Compound 8** [16]. These were each dissolved in 3.0 mL of 0.1 M ammonium acetate (NH_4OAc) at a pH of 4.5. The reactions were conducted either stirring at 50 °C in an oil bath (traditional) or at 400 W in a microwave (CEM MARS 5) at 25% power with a 2 min ramp to temperature and a hold time of 30 min at a maximum temperature of 50 °C. After the reaction was complete, the solutions were freeze-dried. The products were then purified by flash chromatography in 6:4:0.5 $CHCl_3$:MeOH:H_2O, yielding off-white amorphous solids.

Tert-butyl *N*-[3-(2-{(E/Z)-[2-acetamido-2-deoxy-D-glucopyranosyl]oxime}ethoxy)propyl] carbamate (Compound 9): 54.3 mg (0.232 mmol) of **Compound 8** plus 53.2 mg (0.241 mmol) of **Compound 1** were utilized, resulting in 68.9 mg (67.9%) of an off white solid (**Compound 9**). ^1H NMR (500 MHz, D_2O): ^1H NMR (500 MHz, D_2O): δ 7.49 (d, *J* = 6.2 Hz, 0.7H, E isomer), 6.83 (d, *J* = 6.6 Hz, 0.2H, Z isomer), 5.10, (t, *J* = 6.7 Hz, 0.2H, Z isomer), 4.67 (t, *J* = 6.8 Hz, 0.7H, E isomer), 4.32 (d, *J* = 9.8 Hz, 0.1 H, closed ring), 4.30-4.17 (m, overlapping, 2H), 4.17-4.03 (m, overlapping, 1H), 3.39-3.47 (m, overlapping, 9.2H), 3.41 (d, *J* = 3.4 Hz, 0.1H, closed ring), 3.10 (t, *J* = 6.3 Hz, 2H), 2.02 (s, 3H), 1.71 (p, *J* = 6.3, 13.0 Hz, 2H), 1.40 (s, 9H). ^{13}C NMR (125 MHz, D_2O with internal MeOH standard): δ 174.21, 171.20, 149.99, 148.78, 81.03, 72.79, 71.50, 71.07, 70.22, 69.43, 68.65, 68.60, 63.02, 52.07, 49.03, 37.20, 28.84, 23.42, 22.38, 22.14, 22.03. HRMS ESI+: Calc. for $C_{18}H_{36}N_3O_9$ $(M + H)^+$: 438.2416. Found: 438.2455.

Tert-butyl N-[3-(2-{(E/Z)-[β-D-glucopyranosyl-(1→4)-D-glucopyranosyl]oxime}ethoxy)propyl] carbamate (Compound 10-microwave): 43.7 mg (0.187 mmol) of Compound 8 plus 63.9 mg (0.187 mmol) of Compound 2 were utilized, resulting in 64.7 mg (63.1%) of an off white solid (Compound 10). ^{1}H NMR (500 MHz, D$_2$O): δ 7.69 (d, *J* = 5.5 Hz, 0.6H, E isomer), 7.00 (d, *J* = 5.5 Hz, 0.1H, Z isomer), 4.99 (dd, *J* = 4.1, 5.4 Hz, 0.1H, Z isomer), 4.58 (dd, *J* = 5.7, 6.8 Hz, 0.7H, E isomer), 4.56-4.49 (m, overlapping, 0.9H), 4.30 (d, *J* = 9.2 Hz, 0.2H), 4.28-4.21 (m, overlapping, 1.5H), 4.09 (t, *J* = 3.7 Hz, 0.1H, Z isomer), 3.98 (dd, *J* = 1.8, 6.9 Hz, 0.7H, E isomer), 3.96-3.39 (m, overlapping, 14.8 H), 3.46-3.29 (m, overlapping, 1H), 3.17-3.11 (m, overlapping, 2H), 1.75 (p, *J* = 6.5, 12.9 Hz, 2H), 1.43 (s, 9H). ^{13}C NMR (125 MHz, D$_2$O with internal MeOH standard): δ 158.39, 153.22, 152.06, 102.69, 90.25, 81.08, 80.77, 78.64, 78.38, 76.16, 75.97, 75.76, 75.45, 73.51. 73.35, 73.28, 72.81, 71.51, 71.34, 70.59, 69.63, 69.51, 69.52, 68.82, 68.66, 68.53, 68.49, 66.46, 62.27, 62.09, 60.76, 60.66, 60.33, 49.06, 37.29, 28.94, 27.88. HRMS ESI+: Calc. for C$_{22}$H$_{43}$N$_2$O$_{14}$ (M + H)$^+$: 559.2709. Found: 559.2724.

Cellobiose (Compound 10-oil bath, traditional): 55.3 mg (0.236 mmol) of Compound 8 plus 73.3 mg (0.214 mmol) of Compound 2 were utilized, resulting in 67.3 mg (56.1%) of an off white solid (Compound 10).

Tert-butyl N-[3-(2-{(E/Z)-(β-D-glucopyranosyl-(1→6)-D-glucopyranosyl)oxime}ethoxy)propyl] carbamate (Compound 11): 46.6 mg (0.199 mmol) of Compound 8 plus 70.8 mg (0.207 mmol) of Compound 3 were utilized, resulting in 65.8 mg (60.3%) of a fluffy white solid (Compound 11). ^{1}H NMR (500 MHz, D$_2$O): δ 7.49 (d, *J* = 6.5 Hz, 0.7H, E isomer), 6.84 (d, *J* = 6.3 Hz, 0.1H, Z isomer), 4.42 (d, *J* = 9.1 Hz, 1H), 4.39 (d, *J* = 3.7 Hz, 0.7H), 4.39 (t, *J* = 3.7 Hz, 2H), 3.88-3.36 (m, overlapping, 15H), 3.05 (t, *J* = 6.5 Hz, 2H), 1.67 (p, *J* = 6.5, 13.1 Hz, 2H), 1.34 (s, 9H). ^{13}C NMR (125 MHz, D$_2$O with internal MeOH standard): δ 157.48, 151.76, 150.70, 102.10, 89.60, 80.15, 75.94, 75.37, 75.22, 75.16, 74.90, 72.60, 72.47, 72.36, 72.30, 71.94, 70.72, 70.14, 69.80, 69.53, 69.48, 69.07, 69.01, 68.94, 68.66, 68.52, 67.90, 67.74, 67.63, 65.61, 59.99, 48.17, 36.35, 28.02, 27.00, 22.53. HRMS ESI+: Calc. for C$_{22}$H$_{43}$N$_2$O$_{14}$ (M + H)$^+$: 559.2715. Found: 559.2723.

Tert-butyl N-[3-(2-{(E/Z)-(β-D-galactopyranosyl-(1→4)-D-glucopyranosyl)oxime}ethoxy)propyl] carbamate (Compound 12): 45.0 mg (0.192 mmol) of Compound 8 plus 65.8 mg (0.192 mmol) of Compound 4 were utilized, resulting in 68.1 mg (64.6%) of an off white solid (Compound 12). ^{1}H NMR (500 MHz, D$_2$O): δ 7.70 (d, *J* = 5.5 Hz, 0.7H, E isomer), 7.00 (d, *J* = 5.4 Hz, 0.1H, Z isomer), 4.59 (d, *J* = 6.0 Hz, 0.7H), 4.50 (d, *J* = 7.8 Hz, 0.8H), 4.24 (t, *J* = 4.4 Hz, 2H), 3.98-3.54 (m, overlapping, 16H), 3.14 (t, *J* = 6.4 Hz, 2H), 1.76 (p, *J* = 6.5, 13.0 Hz, 2H), 1.43 (s, 9H). ^{13}C NMR (125 MHz, D$_2$O with internal MeOH standard): δ 158.43, 153.38, 152.23, 103.70, 103.26, 103.13, 90.30, 81.08, 80.86, 78.50, 78.35, 76.23, 75.56, 75.43, 75.27, 73.58, 73.32, 72.85, 72.76, 71.52, 71.39, 71.26, 71.18, 70.55, 69.60, 69.48, 68.89, 68.79, 68.71, 68.54, 66.75, 62.31, 62.11, 61.26, 61.09, 61.00, 60.39, 49.12, 37.29, 28.99, 27.95. HRMS ESI+: Calc. for C$_{22}$H$_{43}$N$_2$O$_{14}$ (M + H)$^+$: 559.2715. Found: 559.2727.

Tert-butyl N-[3-(2-{(E/Z)-(α-D-glucopyranosyl-(1→4)-D-glucopyranosyl)oxime}ethoxy)propyl] carbamate (Compound 13): 52.0 mg (0.222 mmol) of Compound 8 plus 80.5 mg (0.223 mmol) of Compound 5 were utilized, resulting in 79.5 mg (65.3%) of a white powdery solid (Compound 13). ^{1}H NMR (500 MHz, D$_2$O): δ 7.51 (d, *J* = 6.1 Hz, 0.7H, E isomer), 6.88 (d, *J* = 5.5 Hz, 0.2H, Z isomer), 5.02 (d, *J* = 4.0 Hz, 1H), 4.44 (t, *J* = 5.5 Hz, 0.7H), 4.16 (t, *J* = 1.7 Hz, 2H), 4.92-3.35 (m, overlapping, 16H), 3.04 (t, *J* = 6.6 Hz, 2H), 1.67 (p, *J* = 6.5, 13.1 Hz, 2H), 1.35 (s, 9H). ^{13}C NMR (125 MHz, D$_2$O with internal MeOH standard): δ 158.38, 153.53, 151.85, 129.60, 128.03, 125.53, 100.73, 100.59, 99.83, 90.27, 81.61, 81.04, 80.34, 77.36, 76.87, 75.94, 73.52, 73.27, 73.12, 73.03, 72.94, 72.86, 72.64, 72.42, 72.29, 71.84, 71.45, 69.59, 69.54, 69.49, 69.43, 68.83, 68.68, 68.66, 68.48, 65.86, 62.48, 62.26, 60.98, 60.64, 60.54, 49.05, 37.27, 28.91, 27.89. HRMS ESI+: Calc. for C$_{22}$H$_{43}$N$_2$O$_{14}$ (M + H)$^+$: 559.2715. Found: 559.2713.

Tert-butyl N-[3-(2-{(E/Z)-(α-D-glucopyranosyl-(1→4)-α-D-glucopyranosyl-(1→4)-D-glucopyranosyl)oxime} ethoxy)propyl] carbamate (Compound 14): 53.4 mg (0.228 mmol) of Compound 8 plus 115.5 mg (0.229 mmol) of Compound 6 were utilized, resulting in 112.2 mg (68.3%) of an off white amorphous solid (**Compound 14**). ¹H NMR (500 MHz, D$_2$O): δ 7.62 (d, J = 6.1 Hz, 0.7 H, E isomer), 6.96 (d, J = 5.5 Hz, 0.1 H, Z isomer), 5.59 (d, J = 3.9 Hz, 1 H), 5.36 (d, J = 4.0 Hz, 0.8 H), 4.54 (t, J = 5.6 Hz, 0.7 H), 4.29 (t, J = 3.7 Hz, 2 H), 4.04-3.61 (m, overlapping, 21H), 3.58 (t, J = 3.5 Hz, 1 H), 3.15 (t, J = 6.3 Hz, 2H), 1.77 (p, J = 6.5, 13.0 Hz, 2H), 1.45 (s, 9H). ¹³C NMR (125 MHz, D$_2$O with internal MeOH standard): δ 158.51, 153.68, 151.96, 100.53, 100.06, 81.84, 81.14, 80.54, 77.46, 77.11, 76.04, 73.69, 73.65, 73.52, 73.20, 72.99, 72.94, 72.51, 72.44, 72.08, 71.77, 71.62, 71.51, 71.30, 69.72, 69.62, 69.52, 68.96, 68.79, 68.60, 65.99, 62.57, 62.36, 61.03, 60.77, 60.65, 49.15, 37.37, 29.04, 27.99. HRMS ESI+: Calc. for C$_{28}$H$_{53}$N$_2$O$_{19}$ (M + H)$^+$: 721.3244. Found: 721.3244.

Tert-butyl *N*-[3-(2-{(E/Z)-(α-D-galactopyranosyl-(1→6)-α-D-glucopyranosyl-(1→4)-D-glucopyranosyl)oxime}ethoxy)propyl] carbamate (**Compound 15**): 46.1 mg (0.197 mmol) of **Compound 8** plus 70.9 mg (0.197 mmol) of **Compound 7** were utilized, resulting in 73.0 mg (67.6%) of an off white amorphous solid (**Compound 15**). ¹H NMR (500 MHz, D$_2$O): δ 7.60 (d, J = 6.5 Hz, 0.7H, E isomer), 6.95 (d, J = 9.4 Hz, 0.1H, Z isomer), 4.99 (d, J = 3.6 Hz, 2H), 4.44 (d, J = 6.8 Hz, 0.7H), 4.26 (d, J = 6.8 Hz, 2H), 4.00-3.51 (m, overlapping, 16H), 1.75 (p, J = 6.6, 13.1 Hz, 2H), 1.44 (s, 9H). ¹³C NMR (125 MHz, D$_2$O with internal MeOH standard): δ 158.44, 152.85, 151.76, 98.58, 81.11, 75.97, 73.27, 72.92, 71.17, 71.12, 71.04, 70.61, 70.49, 70.36, 69.99, 69.77, 69.52, 69.48, 68.94, 68.88, 68.84, 68.72, 68.70, 66.67, 61.37, 61.31, 57.66, 49.12, 37.31, 28.98, 27.96, 22.39, 17.04. HRMS ESI+: Calc. for C$_{22}$H$_{42}$N$_2$NaO$_{14}$ (M + Na)$^+$: 581.2535. Found: 581.2556.

With Aniline

Compounds 9–15 were synthesized using 1 equivalent of the aminooxy linker (**Compound 8**) [16], prepared as a 100 mg/mL solution in methanol. The appropriate volume of this solution was transferred to a flask and evaporated under reduced pressure, then freeze-dried to get an accurate mass of the oil. Next, 1 equivalent of: *N*-acetylglucosamine, cellobiose, gentiobiose, lactose, maltose, maltotriose or melibiose was separately added to each flask containing **Compound 8**. These were each dissolved in 3.0 mL of 0.1 M ammonium acetate (NH$_4$OAc) at a pH of 4.5. Next, 27.3 μL of aniline (0.1 M final concentration) were added to each flask and the pH checked to ensure that it remained at 4.5. The reactions were conducted either stirring at 50 °C in an oil bath (traditional) or at 400 W in a microwave (CEM MARS 5) at 25% power with a 2 min ramp to temperature and a hold time of 30 min at a maximum temperature of 50 °C. After the reaction was complete, the solutions were freeze-dried. The products were then purified by flash chromatography in 6:4:0.5 CHCl$_3$:MeOH:H$_2$O, yielding off white amorphous solids.

N-acetylglucosamine (**Compound 9**): 55.3 mg (0.240 mmol) of **Compound 8** plus 52.2 mg (0.240 mmol) of **Compound 1** were utilized, resulting in 81.4 mg (77.6%) of an off white solid (**Compound 9**).

Cellobiose (**Compound 10-microwave**): 53.1 mg (0.227 mmol) of **Compound 8** plus 77.7 mg (0.227 mmol) of **Compound 2** were utilized, resulting in 96.3 mg (76.1%) of an off white solid (**Compound 10**).

Cellobiose (**Compound 10-oil bath, traditional**): 50.4 mg (0.215 mmol) of **Compound 8** plus 74.2 mg (0.217 mmol) of **Compound 2** were utilized, resulting in 77.8 mg (64.8%) of an off white solid (**Compound 10**).

Gentiobiose (**Compound 11**): 52.0 mg (0.222 mmol) of **Compound 8** plus 80.1 mg (0.222 mmol) of **Compound 3** were utilized, resulting in 90.6 mg (73.1%) of a fluffy white solid (**Compound 11**).

Lactose (**Compound 12**): 56.5 mg (0.241 mmol) of **Compound 8** plus 82.6 mg (0.241 mmol) of **Compound 4** were utilized, resulting in 124.7 mg (92.7%) of an off white solid (**Compound 12**).

Maltose (**Compound 13**): 43.6 mg (0.186 mmol) of **Compound 8** plus 67.0 mg (0.186 mmol) of **Compound 5** were utilized, resulting in 76.4 mg (73.6%) of an off white amorphous solid (**Compound 13**).

Maltotriose (**Compound 14**): 48.1 mg (0.206 mmol) of **Compound 8** plus 103.7 mg (0.206 mmol) of **Compound 6** were utilized, resulting in 137.0 mg (92.3%) of an off white amorphous solid (**Compound 14**).

Melibiose (Compound 15): 47.7 mg (0.204 mmol) of **Compound 8** plus 73.4 mg (0.204 mmol) of **Compound 7** were utilized, resulting in 91.2 mg (80.1%) of an off white amorphous solid (**Compound 15**).

4.2.2. General Procedure for the Large-scale (≥ 0.800 mmol) Synthesis of Sugar-linkers:

Compounds 9–15 were synthesized using 1 equivalent of the aminooxy linker (**Compound 8**), [16] prepared as a 100 mg/mL solution in methanol. The appropriate volume of this solution was transferred to a flask and evaporated under reduced pressure, then freeze-dried to get an accurate mass. Next, 1 equivalent of: N-acetylglucosamine, cellobiose, gentiobiose, lactose, maltose, maltotriose or melibiose was separately added to each flask containing **Compound 8**. These were dissolved in 5.0 mL of 0.1 M ammonium acetate (NH_4OAc) at a pH of 4.5, followed by 45.6 µL of aniline (0.1 M final concentration). The pH was checked after aniline addition to confirm it was still 4.5. The reactions were conducted at 400 W in a microwave (CEM MARS 5) at 25% power with a 2 min ramp to temperature and a hold time of 30 min at a maximum temperature of 50 °C. After the reaction was complete, the solutions were freeze-dried. The products were then purified by flash chromatography in 6:4:0.5 $CHCl_3$:MeOH:H_2O followed by dialysis in 100 molecular weight cutoff (MWCO) tubing against water (for gentiobiose, maltose and maltotriose only), yielding white to off-white solids.

N-acetylglucosamine (Compound 9): 213.5 mg (0.912 mmol) of **Compound 8** plus 201.6 mg (0.912 mmol) of **Compound 1** were utilized, resulting in 315.8 mg (79.2%) of a white amorphous solid (**Compound 9**).

Cellobiose (Compound 10): 186.8 mg (0.798 mmol) of **Compound 8** plus 273.0 mg (0.798 mmol) of **Compound 2** were utilized, resulting in 333.6 mg (74.9%) of a white solid (**Compound 10**).

Gentiobiose (Compound 11): 205.1 mg (0.876 mmol) of **Compound 8** plus 299.8 mg (0.876 mmol) of **Compound 3** were utilized, resulting in 319.4 mg (65.3%) of an off-white solid (**Compound 11**).

Lactose (Compound 12): 196.8 mg (0.841 mmol) of **Compound 8** plus 303.0 mg (0.841 mmol) of **Compound 4** were utilized, resulting in 293.5 mg (62.5%) of an off-white solid (**Compound 12**).

Maltose (Compound 13): 203.2 mg (0.868 mmol) of **Compound 8** plus 312.9 mg (0.868 mmol) of **Compound 5** were utilized, resulting in 299.8 mg (61.9%) of a white powdery solid (**Compound 13**).

Maltotriose (Compound 14): 208.0 mg (0.889 mmol) of **Compound 8** plus 448.4 mg (0.889 mmol) of **Compound 6** were utilized, resulting in 412.4 mg (64.3%) of an off-white solid (**Compound 14**).

Melibiose (Compound 15): 193.8 mg (0.828 mmol) of **Compound 8** plus 298.4 mg (0.828 mmol) of **Compound 7** were utilized, resulting in 275.9 mg (59.7%) of an off-white powdery solid (**Compound 15**).

4.3. Synthesis of Trivalent Glycoclusters

(Cellobiose)$_3$-Glycocluster, Compound 17: **Compound 16** [16] was transferred to a round-bottomed flask as a 10 mg/mL solution in methanol and then evaporated under reduced pressure to give 9.9 mg (0.0183 mmol) of **Compound 16** as an oil. Next, 3 equivalents of **Compound 2** (18.8 mg, 0.0549 mmol) were added to the reaction flask. The solutes were dissolved in 1.5 mL of 0.1 M NH_4OAc buffer, pH 4.5, plus 13.7 µL aniline (0.1 M final concentration) as a catalyst. The pH was confirmed to be 4.5 after aniline addition. The reaction was conducted at 400 W in a microwave (CEM MARS 5) at 25% power for 30 min. After the reaction was complete, the solution was freeze-dried then purified by SEC as described in general methods, yielding **Compound 17** (26 mg, 93.9%) as an off white solid. ^{1}H NMR (500 MHz, D_2O): δ 7.67 (d, J = 5.5 Hz, 0.5 H, E isomer), 7.00 (d, J = 5.5 Hz, 0.1H, Z isomer), 4.61–4.51 (m, 1.4H), 4.31–4.08 (m, 2H), 3.99–3.89 (m, 4H), 3.87-3.66 (m, 7H), 3.65–3.50 (m, 1H), 3.49–3.39 (m, 3H), 2.70 (br s, 2H), 2.53 (app t, 2H). ^{13}C NMR (125 MHz, D_2O with internal MeOH standard): δ 174.39, 152.17, 102.83, 90.39, 78.72, 78.48, 76.30, 76.10, 75.87, 75.81, 75.58, 73.63, 73.59, 73.47, 72.92, 71.42, 69.76, 69.70, 69.63, 69.02, 68.81, 67.09, 66.97, 62.37, 60.89, 60.77, 52.70, 36.27. MALDI-MS: Calc for $C_{57}H_{106}N_7O_{39}$ (M + H)$^+$: 1512.652. Found: 1512.687.

(Sialic Acid)$_3$-Glycocluster, Compound 20: Compound 16 [16] was transferred to a pear shaped flask as a 10 mg/mL solution in methanol, then evaporated, yielding 10.8 mg (0.02 mmol) of the trivalent core. Next, 3 equivalents of sialic acid (Compound 18, Nacalai Tesque, 18.6 mg, 0.06 mmol) were weighed into the flask. The solutes were then dissolved in 1.5 mL of 0.1 M NH$_4$OAc, pH 4.5, plus 13.7 µL aniline (0.1 M final concentration) as a catalyst. The pH was confirmed to be 4.5 after aniline addition. The reaction was conducted at 400 W in a microwave (CEM MARS 5) at 25% power for 30 min. After the reaction was complete, the solution was freeze-dried then purified by SEC as described in general methods, yielding Compound 20 (23 mg, 81.6%) of an off white solid. ^{1}H NMR (500 MHz, D$_2$O): δ 4.41 (m, 1H), 4.28 (app t, 1.5H), 4.15 (app t, 0.5H), 4.01-3.91 (m, 2H), 3.85-3.73 (m, 6H), 3.65-3.56 (m, 3H), 3.47-3.45 (app d, 1H), 3.39-3.36 (m, 2H), 2.82-2.70 (m, 1.5H), 2.58 (app t, 2H), 2.47 (d, J = 6.8 Hz, 0.5H), 2.08 (s, 3H). ^{13}C NMR (125 MHz, D$_2$O with internal MeOH standard): δ 175.10, 175.07, 174.50, 170.44, 170.05, 157.22, 156.15, 73.33, 72.65, 70.72, 69.50, 69.45, 69.02, 68.90, 67.90, 67.86, 66.71, 66.55, 65.97, 63.35, 53.94, 53.56, 53.49, 53.39, 35.90, 35.83, 34.70, 34.64, 30.94, 22.05, 22.01. MALDI-MS: Calc. for C$_{54}$H$_{96}$N$_{10}$O$_{33}$ (M + H)$^+$: 1413.62134. Found: 1413.799.

(Disialic Acid)$_3$-Glycocluster, Compound 21: Compound 16 [16] was transferred to a pear shaped flask as a 10 mg/mL solution in methanol, then evaporated, yielding 5.9 mg (0.011 mmol) of the trivalent core as an oil. Next, the α-2→8 linked dimer of sialic acid (Compound 19, disialic acid, 21.1 mg, 0.033 mmol) [35] was added. The solutes were then dissolved in 1.5 mL of 0.1 M NH$_4$OAc, pH 4.5, plus 13.7 µL of aniline (0.1 M final concentration) as a catalyst. The pH was confirmed to be 4.5 after aniline addition. The reaction was conducted at 400 W in a microwave (CEM MARS 5) at 25% power for 90 min with a temperature maximum set at 50 °C. After the reaction was complete, the solution was freeze-dried then purified by FPLC as described in general methods, yielding Compound 21 (22 mg, 87.6%) as an off white solid. ^{1}H NMR (500 MHz, D$_2$O): δ 4.46-4.40 (m, 1H), 4.29 (app t, 1.5H), 4.15 (app t, 0.5H), 3.99-3.91 (m, 4H), 3.89-3.74 (m, 9.5H), 3.70-3.61 (m, 4H), 3.57-3.53 (m, 3H), 3.26 (br s, 2H), 2.83-2.67 (m, 2.5H), 2.57 (t, J = 5.9 Hz, 2H), 2.47 (m, 0.5H), 2.09 (s, 3H), 2.03 (s, 3H), 1.78 (t, J = 12.2 Hz, 1H). ^{13}C NMR (125 MHz, D$_2$O with internal MeOH standard): δ 175.20, 174.89, 174.36, 173.47, 101.84, 74.30, 74.24, 72.71, 72.51, 71.80, 71.73, 68.96, 68.77, 68.21, 68.05, 67.75, 67.70, 67.49, 67.45, 66.57, 66.28, 65.79, 62.66, 61.14, 53.72, 53.40, 53.36, 53.31, 51.65, 40.05, 35.79, 35.75, 35.68, 34.42, 30.82, 21.97, 21.95. MALDI-MS: Calc. for C$_{87}$H$_{147}$N$_{13}$O$_{57}$ (M + H)$^+$: 2286.90755. Found: 2286.791.

Supplementary Materials: The following are available online at http://www.mdpi.com/1424-8247/12/1/39/s1, Figures S1–S20: ^{1}H (odd) and ^{13}C (even) NMR spectra, Table S1: Summary of the E/Z ratios and % ring open oxime for all products.

Author Contributions: Conceptualization, K.M.; methodology, K.M., D.D., G.F.; validation, K.M., D.D., G.F., K.Z.; formal analysis, K.M., D.D., G.F., K.Z.; investigation, K.M., D.D., G.F., K.Z.; resources, K.M.; data curation, K.M.; writing—original draft preparation, K.M., D.D., G.F.; writing—review and editing, K.M., D.D., G.F., K.Z.; visualization, K.M., D.D., G.F., K.Z.; supervision, K.M.; project administration, K.M.; funding acquisition, K.M.

Funding: This work was financially supported by a Research Development grant from California State University Program for Research and Education in Biotechnology (CSUPERB).

Acknowledgments: The authors would like to thank Lucia Gwarada and Juan Gonzalez for their technical assistance. Mass spectrometry was carried out at Campus Chemical Instrument Center (CCIC) Mass Spectrometry and Proteomics Facility at The Ohio State University (OSU) (NIH grants: P30CA016058, 1S10RR025660-01A1, 1S10OD018507).

Conflicts of Interest: The authors declare no conflict of interest. The funders had no role in the design of the study; in the collection, analyses or interpretation of data; in the writing of the manuscript or in the decision to publish the results.

References

1. Kottari, N.; Chabre, Y.M.; Sharma, R.; Roy, R. Applications of glyconanoparticles as "sweet" glycobiological therapeutics and diagnostics. *Adv. Polym. Sci.* **2013**, *254*, 297–342.

2. Mellet, C.O.; Mendez-Ardoy, A.; Ferenandez, J.M.G. Click multivalent glycomaterials: Glycoclusters, glycodendrimers, glycopolymers, hybrid glycomaterials and glycosurfaces. In *Click Chemistry in Glycoscience: New Developments and Strategies*, 1st ed.; Witczak, Z.J., Bielski, R., Eds.; John Wiley and Sons, Inc.: Hoboken, NJ, USA, 2013; pp. 143–182.
3. Adak, A.K.; Yu, C.-C.; Lin, C.-C. Synthesis and applications of glyconanoparticles, glycodendrimers, and glycoclusters in biological systems. In *Glycochemical Synthesis: Strategies and Applications*; Hung, S.-C., Zulueta, M.M.L., Eds.; John Wiley and Sons, Inc.: Hoboken, NJ, USA, 2016; pp. 425–454.
4. Jebali, A.; Nayeri, E.K.; Roohana, S.; Aghaei, S.; Ghaffari, M.; Daliri, K.; Fuente, G. Nano-carbohydrates: Synthesis and application in genetics, biotechnology, and medicine. *Adv. Colloid Interface* **2017**, *240*, 1–14. [CrossRef] [PubMed]
5. Ramella, D.; Polito, L.; Mazzini, S.; Ronchi, S.; Scaglioni, L.; Marelli, M.; Lay, L. A strategy for multivalent presentation of carba analogues from *N. meningitidis* a capsular polysaccharide. *Eur. J. Org. Chem.* **2014**, *2014*, 5915–5924. [CrossRef]
6. Lee, Y.-C.; Lee, R.T. Carbohydrate-protein interactions: Basis of glycobiology. *Acc. Chem. Res.* **1995**, *28*, 321–327. [CrossRef]
7. Clayton, R.; Hardman, J.; LaBranche, C.C.; McReynolds, K.D. Evaluation of the synthesis of sialic acid-PAMAM glycodendrimers without the use of sugar protecting groups, and the anti-HIV-1 properties of these compounds. *Bioconj. Chem.* **2011**, *22*, 2186–2197. [CrossRef] [PubMed]
8. Cecioni, S.; Praly, J.-P.; Matthews, S.E.; Wimmerova, M.; Imberty, A.; Vidal, S. Rational design and synthesis of optimized glycoclusters for multivalent lectin-carbohydrate interactions: Influence of the linker arm. *Chem. Eur. J.* **2012**, *18*, 6250–6263. [CrossRef]
9. Yang, Z.-L.; Zeng, X.-F.; Liu, H.-P.; Yu, Q.; Meng, X.; Yan, Z.-L.; Fan, Z.-C.; Xiao, S.S.; Yang, Y.; Yu, P. Synthesis of multivalent difluorinated zanamivir analogs as potent antiviral inhibitors. *Tetrahedron Lett.* **2016**, *57*, 2579–2582. [CrossRef]
10. Bagul, R.S.; Hosseini, M.; Shiao, T.C.; Saadeh, N.K.; Roy, R. Heterolayered hybrid dendrimers with optimized sugar head groups for enhancing carbohydrate-protein interactions. *Polym. Chem.* **2017**, *8*, 5354–5366. [CrossRef]
11. Villadson, K.; Martos-Maldonado, M.C.; Jensen, K.J.; Thygesen, M.B. Chemoselective reactions for the synthesis of glycoconjugates from unprotected carbohydrates. *ChemBioChem* **2017**, *18*, 574–612. [CrossRef]
12. Kolmel, D.K.; Kool, E.T. Oximes and hydrazones in bioconjugation: Mechanism and catalysis. *Chem. Rev.* **2017**, *117*, 10358–10376. [CrossRef]
13. Kalia, J.; Raines, R.T. Hydrolytic stability of hydrazones and oximes. *Angew. Chem. Int. Ed. Engl.* **2008**, *47*, 7523–7526. [CrossRef]
14. Gudmundsdottir, A.V.; Paul, C.E.; Nitz, M. Stability studies of hydrazide and hydroxylamine-based glycoconjugates in aqueous solution. *Carbohydr. Res.* **2009**, *344*, 278–284. [CrossRef]
15. Iqbal, A.; Chibli, H.; Hamilton, C.J. Stability of aminooxy glycosides to glycosidase catalyzed hydrolysis. *Carbohydr. Res.* **2013**, *377*, 1–3. [CrossRef]
16. McReynolds, K.D.; Dimas, D.; Le, H. Synthesis of hydrophilic aminooxy linkers and multivalent cores for chemoselective aldehyde/ketone conjugation. *Tetrahedron Lett.* **2014**, *55*, 2270–2273. [CrossRef]
17. Chen, N.; Xie, J. N-O linkage in carbohydrates and glycoconjugates. *Org. Biomol. Chem.* **2016**, *14*, 11028–11047. [CrossRef]
18. Pifferi, C.; Daskhan, G.C.; Fiore, M.; Shiao, T.C.; Roy, R. Aminooxylated carbohydrates: Synthesis and applications. *Chem. Rev.* **2017**, *117*, 9839–9873. [CrossRef]
19. Thygesen, M.B.; Sauer, J.; Jensen, K.J. Chemoselective capture of glycans for analysis on gold nanoparticles: Carbohydrate oxime tautomers provide functional recognition by proteins. *Chem. Eur. J.* **2009**, *15*, 1649–1660. [CrossRef]
20. Rathi, A.K.; Gawande, M.B.; Zboril, R.; Varma, R.S. Microwave-assisted synthesis-catalytic applications in aqueous media. *Coord. Chem. Rev.* **2015**, *291*, 68–94. [CrossRef]
21. Corsaro, A.; Pistaria, V.; Chiacchio, M.A.; Romeo, G. A journey into recent microwave-assisted carbohydrate chemistry. In *Microwaves in Organic Synthesis*, 3rd ed.; de la Hoz, A., Loupy, A., Eds.; Wiley-VCH Verlag GmbH and Co.: Weinheim, Germany, 2012; pp. 961–1011.

22. Joosten, J.A.F.; Tholen, N.T.H.; El Maate, F.A.; Brouwer, A.J.; van Esse, G.W.; Rijkers, D.T.S.; Liskamp, R.M.J.; Pieters, R.J. High-yielding microwave-assisted synthesis of triazole-linked glycodendrimers by copper-catalyzed [3+2] cycloaddition. *Eur. J. Org. Chem.* **2005**, *2005*, 3182–3185. [CrossRef]
23. Brun, M.A.; Disney, M.D.; Seeberger, P.H. Miniaturization of microwave assisted carbohydrate functionalization to create oligosaccharide microarrays. *ChemBioChem* **2006**, *7*, 421–424. [CrossRef]
24. Cecioni, S.; Faure, S.; Darbost, U.; Bonnamour, I.; Parrot-Lopez, H.; Roy, O.; Taillefumier, C.; Wimmerova, M.; Praly, J.-P.; Imberty, A.; et al. Selectivity among two lectins: Probing the effect of topology, multivalency and flexibility of "clicked" multivalent glycoclusters. *Chem. Eur. J.* **2011**, *17*, 2146–2159. [CrossRef]
25. Cagnoni, A.J.; Varela, O.; Gouin, S.G.; Kovensky, J.; Uhrig, M.L. Synthesis of multivalent glycoclusters from 1-thio-β-D-galactose and their inhibitory activity agains the β-galactosidase from *E. coli*. *J. Org. Chem.* **2011**, *76*, 3064–3077. [CrossRef]
26. Cecioni, S.; Matthews, S.E.; Blanchard, H.; Praly, J.-P.; Imberty, A.; Vidal, S. Synthesis of lactosylated glycoclusters and inhibition studies with plant and human lectins. *Carbohydr. Res.* **2012**, *356*, 132–141. [CrossRef]
27. Cagnoni, A.J.; Kovensky, J.; Uhrig, M.L. Design and synthesis of hydrolytically stable multivalent ligands bearing thiodigalactoside analogues for peanut lectin and human galectin-3 binding. *J. Org. Chem.* **2014**, *79*, 6456–6467. [CrossRef]
28. Ding, F.; Ji, L.; William, R.; Chai, H.; Liu, X.-W. Design and synthesis of multivalent neoglycoconjugates by click conjugations. *Beilstein J. Org. Chem.* **2014**, *10*, 1325–1332. [CrossRef]
29. Chuang, Y.-J.; Zhou, X.; Pan, Z.; Turchi, C. A convenient method for synthesis of glyconanoparticles for calorimetric measuring carbohydrate-protein interaction. *Biochem. Biophys. Res. Commun.* **2009**, *389*, 22–27. [CrossRef]
30. Seo, J.; Michaelian, N.; Owens, S.C.; Dashner, S.T.; Wong, A.J.; Barron, A.E.; Carrasco, M.R. Chemoselective and microwave-assisted synthesis of glycopeptoids. *Org. Lett.* **2009**, *11*, 5210–5213. [CrossRef]
31. Thygesen, M.B.; Munch, H.; Sauer, J.; Cló, E.; Jorgensen, M.R.; Hindsgaul, O.; Jensen, K.J. Nucleophilic catalysis of carbohydrate oxime formation by anilines. *J. Org. Chem.* **2010**, *75*, 1752–1755. [CrossRef]
32. Ray, G.J.; Siekman, J.; Scheinecker, R.; Zhang, Z.; Gerasimov, M.V.; Szabo, C.M.; Kosma, P. Reaction of oxidized polysialic acid and a diaminooxy linker: Characterization and process optimization using nuclear magnetic resonance spectroscopy. *Bioconj. Chem.* **2016**, *27*, 2071–2080. [CrossRef]
33. Berthet, N.; Thomas, B.; Bossu, I.; DuFour, E.; Gillon, E.; Garcia, J.; Spinelli, N.; Imberty, A.; Dumy, P.; Renaudet, O. High affinity glycodendrimers for the lectin LecB from *Pseudomonas aeruginosa*. *Bioconj. Chem.* **2013**, *24*, 1598–1611. [CrossRef]
34. Dirksen, A.; Dawson, P.E. Rapid oxime and hydrazone ligations with aromatic aldehydes for biomolecular labeling. *Bioconj. Chem.* **2008**, *19*, 2543–2548. [CrossRef]
35. Patane, J.; Trapani, V.; Villavert, J.; McReynolds, K.D. Preparative production of colominic acid oligomers via a facile microwave hydrolysis. *Carbohydr. Res.* **2009**, *344*, 820–824. [CrossRef]
36. Sato, C.; Kitajima, K. Disialic, oligosialic and polysialic acids: Distribution, functions and related disease. *J. Biochem.* **2013**, *154*, 115–136. [CrossRef]
37. Bhide, G.P.; Colley, K.J. Sialylation of *N*-glycans: Mechanism, cellular compartmentalization and function. *Histochem. Cell Biol.* **2017**, *147*, 149–174. [CrossRef]

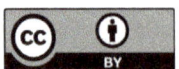 © 2019 by the authors. Licensee MDPI, Basel, Switzerland. This article is an open access article distributed under the terms and conditions of the Creative Commons Attribution (CC BY) license (http://creativecommons.org/licenses/by/4.0/).

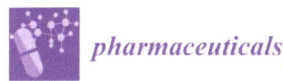

Article

Development and Characterization of Chitosan Microparticles-in-Films for Buccal Delivery of Bioactive Peptides

Patrícia Batista [1], Pedro Castro [1], Ana Raquel Madureira [1], Bruno Sarmento [2,3,4] and Manuela Pintado [1,*]

1. Escola Superior de Biotecnologia, Centro de Biotecnologia e Química Fina, Rua Arquiteto Lobão Vital, 172, 4200-374 Porto, Portugal; pbatista@porto.ucp.pt (P.B.); pedro.joao.castro@gmail.com (P.C.); rmadureira@porto.ucp.pt (A.R.M.)
2. CESPU, Instituto de Investigação e Formação Avançada em Ciências e Tecnologias da Saúde, Rua Central de Gandra 1317, 4585-116 Gandra-PRD, Portugal; bruno.sarmento@ineb.up.pt
3. i3S—Instituto de Investigação e Inovação em Saúde, Universidade do Porto, Rua Alfredo Allen 208, 4200-393 Porto, Portugal
4. INEB—Instituto Nacional de Engenharia Biomédica, Universidade do Porto, Rua Alfredo Allen 208, 4200-393 Porto, Portugal
* Correspondence: mpintado@porto.ucp.pt; Tel.: +351-225580097

Received: 17 January 2019; Accepted: 11 February 2019; Published: 20 February 2019

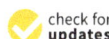

Abstract: Nowadays, bioactive peptides are used for therapeutic applications and the selection of a carrier to deliver them is very important to increase the efficiency, absorption, release, bioavailability and consumer acceptance. The aim of this study was to develop and characterize chitosan-based films loaded with chitosan microparticles containing a bioactive peptide (sequence: KGYGGVSLPEW) with antihypertensive properties. Films were prepared by the solvent casting method, while the microparticles were prepared by ionic gelation. The final optimized chitosan microparticles exhibited a mean diameter of 2.5 µm, a polydispersity index of 0.46, a zeta potential of +61 mV and a peptide association efficiency of 76%. Chitosan films were optimized achieving the final formulation of 0.79% (w/v) of chitosan, 6.74% (w/v) of sorbitol and 0.82% (w/v) of citric acid. These thin (±0.100 mm) and transparent films demonstrated good performance in terms of mechanical and biological properties. The oral films developed were flexible, elastic, easy to handle and exhibited rapid disintegration (30 s) and an erosion behavior of 20% when they came into contact with saliva solution. The cell viability (75–99%) was proved by methylthiazolydiphenyl-tetrazolium bromide (MTT) assay with TR146 cells. The chitosan mucoadhesive films loaded with peptide–chitosan microparticles resulted in an innovative approach to perform administration across the buccal mucosa, because these films present a larger surface area, leading to the rapid disintegration and release of the antihypertensive peptide under controlled conditions in the buccal cavity, thus promoting bioavailability.

Keywords: bioactive peptides; buccal delivery; chitosan; microparticles; oral films

1. Introduction

In the last decade, protein and peptide delivery has become an important area of research for therapeutic applications [1–4]. Bioactive peptides are defined as specific protein fragments that have a positive impact on body functions or conditions, presenting many beneficial health effects (e.g., antimicrobial, antioxidant, antithrombotic and antihypertensive properties) [5,6]. The activity of bioactive peptides is based on their inherent amino acid composition and sequence. The peptide sequence KGYGGVSLPEW was identified in a whey protein hydrolysate and was recognized as a bioactive peptide with antihypertensive properties [7]. This peptide can be administered by parenteral route to avoid biological barriers that can hinder permeability. Nonetheless, the oral delivery of peptides and proteins remains an easier, more attractive and convenient alternative [8,9]. The buccal mucosa represents an important non-invasive alternative route for protein and peptide delivery, due to its ease of administration, evasion from the first pass hepatic metabolism, high relative permeability of many therapeutic agents and rich vascularization [10,11].

However, a number of factors limit the absorption of peptides, due to their relatively large molecular size, physical/chemical barriers, involuntary swallowing of dosage forms and continuous dilution of dissolved molecules by saliva [2]. Indeed, the absolute buccal bioavailability levels of most peptides and proteins are less than 1% [6,12,13]. So, numerous approaches have been attempted with the aim of improving the permeability of peptides. The development of delivery systems such as micro/nanoparticles (MPs/NPs) and their use as carriers coupled to other systems represents a valid approach to overcome these drawbacks. Such systems have attracted growing scientific and commercial attention as bioactive protein/peptide carriers during the last few years [6,14]. The encapsulation of bioactive peptides presents many advantages, such as improved efficiency and absorption, enhanced protection from enzymatic and pH degradation, controlled release of loaded peptide, increased bioavailability and enhanced patient compliance [10,14,15]. The development of nano/micro carriers and the use of the buccal route for mucosal (local) and transmucosal (systemic) delivery of therapeutic macromolecules is an interesting and promising combination. The association of mucoadhesive oral films with MPs/NPs represents a promising strategy to overcome these obstacles [10].

In the development of these delivery systems, polymers are often used as a matrix for peptide loading. Thus, chitosan (CH) was chosen as the polymer to be used, because previous studies have shown it to possess diverse biological activities, including biocompatible, biodegradable, non-toxic, antihypertensive, anti-inflammatory and antimicrobial properties, and it has shown great potential in applications of drug delivery [14,16–19]. Chitosan is a mucoadhesive polymer due to its ability to form ionic, pH-dependent interactions with mucin and its ability to enhance the penetration of large molecules across the mucosal surface. Therefore, it is a good candidate for buccal delivery [20,21]. So, chitosan has attracted attention as a potential food preservative of natural origin and was approved by the United States Food and Drug Administration (USFDA) as a Generally Recognized as Safe (GRAS) food additive and as a delivery system to the human body, more specifically as an oral delivery system [22].

This paper reports the development and characterization of chitosan microparticles loaded with an antihypertensive peptide with subsequent incorporation into chitosan films, aiming to achieve the administration of peptides across the buccal mucosa. This delivery system (film-MPs) is interesting because the mucoadhesive films administered to the mucosal surface could represent a delivery device with multifunctionalities such as mucoadhesion, control release and drug protection by avoiding or reducing passage through the gastrointestinal tract, and a conveyor system of MPs with bioactive peptides. The MPs exert their function by protecting the bioactive peptides from degradation and acting as a controlled release system because chitosan mucoadhesive properties are able to promote enhanced bioactive molecules delivery.

This study intends to have an impact on the nutraceutical and pharmaceutical industry. The development of an oral film incorporating microparticles enhances the advantages of oral films in terms of administration (reported in many studies) with the controlled delivery. The fact that the transported molecule is a peptide resulting from whey protein hydrolysate enhances its nutritional value and associated therapeutic potential. Therefore, this new delivery system may prove to be an enhancer of controlled release delivery of bioactive molecules with potential therapeutic effect, although clinical studies are needed.

2. Materials and Methods

2.1. Materials and Cell Line

KGYGGVSLPEW peptide was purchased from GenScript (Piscataway, USA). Low-molecular-weight chitosan (50,000–190,000 Da, 75–85% of deacetylation), ethyl acetate, pentasodium tripolyphosphate (TPP), α-amylase, pepsin, bovine bile salts, pancreatin, trifluoroacetic acid (TFA) and D-sorbitol (assay purity ≥ 98%) and phosphate-buffered saline tablets (PBS) were purchased from Sigma-Aldrich (Steinheim, Germany). Citric acid monohydrate, potassium phosphate monobasic anhydrous and sodium phosphate dibasic were obtained from Merck (Darmstadt, Germany). Sodium chloride was purchased from Panreac (Barcelona, Spain). Glacial acetic acid, sodium hydroxide and all other chemicals were of analytical grade, purchased from Sinopharm Chemical Reagent Co., Ltd., Shanghai, China. Methanol and acetonitrile (HPLC gradient grade) were purchased from Fisher (Loughborough, UK). Ultrapure water was used to prepare all formulations.

TR146 cell line was purchased from Sigma-Aldrich (Stenheim, Germany). Fetal bovine serum (FBS), HAMS-F12 culture medium and Pen-Strep (10,000 U Penicillin, 10,000 U Streptomycin) were purchased from Lonza® (Verviers, Belgium). TrypLE™ express was purchased from Gibco® (Taastrup, Denmark). Thiazolyl Blue Tetrazolium Bromide (MTT) was purchased from VWR (Solon, USA). Dimethyl sulphoxide (DMSO) 99.7% was purchased from Fisher Bioreagents™ (Pennsylvania, USA). Lastly, 96-well plates were purchased from Thermo Scientific (Hvidovre, Denmark).

2.2. Formulation of Chitosan Microparticles Loaded with the Antihypertensive Peptide

Chitosan microparticles (CH MPs) were prepared by the ionic gelation method of chitosan with TPP [23]. Chitosan solutions were prepared by dissolving 40 mg of chitosan (0.4–0.1 M) in 2 mL of a 1% (*v/v*) glacial acetic acid solution [24]. Afterwards, the peptide was dissolved in the chitosan solution and 1.5 mg of TPP (cross-linker) was added and left under magnetic stirring at 1000 rpm for 90 min at room temperature. Microparticles were formed spontaneously upon the incorporation of TPP into the CH solution.

Preliminary Optimization and Factorial Design

Experimental design for chitosan microparticles was performed using SAS JMP® 9 software [25]. Factorial design allowed all the factors to be varied simultaneously, enabling the evaluation of the effects of each variable at each level and showing the interrelationship among them. The number of experiments required for these studies was dependent on the number of independent variables selected. Each design was performed considering five dependent variables (size, zeta potential, polydispersity index (PDI), association efficiency and loading degree) as well as two independent variables (polymer and TPP concentration). Every response test was performed in triplicate. When responses were determined, independent variables that influenced the behavior of evaluated dependent variables were selected for the elaboration of the predictive statistic model, according to RSquare and RSquare adjusted values. Finally, optimal formulations for each polymer were obtained by maximizing desirability values.

2.3. Characterization of Chitosan Microparticles

After production, MPs were characterized for their mean particle size and PDI by dynamic light scattering. Zeta potential was determined by phase analysis light scattering. All measurements were performed using a Malvern Zetasizer Nano ZS instrument (Malvern Instruments Ltd., Malvern, UK). For these measurements, samples were diluted in saline solution.

2.4. Association Efficiency and Loading Degree

The CH MPs association efficiency was determined upon the separation of MPs from the aqueous preparation medium containing the non-associated protein by centrifugation (15,000× g, 45 min, 15 °C). The amount of free peptide was determined in the supernatant by a HPLC-UV (Waters Alliance® instrument (Milford, MA, USA)) method. In this method, a Kromasil® C18 column (AkzoNobel, Bohus, Sweden) was used and the UV detector wavelength was set to 280 nm. The mobile phases consisted of acetonitrile and 0.1% TFA, and water and 0.1% TFA. The ratio was initially set at the ratio of 80:20 (acetonitrile: 0.1% TFA, v/v), which linearly changed to a 40:60 (v/v) gradient over 10 min. The flow rate was 0.8 mL/min and the injected volume of the sample was 20 µL. The UV detector wavelength was set at 280 nm. The total area under the peak was used to quantify the KGYGGVSLPEW peptide sequence. Each sample was assayed in triplicate ($n = 3$). The CH MPs peptide association efficiency (AE) and loading degree (LD) were calculated as follows (Equations (1) and (2)):

$$AE\ (\%) = \frac{total\ peptide\ amount - free\ peptide\ amount}{total\ peptide\ amount} \times 100, \quad (1)$$

$$LD\ (\%) = \frac{total\ peptide\ amount - free\ peptide\ amount}{peptide\ loaded\ CH\ MPs\ dry\ weight} \times 100, \quad (2)$$

2.5. Preparation of Chitosan Oral Films

Chitosan films were prepared by the solvent casting method with some modifications [26]. The composites (78.6 mg chitosan (0.15–0.04 M), 82.5 mg of citric acid (0.039 M) and 674 mg of sorbitol (0.37 M)) were added to 10 mL of deionized water. The mixture was covered and stirred (magnetic stirring, 300 rpm, at room temperature for 120 min) until chitosan was totally dissolved. Subsequently, the solution (10 mL) was dispensed into Petri dishes (90 × 15 mm) and dried for 48 h in an incubator set to 30 °C. After drying, films were then cut into squares (2 × 2 cm).

Chitosan Films Experimental Design Testing

The experimental design employed SAS JMP® 9 software (JMP Statistical Discovery™, Marlow, UK), using a similar procedure to that described in microparticles section. Each design was performed considering five dependent variables: elongation at break, tensile strength, Young's modulus, water uptake and erosion. For each polymer tested, three independent variables were considered (polymer concentration (chitosan 0.5, 1, 1.5 (%, w/v)), plasticizers (sorbitol) concentration (32.5, 56.3, 75 mg/mL) and citric acid concentration (7.5, 10, 12.4 mg/mL)). Citric acid was used to induce the production of saliva in order to promote the disintegration of oral films the oral cavity [15]. Sorbitol concentration was stipulated according to polymer dry weight.

Each sample was tested in triplicate ($n = 3$). When the results were obtained, a screening design was executed, and independent variables that influenced the behavior of the evaluated dependent variables were selected for the elaboration of the predictive statistic model (with RSquare and RSquare adjusted values). Thus, optimal formulations were obtained by setting desirability values to each response type to obtain maximum desirability.

2.6. Chitosan Films Characterization

2.6.1. Film Appearance

The appearance of films was evaluated by visual observation using parameters such as the transparency and semi-transparency nature of the strip [26].

2.6.2. Film Weight and Thickness

Films strips were weighed on a calibrated analytical scale and the thickness was measured using a calibrated Vernier gauge caliper micrometer [15].

2.6.3. Determination of the Mechanical Properties

The main mechanical properties such as tensile strength (MPa), strain at tensile strength (%), Young's modulus and strain energy (MPa) (Equations (3) and (4), respectively) were evaluated. For that purpose, the developed films were cut in squares (2 × 2 cm) and these properties were measured using a texturometer (TA.XT plus Texture Analyser, Stable Micro Sydtems, Cardiff, UK) [15]. All measurements were performed in three films for each formulation.

$$Young's\ modulus\ (MPa) = \frac{Force\ at\ corresponding\ strain}{Cross-sectional\ area\ of\ the\ film\ \times\ Corresponding\ strain} \times 100, \quad (3)$$

$$Strain\ Energy\ (MPA) = \frac{1}{2} \times \frac{volume}{Young's\ modulus} \times Stress^2, \quad (4)$$

2.6.4. Swelling and Erosion Studies

Plain films were characterized for their swelling properties and erosion features by calculating the percentage of hydration and matrix erosion of the films. Films (2 × 2 cm) were cut and weighed (W_0). Subsequently, films were immersed in the artificial salivary solution (pH 6.8) for a consecutive series of 30 s each, over 1 min. At these time intervals, the films were wiped off using filter paper and weighed (W_1). The swelling of the films was determined using the following relation (Equation (5)):

$$Swelling\ (\%) = \frac{W_1 - W_0}{W_0} \times 100, \quad (5)$$

where W_1 is the weight of swollen film after time t and W_0 is the weight of the film at time zero.

After complete hydration, films were dried at 37 °C for 24 h. The dried films were taken and their weight was registered (W_2). Erosion was calculated using the following relation (Equation (6)):

$$Erosion\ (\%) = \frac{W_1 - W_2}{W_1} \times 100, \quad (6)$$

where W_1 is the weight of swollen film after time t and W_2 is the weight of dry film after erosion.

2.7. Chitosan Films with Chitosan Microparticles

Chitosan MPs (0.4–0.1 M) were incorporated into CH film solutions (15.7 mg of chitosan (0.157–0.041 M), 16.5 mg of citric acid (0.039 M) and 134.8 mg of sorbitol (0.37 M) in 2 mL of deionized water for 30 min in order to uniformly disperse MPs. The CH films with CH MPs were prepared by the solvent casting method.

Chitosan films with CH MPs were poured on Petri dishes and placed to dry for 48 h in an incubator at 37 °C. After drying, films were cut into squares (2 × 2 cm). Each formulated film was prepared in triplicate.

2.8. Cell Culture

Cell culture systems are important for the examination the biological properties, such as the bioavailability or toxicity of bioactive molecules. The TR146 cell culture model was selected as an in vitro model of the human buccal epithelium. The TR146 cell line originated from a human buccal carcinoma. After culturing, the TR146 cell line forms a stratified epithelium similar to the buccal epithelium [27,28].

The TR146 cells were grown in HAMS F-12 Medium with supplements of 10% (v/v) fetal bovine serum (FBS) and 1% (v/v) antibiotic/antimitotic mixture (final concentration of 100 U/mL penicillin and 100 U/mL streptomycin). Culture conditions were maintained at 37 °C, 5% CO_2 and 95% relative humidity. Sub-cultivation was performed at approximately 80% confluence with 0.25% trypsin-EDTA to detach the cells from the flasks. Cells were then seeded at a density of 1×10^6 cells per 75 cm^2 flask. The culture medium was replaced every other day. Cells were maintained in an incubator (BB 16 gas incubator, Heraeus Instruments GmbH) at 37 °C, 5% CO_2 and 95% relative humidity.

Cell Viability Studies

The cell viability of TR146 cell line, after 24 h treatment with CH MPs, CH films, with or without peptide (with concentration 5 µg/mL), was measured using the methylthiazolydiphenyl-tetrazolium bromide conversation (MTT) assay [23].

Cells were seeded in 96-well plates at 2×10^5/well in 300 µL culture medium and incubated for 24 h at 37 °C in a 5% CO_2 environment. The medium was then changed and the cells were treated with test samples (peptide, CH MPs, CH MPs with peptide; CH films; CH films with peptide; CH films with MPs with peptide or free) for 24 h. Each treatment was tested in six individual wells. After 24 h, the supernatant was removed and 200 µL of MTT solution (5 mg/mL in the cellular culture medium) was added to each well of the 96-well plates. They were then incubated for 4 h at 37 °C to allow the formation of formazan crystal. The medium was then removed, and the blue formazan was eluted from cells using 150 µL of DMSO. The negative control used was also DMSO. The plates were shaken on an orbital shaker to solubilize the crystals of formazan. The dark blue crystals were aspirated to another new 96-well microplate and the optical density (OD) was measured directly in the microplate reader at 570 and 690 nm for background reduction. All samples were tested for $n = 5$ experiments with comparable results.

The cell viability of the tested delivery systems was calculated from the average OD values (Equation (7)).

$$Cell\ viability\ (\%) = \frac{OD\ value\ of\ specimen\ suspension}{OD\ value\ of\ negative\ control\ suspension} \times 100, \quad (7)$$

2.9. Statistical Analysis

Statistical analysis was performed using SPSS® for Windows version 22 (IBM SPSS, Chicago, IL). The average percentage of peptide released from CH films was calculated for each time point, along with respective standard deviation values.

The *t*-test was used to verify the existence of statistically significant differences between predictive models and experimental results. Chitosan MPs experimental data were obtained from three samples and the mean values were compared with the values predicted in the model.

Prediction formulas that describe the statistically significant influence of independent variables on dependent variables were obtained using SAS JMP® software. From the analysis of RSquared and adjusted RSquared, the best models were chosen and prediction formulas were obtained. From the predictive models, predictive profilers were obtained and optimal formulations were determined for each formulation of the CH oral film.

3. Results and Discussion

3.1. Preparation and Characterization of Chitosan Microparticles

Chitosan MPs were prepared by the ionic gelation method by auto-aggregation between a positively charged amino group of chitosan and the negatively charged phosphate groups of TPP (cross-linking agent) [19,29,30]. Chitosan MPs cross-linked with TPP have been employed in many studies for drug delivery systems because TPP is used to improve the mechanical properties and stability of CH MPs [8,29]. The parameters, type of cross-linking agent and polymer were optimized in preliminary studies. The CH MPs optimized formulation was set as 40 mg chitosan (polymer) and 1.5 mg TPP (cross-linker). Figure 1 outlines the factorial design and values of the formulation parameters.

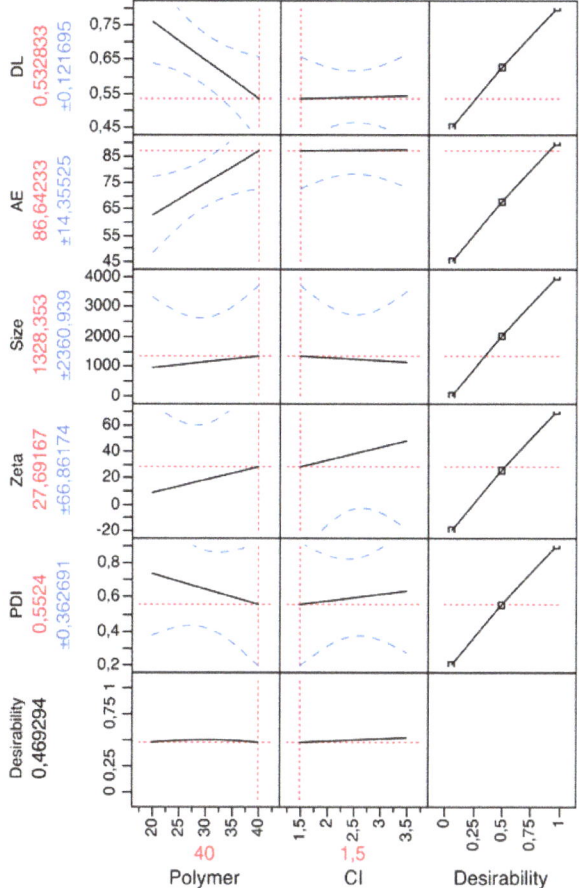

Figure 1. Prediction profiler for chitosan (CH) microparticles (MPs). X-axis: polymer (CH) (mg), counter-ion (TPP) (mg); Y-axis: polydispersity index (PDI), zeta potential (mV), size (nm), association efficiency (AE), drug loading (DL).

In order to achieve theoretical optimization to validate the results, the formulations of CH MPs were further assessed for mean size, polydispersity index, zeta potential and association efficiency. The obtained results were individually compared with the theoretical (predicted) values by Student t-tests. No statistically differences ($P > 0.05$) were found between predicted and experimental values.

After the optimization of the CH MPs, peptide-loaded CH MPs were prepared and parameters such as particle size, zeta potential, PDI, association efficiency and loading capacity were analyzed because those properties are important for therapeutic properties.

The mean size of CH MPs is dependent on both chitosan molecular weight and concentration and on TPP concentrations. Particle size can influence the biopharmaceutical properties of microparticles, their biodistribution and the particle content uptake [8,31]. Particle size was the leading assessed property during formulation optimization studies, oriented towards obtaining microparticles with a mean diameter of about 2.5 µm with a reproducible size distribution. As shown in Table 1, unloaded CH MPs presented a size of 2.544 ± 0.97 µm and peptide-loaded CH MPs had a size 2.582 ± 0.87 µm. The determined size of chitosan microparticles was in agreement with results reported in the literature [32].

Peptide loading by the encapsulation method did not induced an increase in particle size when compared with empty CH MPs (Table 1). So, the incorporation of the peptide into CH MPs did not have a significant effect on particle size.

Table 1. Characteristics of unloaded CH MPs and peptide-loaded CH MPs (CH MPs + peptide) (mean ± sd (n = 3)).

Caption	Size (µm)	Polydispersity Index	Zeta Potential (mV)	Association Efficiency (%)	Loading Capacity (%)
CH MPs	2.544 ± 0.97	0.66 ± 0.18	50.38 ± 7.18	-	-
CH MPs + Peptide	2.582 ± 0.87	0.45 ± 0.18	60.97 ± 9.20	76.16 ± 1.96	0.46 ± 0.01

The particle size and surface charge of MPs/NPs regulate the biodistribution and pharmacokinetic properties of the MPs/NPs in the body. Therefore, the zeta potential is another important parameter and useful indicator of the electronic charge, which can be used to predict and control the stability of colloidal suspensions or emulsions [8,31]. The greater the zeta potential, the more likely the suspension is to be stable because the charged particles repel one another and thus overcome the natural tendency to aggregate. Microparticles with a zeta potential above ± 30 mV have been shown to be stable in suspension, as the surface charge prevents the aggregation of the particles [33]. According to the results obtained (Table 1), all the batches prepared showed a zeta potential more than + 30 mV, confirming that microspheres exhibited good stability and no aggregation in the suspension. The positive value of the zeta potential might be due to the positive charge of chitosan and the high positive zeta potential indicated that the electrostatic repulsion between particles prevented aggregation and increased their stability. The positive value of the zeta potential is important for buccal drug delivery since it can facilitate adhesion to the mucosal epithelial surface, thus prolonging the peptide release and enhancing the peptide bioavailability. The results showed that the addition of peptide has no significant effect on the microparticles zeta potential.

The PDI values of CH MPs and peptide-loaded CH MPs were around 0.5 (the index is a measure of dispersion homogeneity; values closer to zero indicate a homogeneous dispersion), indicating uniformity of particle size and monodispersity distribution, with low variability and no aggregation, as reported in the literature [30,34]. If a scale from 0 to 1 is considered, a PDI lower than 0.1 might be associated with a high homogeneity in the particle population, whereas high PDI values suggest a broad size distribution or even several populations. The calculation of PDI takes into account the mean particle size, the refractive index of the solvent, the measurement angle and the variance of the distribution. So, the PDI affects the mechanical strength of the polymer and its ability to be formulated as a delivery device, and these properties may control the polymer biodegradation rate [35].

Association efficiency and loading capacity are other characteristics that should be calculated for controlled delivery systems [8]. The association of bioactive peptides with the delivery systems components conditions the delivery system success, because it can protect biomolecules against metabolic degradation and improve protein absorption into the intestinal epithelium with better bioavailability. CH MPs were successfully prepared via the ionic gelation method and ensured encapsulation of the peptide. Although the association efficiency of hydrophilic molecules is usually low, in this study we obtained high encapsulation efficiency values, similar to other studies. Table 1 shows the association efficiency and loading capacity of peptide-loaded CH MPs. The CH MPs with peptide showed an encapsulation efficiency of 76%, achieving a particle loading degree of 0.46% (n = 3). The antihypertensive peptide was successfully entrapped into the CH MPs with a high association efficiency, indicating the good potential of CH MPs as a delivery system. The AE was optimized by varying some parameters, including the amount of chitosan and TPP concentrations. The AE and size are important indexes for evaluating the quality of delivery systems. The high AE% can improve the utilization of the peptide and a smaller size could enhance the absorption of buccal cells [36,37]. Indeed, other authors [33,36,38] have already proven that CH MPs are natural materials with excellent physicochemical properties, good carriers for encapsulating proteins, which can achieve high protein loading efficiency and protect them from degradation.

3.2. Chitosan Films Characterization

Various methods have been described in the literature as appropriate to prepare CH films for delivery systems [26]. The solvent casting method was selected because it is the method most commonly reported in the literature due to its inherent simplicity and robustness. It is a feasible and cost-effective technique which ensures greater commercial viability.

Firstly, a CH film experimental design was performed in order to obtain optimized formulations and understand how excipients influence the mechanical characteristics of the films. Figure 2 shows the prediction profilers used in the optimization of the formulations of CH films.

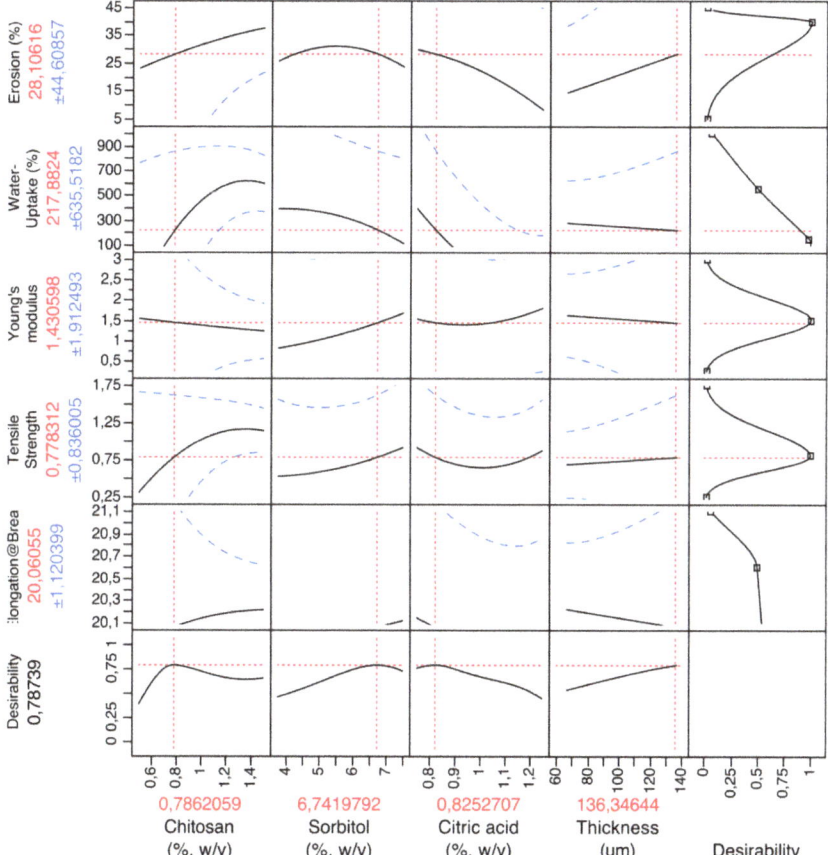

Figure 2. Prediction profiler for CH films. X-axis: excipients (chitosan, sorbitol, citric acid) and thickness; Y-axis: mechanical properties (elongation at break (%), tensile strength (MPa), Young's modulus (MPa)), water uptake (%) and erosion (%).

By setting the desirability of dependent variables to maximum, it was possible to obtain the best possible formulations. So, the optimized formulation of the CH films was set as 0.79% (w/v) of chitosan (polymer), 6.74% (w/v) of sorbitol (plasticizer), 0.82% (w/v) of citric acid (salivary stimulator) and an ideal thickness of 136 µm.

Chitosan is commonly used for producing MPs/NPs thanks to their excellent properties (biocompatible, biodegradable, non-toxic, antihypertensive, anti-inflammatory, antimicrobial, mucoadhesive). However, the properties of these carriers can be further improved by the addition of plasticizers; for example, in this case sorbitol was used. The plasticizer molecules interposing between the polymer chains and interacting with their functional groups increased polymer chain mobility and flexibility and improved mechanical properties. Specifically, they reduced brittleness, improved flow, imparted flexibility and increased the toughness of films [17].

For the preparation of the films, citric acid was also added as a saliva stimulating agent [26]. The purpose of using citric acid is to increase the rate of production of saliva, which would aid in the faster disintegration and consequently the rapid dissolution of the film.

After optimized CH films composition, the films were produced at the same time as CH MPs. That way, the constituents of the films were added to the microparticle solution. Finally, the final solution was dried at room temperature and the optical and morphological properties were evaluated. These films were transparent, flexible and homogeneous, and their surfaces appeared to be smooth without pores and cracks [39,40]. The films were thin, with a thickness ranging between 0.085 and 0.117 mm, evaluated using a digital Vernier caliper [40]. The thickness, flexibility, elasticity and easy handling are important properties for oral films application and consumer acceptance [17]. So, we needed to evaluate mechanical properties: the elastic modulus, to evaluate the film's rigidity; the tensile strength, to determine the brittleness of the film; the elongation at break, to know the flexibility and elasticity. These properties needed to be investigated as they condition the film's integrity and its performance [38]. The Young's modulus, tensile strength and elongation at break were measured and are shown in Table 2.

Table 2. Mechanical properties of CH films incorporated with peptide-loaded CH MPs.

Caption	Young's Modulus (MPa)	Tensile Strength (MPa)	Elongation at Break (%)
CH MPs	2.12 ± 0.93	0.71 ± 0.09	20.06 ± 0.68
CH MPs + Peptide	2.29 ± 0.81	0.77 ± 0.09	20.27 ± 0.72

The tensile strength is an important mechanical property to avoid damage (release of the carrier molecule) during post-production storage and transporting. Basically, this test is performed to measure of the maximum strength of a film to withstand applied tensile stress, and the percent elongation represents the ability of a film to stretch [41]. In optimized CH films, the tensile strength obtained was 0.767 ± 0.091 (MPa). This result is very low when compared with the tensile strength of the pure CH film in other studies, such as 8 MPa [41], 10.97 MPa [40] and 98 MPa [39]. The different results may be due to differences in chitosan type, plasticizer presence, film formation method or analytical methods used [39,40].

Another mechanical property is the Young's modulus, which is an indicator of the stiffness (rigidity) of the film. It is reported to offer a sharp burst release of carrier molecules. The elongation at break is an indicator of its extensibility. The Young's modulus for CH films incorporated with peptide-loaded CH MPs are higher than CH films (Table 2), because the Young's modulus increased with the increase of filler content [42], but no statistically significant differences ($P > 0.05$) were found. The values obtained were low when compared with those of other oral films [43], but the composition and the evaluation methods were not the same. The low Young's modulus obtained in our films indicates softer networks, lower water sorption and higher solubility.

The tensile strength and elongation at break values obtained for the peptide-loaded CH MPs indicate that the incorporation of the peptide into the films did not significantly alter the tensile strength compared with that of uncoated films, corroborating the findings of Aguilar and collaborators [44].

Films were also analyzed regarding disintegration capacity. Effectively, orodispersible films have a high delivery potential because when placed on the tongue, they are immediately hydrated by saliva, followed by disintegration and/or dissolution and the release of the bioactive peptide [45]. This CH film with peptide-loaded CH MPs, when contacted with saliva solution, showed a quickly swelling (217.05 ± 122.36%) and erosion (17.25 ± 12.21%) due to the disentanglement of the loosely bound chitosan molecules, which allowed a facile diffusion of the peptide-loaded CH MPs from the matrix (see Table 3) [46]. The swelling of the films first increased dramatically due to the porous structure and the hydrophilicity of the CH film, indicating a strong hydration of chitosan, which facilitates the rapid mucoadhesion to the absorptive epithelia [46]. Mucoadhesion occurs when the CH film comes in contact with buccal epithelial cells; a double layer of electrical charge forms at the interface to promote the adhesion [46]. The data obtained in this study confirm other reports in the literature; that is, the optimized CH film provides rapid disintegration (30 s) and the release of actives when the strip comes into contact with saliva in the mouth. These results agree with the range of values indicated by the Guidance for Industry [47,48].

Table 3. Swelling and erosion behavior of CH films incorporated with peptide-loaded CH MPs.

Erosion (%)	Swelling (%)	Disintegration Time (s)
20.03 ± 1.3	257 ± 56	30

3.3. In Vitro Cell Viability

In addition to the preparation and characterization, the in vitro evaluations of CH films with peptide-loaded CH MPs are important for understanding the behavior of these delivery systems in biological systems, as well as for elucidating the nature of interaction between the delivery system and tissues, i.e., the biocompatibility. Among the biocompatibility tests, cytotoxicity is preferred as it is simple, fast and has a high sensitivity. The cytotoxicity test is one of the most important methods for biological evaluation. In order to evaluate the cytotoxicity of developed formulations, the MTT assay was performed. The effect of CH films with peptide-loaded CH MPs on TR146 cells was tested in vitro.

Cytotoxicity ratios and viability were classified according to the following criteria for cytotoxicity: (a) if viability > 100%, the corresponding cytotoxicity type was class 0, indicating no toxicity; (b) if viability = 0%, the corresponding cytotoxicity type was class 5, indicating the highest toxicity; (c) 75–99%, 50–74%, 24–49% and 1–25% viability were categorized as classes 1, 2, 3 and 4, respectively [49].

Figure 3 outlines the results obtained from the MTT assay of TR146 cells after being exposed to developed formulations for a period of 24 h. The results indicate that all experimental conditions (CH MPs; peptide-loaded CH MPs; CH films; peptide CH films; CH films with CH MPs; CH films with peptide-loaded CH MPs) assured high cell viability. Hence, the cytotoxicity could be categorized as class 1 (Figure 3), which demonstrates that the CH films with peptide-loaded CH MPs have excellent cell biocompatibility. The results were obtained in conformity with other studies in which chitosan did not interfere with cell viability [20].

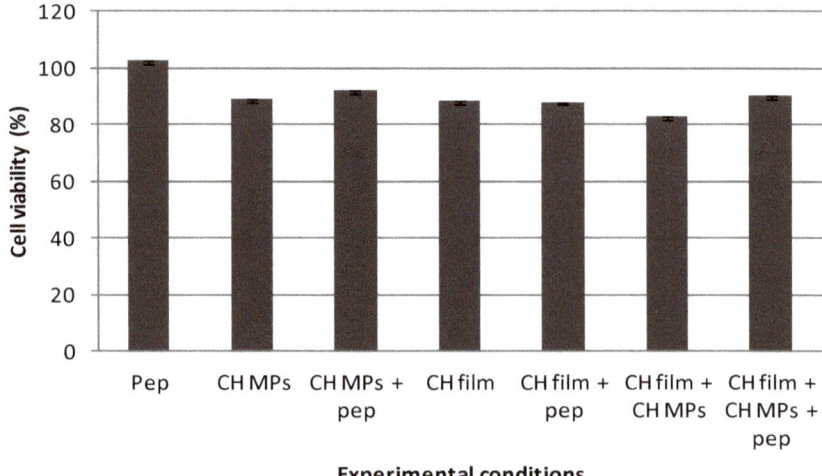

Figure 3. Cell viability under effect of peptide (5 μg/mL); CH MPs, CH film and CH MPs incorporated into CH film with and without peptide (5 μg/mL), measured by MTT assay and expressed as the mean ± SD ($n = 5$).

4. Conclusions

The present study presented an innovative approach focused on combining CH MPs with CH films as delivery systems for the potential administration of peptide/proteins across the buccal mucosa. CH MPs loaded with antihypertensive peptide were successfully prepared using the ionic gelation method and showed desirable pharmaceutical properties including small size and high AE%. Encapsulation of the peptide into CH MPs enhanced the peptide stability and the controlled release.

Chitosan MPs with peptide were incorporated into CH films by solvent casting. The method used for film production is practical, simple, safe and reproducible. These mucoadhesive films have the ability to enhance the penetration of large molecules across the oral mucosal surface and have a protective effect of the MPs, which can elevate the peptide bioavailability.

Therefore, the developed system has ample potential for the delivery of drugs or/and bioactive molecules (bioactive peptides) by the oral route. It constitutes a good solution for the oral delivery of antihypertensive small peptides, and might be a potential strategy for hypertension control in the future.

Author Contributions: All authors contributed for this paper. P.B. and P.C. contributed equally to the paper in investigation and writing. A.R.M.; B.S. and M.P. writing and review. M.P. was the supervisor.

Funding: This research was funded by national funds from FCT through project PTDC/BBB-NAN/3249/2014.

Acknowledgments: The authors acknowledge the support granted by national funds from FCT through project PTDC/BBB-NAN/3249/2014.

Conflicts of Interest: The authors declare no conflict of interest.

References

1. Batista, P.; Castro, P.M.; Madureira, A.R.; Sarmento, B.; Pintado, M. Recent insights in the use of nanocarriers for the oral delivery of bioactive proteins and peptides. *Peptides* **2018**, *101*, 112–123. [CrossRef] [PubMed]
2. Giovino, C.; Ayensu, I.; Tetteh, J.; Boateng, J.S. An integrated buccal delivery system combining chitosan films impregnated with peptide loaded PEG-b-PLA nanoparticles. *Colloids Surf. B Biointerfaces* **2013**, *112*, 9–15. [CrossRef] [PubMed]

3. Patel, A.; Cholkar, K.; Mitra, A.K. Recent developments in protein and peptide parenteral delivery approaches. *Ther. Deliv.* **2014**, *5*, 337–365. [CrossRef] [PubMed]
4. Yu, M.; Wu, J.; Shi, J.; Farokhzad, O.C. Nanotechnology for protein delivery: Overview and perspectives. *J. Control. Release* **2016**, *240*, 24–37. [CrossRef] [PubMed]
5. Moutinho, C.G.; Matos, C.M.; Teixeira, J.A.; Balcão, V.M. Nanocarrier possibilities for functional targeting of bioactive peptides and proteins: State-of-the-art. *J. Drug Target.* **2012**, *20*, 114–141. [CrossRef] [PubMed]
6. Brandelli, A.; Daroit, D.J.; Corrêa, A.P.F. Whey as a source of peptides with remarkable biological activities. *Food Res. Int.* **2015**, *73*, 149–161. [CrossRef]
7. Tavares, T.; del Mar Contreras, M.; Amorim, M.; Pintado, M.; Recio, I.; Malcata, F.X. Novel whey-derived peptides with inhibitory effect against angiotensin-converting enzyme: In vitro effect and stability to gastrointestinal enzymes. *Peptides* **2011**, *32*, 1013–1019. [CrossRef]
8. Ahmed, T.A.; Aljaeid, B.M. Preparation, characterization, and potential application of chitosan, chitosan derivatives, and chitosan metal nanoparticles in pharmaceutical drug delivery. *Drug Des. Dev. Ther.* **2016**, *10*, 483–507. [CrossRef]
9. Morishita, M.; Peppas, N.A. Is the oral route possible for peptide and protein drug delivery? *Drug Discov. Today* **2006**, *11*, 905–910. [CrossRef]
10. Castro, P.M.; Fonte, P.; Sousa, F.; Madureira, A.R.; Sarmento, B.; Pintado, M.E. Oral films as breakthrough tools for oral delivery of proteins/peptides. *J. Control. Release* **2015**, *211*, 63–73. [CrossRef]
11. Rossi, S.; Sandri, G.; Caramella, C.M. Buccal drug delivery: A challenge already won? *Drug Discov. Today Technol.* **2005**, *2*, 59–65. [CrossRef]
12. Mahato, R.I.; Narang, A.S.; Thoma, L.; Miller, D.D. Emerging trends in oral delivery of peptide and protein drugs. *Crit. Rev.™ Ther. Drug Carr. Syst.* **2003**, *20*. [CrossRef]
13. Shaji, J.; Patole, V. Protein and Peptide Drug Delivery: Oral Approaches. *Indian J. Pharm. Sci.* **2008**, *70*, 269–277. [CrossRef] [PubMed]
14. Giovino, C.; Ayensu, I.; Tetteh, J.; Boateng, J.S. Development and characterisation of chitosan films impregnated with insulin loaded PEG-b-PLA nanoparticles (NPs): A potential approach for buccal delivery of macromolecules. *Int. J. Pharm.* **2012**, *428*, 143–151. [CrossRef] [PubMed]
15. Castro, P.M.; Fonte, P.; Oliveira, A.; Madureira, A.R.; Sarmento, B.; Pintado, M.E. Optimization of two biopolymer-based oral films for the delivery of bioactive molecules. *Mater. Sci. Eng. C* **2017**, *76*, 171–180. [CrossRef]
16. Andrade, F.; Antunes, F.; Vanessa Nascimento, A.; Baptista da Silva, S.; das Neves, J.; Ferreira, D.; Sarmento, B. Chitosan formulations as carriers for therapeutic proteins. *Curr. Drug Discov. Technol.* **2011**, *8*, 157–172. [CrossRef] [PubMed]
17. Boateng, J.S.; Stevens, H.N.; Eccleston, G.M.; Auffret, A.D.; Humphrey, M.J.; Matthews, K.H. Development and mechanical characterization of solvent-cast polymeric films as potential drug delivery systems to mucosal surfaces. *Drug Dev. Ind. Pharm.* **2009**, *35*, 986–996. [CrossRef]
18. Ngo, D.-H.; Vo, T.-S.; Ngo, D.-N.; Kang, K.-H.; Je, J.-Y.; Pham, H.N.-D.; Byun, H.-G.; Kim, S.-K. Biological effects of chitosan and its derivatives. *Food Hydrocoll.* **2015**, *51*, 200–216. [CrossRef]
19. Wang, J.J.; Zeng, Z.W.; Xiao, R.Z.; Xie, T.; Zhou, G.L.; Zhan, X.R.; Wang, S.L. Recent advances of chitosan nanoparticles as drug carriers. *Int. J. Nanomed.* **2011**, *6*, 765.
20. Caetano, L.; Almeida, A.; Gonçalves, L. Effect of Experimental Parameters on Alginate/Chitosan Microparticles for BCG Encapsulation. *Mar. Drugs* **2016**, *14*, 90. [CrossRef]
21. Verma, S.; Kumar, N.; Sharma, P.K. Buccal film: An advance technology for oral drug delivery. *Adv. Biol. Res.* **2014**, *8*, 260–267.
22. FDA, Food and Drug Administration. GRAS Notice Inventory. Available online: https://www.fda.gov/Food/IngredientsPackagingLabeling/GRAS/ (accessed on 17 January 2019).
23. Calvo, P.; Remunan-Lopez, C.; Vila-Jato, J.L.; Alonso, M. Novel hydrophilic chitosan-polyethylene oxide nanoparticles as protein carriers. *J. Appl. Polym. Sci.* **1997**, *63*, 125–132. [CrossRef]
24. Araújo, F.; Shrestha, N.; Shahbazi, M.-A.; Fonte, P.; Mäkilä, E.M.; Salonen, J.J.; Hirvonen, J.T.; Granja, P.L.; Santos, H.A.; Sarmento, B. The impact of nanoparticles on the mucosal translocation and transport of GLP-1 across the intestinal epithelium. *Biomaterials* **2014**, *35*, 9199–9207. [CrossRef] [PubMed]

25. Castro, P.M.; Baptista, P.; Madureira, A.R.; Sarmento, B.; Pintado, M.E. Combination of PLGA nanoparticles with mucoadhesive guar-gum films for buccal delivery of antihypertensive peptide. *Int. J. Pharm.* **2018**, *547*, 593–601. [CrossRef] [PubMed]
26. Cardelle-Cobas, A.; Madureira, A.R.; Costa, E.; Barros, R.; Tavaria, F.K.; Pintado, M.E. Development of Oral Strips Containing Chitosan as Active Ingredient: A Product for Buccal Health. *Int. J. Polym. Mater. Polym. Biomater.* **2015**, *64*, 906–918. [CrossRef]
27. Nielsen, H.M.; Rassing, M.R. TR146 cells grown on filters as a model of human buccal epithelium: IV. Permeability of water, mannitol, testosterone and β-adrenoceptor antagonists. Comparison to human, monkey and porcine buccal mucosa. *Int. J. Pharm.* **2000**, *194*, 155–167. [CrossRef]
28. Portero, A.; Remuñán-López, C.; Nielsen, H.M. The potential of chitosan in enhancing peptide and protein absorption across the TR146 cell culture model—An in vitro model of the buccal epithelium. *Pharm. Res.* **2002**, *19*, 169–174. [CrossRef] [PubMed]
29. Ahsan, S.M.; Thomas, M.; Reddy, K.K.; Sooraparaju, S.G.; Asthana, A.; Bhatnagar, I. Chitosan as biomaterial in drug delivery and tissue engineering. *Int. J. Biol. Macromol.* **2017**, *110*, 97–109. [CrossRef]
30. Jain, A.; Thakur, K.; Sharma, G.; Kush, P.; Jain, U.K. Fabrication, characterization and cytotoxicity studies of ionically cross-linked docetaxel loaded chitosan nanoparticles. *Carbohydr. Polym.* **2016**, *137*, 65–74. [CrossRef]
31. Shah, U.; Joshi, G.; Sawant, K. Improvement in antihypertensive and antianginal effects of felodipine by enhanced absorption from PLGA nanoparticles optimized by factorial design. *Mater. Sci. Eng. C* **2014**, *35*, 153–163. [CrossRef]
32. Oliveira, P.M.; Matos, B.N.; Pereira, P.A.; Gratieri, T.; Faccioli, L.H.; Cunha-Filho, M.S.; Gelfuso, G.M. Microparticles prepared with 50–190 kDa chitosan as promising non-toxic carriers for pulmonary delivery of isoniazid. *Carbohydr. Polym.* **2017**, *174*, 421–431. [CrossRef] [PubMed]
33. Walke, S.; Srivastava, G.; Nikalje, M.; Doshi, J.; Kumar, R.; Ravetkar, S.; Doshi, P. Fabrication of chitosan microspheres using vanillin/TPP dual crosslinkers for protein antigens encapsulation. *Carbohydr. Polym.* **2015**, *128*, 188–198. [CrossRef] [PubMed]
34. Sipoli, C.C.; Santana, N.; Shimojo, A.A.M.; Azzoni, A.; de la Torre, L.G. Scalable production of highly concentrated chitosan/TPP nanoparticles in different pHs and evaluation of the in vitro transfection efficiency. *Biochem. Eng. J.* **2015**, *94*, 65–73. [CrossRef]
35. Jain, R.A. The manufacturing techniques of various drug loaded biodegradable poly (lactide-co-glycolide)(PLGA) devices. *Biomaterials* **2000**, *21*, 2475–2490. [CrossRef]
36. Tao, C.; Huang, J.; Lu, Y.; Zou, H.; He, X.; Chen, Y.; Zhong, Y. Development and characterization of GRGDSPC-modified poly (lactide-co-glycolide acid) porous microspheres incorporated with protein-loaded chitosan microspheres for bone tissue engineering. *Colloids Surf. B Biointerfaces* **2014**, *122*, 439–446. [CrossRef] [PubMed]
37. Yu, T.; Zhao, S.; Li, Z.; Wang, Y.; Xu, B.; Fang, D.; Wang, F.; Zhang, Z.; He, L.; Song, X. Enhanced and Extended Anti-Hypertensive Effect of VP5 Nanoparticles. *Int. J. Mol. Sci.* **2016**, *17*, 1977. [CrossRef] [PubMed]
38. Dammak, I.; Bittante, A.M.Q.B.; Lourenço, R.V.; do Amaral Sobral, P.J. Properties of gelatin-based films incorporated with chitosan-coated microparticles charged with rutin. *Int. J. Biol. Macromol.* **2017**, *101*, 643–652. [CrossRef] [PubMed]
39. Chen, H.; Hu, X.; Chen, E.; Wu, S.; McClements, D.J.; Liu, S.; Li, B.; Li, Y. Preparation, characterization, and properties of chitosan films with cinnamaldehyde nanoemulsions. *Food Hydrocoll.* **2016**, *61*, 662–671. [CrossRef]
40. Ojagh, S.M.; Rezaei, M.; Razavi, S.H.; Hosseini, S.M.H. Development and evaluation of a novel biodegradable film made from chitosan and cinnamon essential oil with low affinity toward water. *Food Chem.* **2010**, *122*, 161–166. [CrossRef]
41. Park, S.-I.; Zhao, Y. Incorporation of a high concentration of mineral or vitamin into chitosan-based films. *J. Agric. Food Chem.* **2004**, *52*, 1933–1939. [CrossRef] [PubMed]
42. Frindy, S.; Primo, A.; el kacem Qaiss, A.; Bouhfid, R.; Lahcini, M.; Garcia, H.; Bousmina, M.; El Kadib, A. Insightful understanding of the role of clay topology on the stability of biomimetic hybrid chitosan-clay thin films and CO_2-dried porous aerogel microspheres. *Carbohydr. Polym.* **2016**, *146*, 353–361. [CrossRef] [PubMed]

43. Chonkar, A.D.; Rao, J.V.; Managuli, R.S.; Mutalik, S.; Dengale, S.; Jain, P.; Udupa, N. Development of fast dissolving oral films containing lercanidipine HCl nanoparticles in semicrystalline polymeric matrix for enhanced dissolution and ex vivo permeation. *Eur. J. Pharm. Biopharm.* **2016**, *103*, 179–191. [CrossRef] [PubMed]
44. Aguilar, K.C.; Tello, F.; Bierhalz, A.C.; Romo, M.G.G.; Flores, H.E.M.; Grosso, C.R. Protein adsorption onto alginate-pectin microparticles and films produced by ionic gelation. *J. Food Eng.* **2015**, *154*, 17–24. [CrossRef]
45. Irfan, M.; Rabel, S.; Bukhtar, Q.; Qadir, M.I.; Jabeen, F.; Khan, A. Orally disintegrating films: A modern expansion in drug delivery system. *Saudi Pharm. J.* **2016**, *24*, 537–546. [CrossRef] [PubMed]
46. Tang, C.; Guan, Y.-X.; Yao, S.-J.; Zhu, Z.-Q. Preparation of ibuprofen-loaded chitosan films for oral mucosal drug delivery using supercritical solution impregnation. *Int. J. Pharm.* **2014**, *473*, 434–441. [CrossRef] [PubMed]
47. US Food and Drug Administration. *American Guidance for Industry: Orally Disintegrating Tablets*; US Food and Drug Administration: Washington, DC, USA, 2008.
48. Dahiya, M.; Saha, S.; Shahiwala, A.F. A review on mouth dissolving films. *Curr. Drug Deliv.* **2009**, *6*, 469–476. [CrossRef] [PubMed]
49. Shi, R.; Zhu, A.; Chen, D.; Jiang, X.; Xu, X.; Zhang, L.; Tian, W. In vitro degradation of starch/PVA films and biocompatibility evaluation. *J. Appl. Polym. Sci.* **2010**, *115*, 346–357. [CrossRef]

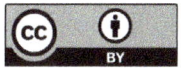 © 2019 by the authors. Licensee MDPI, Basel, Switzerland. This article is an open access article distributed under the terms and conditions of the Creative Commons Attribution (CC BY) license (http://creativecommons.org/licenses/by/4.0/).

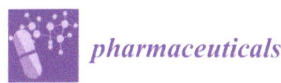

Article

Conformation and Cross-Protection in Group B Streptococcus Serotype III and *Streptococcus pneumoniae* Serotype 14: A Molecular Modeling Study

Michelle M. Kuttel [1],* and Neil Ravenscroft [2]

1 Department of Computer Science, University of Cape Town, Cape Town 7701, South Africa
2 Department of Chemistry, University of Cape Town, Cape Town 7701, South Africa; neil.ravenscroft@uct.ac.za
* Correspondence: mkuttel@cs.uct.ac.za; Tel.: +27-21-6505107

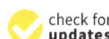

Received: 19 January 2019; Accepted: 9 February 2019; Published: 13 February 2019

Abstract: Although the branched capsular polysaccharides of *Streptococcus agalactiae* serotype III (GBSIII PS) and *Streptococcus pneumoniae* serotype 14 (Pn14 PS) differ only in the addition of a terminal sialic acid on the GBSIII PS side chains, these very similar polysaccharides are immunogenically distinct. Our simulations of GBSIII PS, Pn14 PS and the unbranched backbone polysaccharide provide a conformational rationale for the different antigenic epitopes identified for these PS. We find that side chains stabilize the proximal βDGlc(1→6)βDGlcNAc backbone linkage, restricting rotation and creating a well-defined conformational epitope at the branch point. This agrees with the glycotope structure recognized by an anti-GBSIII PS functional monoclonal antibody. We find the same dominant solution conformation for GBSIII and Pn14 PS: aside from the branch point, the backbone is very flexible with a "zig-zag" conformational habit, rather than the helix previously proposed for GBSIII PS. This suggests a common strategy for bacterial evasion of the host immune system: a flexible backbone that is less perceptible to the immune system, combined with conformationally-defined branch points presenting human-mimic epitopes. This work demonstrates how small structural features such as side chains can alter the conformation of a polysaccharide by restricting rotation around backbone linkages.

Keywords: capsular polysaccharide; carbohydrate antigen; molecular modeling; Group B Streptococcus; *Streptococcus pneumoniae*; conjugate vaccines

1. Introduction

The bacterium *Streptococcus agalactiae*, usually termed Group B Streptococcus, is a primary cause of neonatal sepsis and meningitis, particularly in infants born to carriers of the pathogen. The *Streptococcus pneumoniae* bacterium is another common cause of serious infections in young infants, including meningitis and pneumonia. Ten serotypes of Group B Streptococcus have been characterized, of which serotype III (GBSIII) is currently the most prevalent [1]. Over 90 serotypes of *Streptococcus pneumoniae* have been identified, with serotype 14 (Pn14) being the most common cause of invasive pneumococcal disease in children prior to the introduction of conjugate vaccines [2].

Both of these gram-positive bacteria are encapsulated by polysaccharides that vary in structure according to bacterial serotype and are essential for bacterial virulence: vaccination with carbohydrate-protein conjugates can provide effective serotype-specific protection. The Pn14 capsular polysaccharide (PS) is a component of all licensed conjugate vaccines since the introduction of the

7-valent Prevenar vaccine. GBSIII PS is present in a trivalent conjugate vaccine targeting serotypes Ia, Ib, and III that has completed phase-2 trials [3,4] and a hexavalent vaccine currently in clinical trials.

The similarity of the branched GBSIII PS and Pn14 PS has long been of interest [5]: they are identical except that the GBSIII PS carries a terminal $\alpha(2\rightarrow3)$-linked sialic acid (αDNeu5Ac) on the galactose side chain. The Pn14 PS thus has a four-residue repeat unit (RU) and the GBSIII PS a five-residue RU, as follows.

Pn14 PS : →6)[βDGal$p$(1→4)]βDGlc$p$NAc(1→3)βDGal$p$(1→4)βDGlc$p$(1→
GBSIII PS: →6) [α**DNeu5Ac(2→3)**βDGal$p$(1→4)]βDGlc$p$NAc(1→3)βDGal$p$(1→4)βDGlc$p$(1→

This structural similarity of the GBSIII PS and Pn14 PS raises the possibility that type-specific antibodies induced by one of these organisms might protect against disease caused by the other, a phenomenon referred to as cross-protection. Indeed, vaccination with GBSIII PS has been shown to raise two types of anti-carbohydrate antibody: a major population recognising the native PS but not the desialylated PS (equivalent to Pn14 PS) and a minor population that cross-reacts with Pn14 PS. However, the converse has not been found to be true: antibodies elicited by Pn14 PS are not protective against GBSIII bacteria, although desialylation of the GBSIII PS significantly increases the cross-reactivity with Pn14 antibodies [6,7]. Evidence for serotype cross-protection is necessarily indirect and complicated by the fact that cross-reaction of a PS with antibody raised by a different PS does not reliably predict cross-protection: vaccination raises families of antibodies against various PS epitopes, not all of which are of high avidity and thus effective opsonophagocytic (killing) antibodies. Indeed, effective cross-protection between GBSIII and Pn14 has not been demonstrated: antibodies elicited by Pn14 PS (desialylated GBSIII PS) are not protective against GBSIII bacteria and there is considerable evidence that the presence of the terminal sialic acid residue is essential for the elicitation of protective antibodies against GBSIII PS [6–9].

The native PS produced by GBSIII and Pn14 contains between 50 and 300 RU, which is far longer that the epitope bound by an antibody. There has been some effort expended into identification of the minimal epitope for both GBSIII PS and Pn14 PS, with some conflicting results (Figure 1). Originally, on the basis of NMR measurements and molecular modeling, a long 3–4 RU helical conformational epitope for GBSIII PS was proposed (Figure 1a), with the Pn14 PS being comparatively flexible and disordered. The antigenic differences between GBSIII and Pn14 were thus originally attributed to significantly different PS conformations (and hence conformational epitopes), rather than direct interaction of the antibody with the sialic acid side chain in GBSIII PS [9–12]. The hypothesis was that anti-GBSIII antibodies bind the helical GBSIII PS backbone (stabilized by the sialic acid residues on the exterior surface of the helix) and not the sialylated side chain, with a 3 to 4 RU epitope necessary for raising protective antibodies.

However, this hypothesis is challenged by later work that provides evidence that a helical conformational epitope of GBSIII PS is not required for antigen recognition and that the sialic acid participates directly in antibody recognition of GBSIII. Safari et al. investigated the epitope specificity of GBSIII and showed that human anti-GBSIII PS antibodies recognized the linear backbone epitope common to Pn14 PS and GBSIII PS: -Glc-GlcNAc-Gal- (Figure 1b) [7]. However, although conjugates of linear oligosaccharides of GBSIII PS (such as Gal-Glc-GlcNAc, Glc-GlcNAc-Gal, and GlcNAc-Gal-Glc) did evoke specific oligosaccharide antibodies in mice, these antibodies bound neither native nor desialylated GBSIII PS. Therefore, it was assumed that they are too small or flexible to raise antibody and longer chain lengths exhibiting this epitope are required. Furthermore, the recent elucidation of the crystal structure of a short six-sugar GBSIII epitope in complex with a functional antibody showed a branched hexasaccharide functional epitope with sialic acid participating directly in antigen binding [13]. Identification of a short epitope for GBSIII is valuable information for the development of synthetic vaccines, due to the difficulty and cost associated with synthesis of longer oligosaccharides.

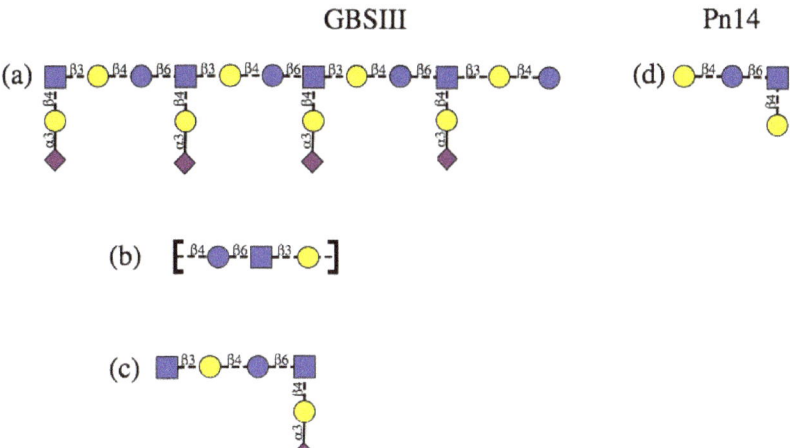

Figure 1. Schematic representation of the protective epitopes previously identified for GBS PS (left column) and Pn14 PS (right column). GBSIII: (**a**) 3–4 RU helical conformational epitope postulated for GBSIII PS [10,11]; (**b**) the linear backbone epitope identified from fragment binding to GBSIII antibodies [14] and (**c**) a 6-residue epitope identified from a DP2-Fab crystal structure [13]. Pn14: (**d**) the tetrasaccharide epitope first identifed by Safari et al. [7,14] and then by Kurbatova et al. [15] from antibody studies. Structures are depicted using the ESN symbol set [16] with yellow circle: Gal, blue circle: Glc, blue square: GlcNAc, purple diamond: Neu5Ac.

Effective short, branched epitopes have also been identified for the Pn14 PS: Safari et al. demonstrated that one RU of the Pn14 PS (Figure 1c) is essential and sufficient for inducing protective Pn14-specific antibodies: the presence of the trisaccharide branch point in an epitope is crucial for anti-Pn14 antibody recognition and the extra galactose contributes to the immunogenicity of the epitope [14]. Kurbatova et al. recently identified a similar branched tetrasaccharide as the most effective epitope for Pn14 PS [15]. In contrast, linear Pn14 PS fragments were found to be completely ineffective: none of a range of short linear epitopes of the PS backbone were recognized by Pn14 antibodies [7]. Only branched fragments containing the Gal-Glc-(Gal-)GlcNAc moiety were found to provide significant protection.

Identification of the capsular polysaccharide epitopes recognized by protective antibodies (or glycotopes) and their conformation is crucial for understanding the affinity and specificity of carbohydrate-antibody interactions and, ultimately the cross-protection mechanisms. Furthermore, identification of the conformational effect of side chains on PS conformation may usefully inform optimal antigen design and the development of effective conjugate vaccines. However, as direct experimental evidence of the key PS epitopes is difficult to obtain, systematic molecular modeling protocols have been developed to provide a theoretical estimate of carbohydrate conformation and dynamics [17]. In the last decade, a considerable improvement in both carbohydrate force fields [18–21] and computer hardware has facilitated far larger, longer and more accurate computer simulations of polysaccharides than was possible when the previous simulations of GBSIII/Pn14 PS were performed. Therefore, we considered it timely to embark on more extensive modeling of these capsular polysaccharides. Our aim is to shed light on the remaining unanswered questions on the conformations of the GBSIII and Pn14 PS, including the following. Does the GBSIII PS have a helical conformation? Are the conformation and dynamics of the GBSIII PS significantly different to Pn14 PS? What are the likely minimal epitopes for these two PS? Why are some fragments more effective antigens than others?

To answer these questions, we compare the solution conformation and dynamics of the GBSIII and Pn14 PS, as well as the corresponding unbranched saccharide, to determine the effects of the side chains on the polysaccharide backbone conformation. We ran long simulations of 1 µs, an order of magnitude more than the previous simulations of 50 ns.

We do not consider O-acetylation of the terminal αDNeu5Ac sialic acid residues [22], as O-acetylation was not found to be necessary for elicitation of functional antibodies against GBSIII [23]. We find that contrary to previous simulations, the polysaccharide backbone dynamics is almost identical in the GBSIII and Pn14 polysaccharides. The backbone is not helical, but rather has a highly flexible zig-zag conformation, whereas the branch points are relatively inflexible with well-defined conformational epitopes. In contrast, the unbranched PS is highly flexible and conformationally varied. Our results are supported by NMR NOESY experiments performed on the GBSIII polysaccharide.

2. Materials and Methods

Our established systematic approach to modeling of polysaccharide antigens involves first determining the preferred conformations of each of the glycosidic linkages in the polysaccharide by calculation of the ϕ, ψ potential of mean force (PMF) for the corresponding disaccharides and then progresses to molecular dynamics simulations of three- and six-RU oligosaccharides in aqueous solution to establish the preferred conformations and dynamics of the carbohydrate chains [24–26].

2.1. Disaccharide PMF Calculations

We identified the preferred conformations of the each of the glycosidic linkages in isolation by calculation of the potential of mean force (PMF) for rotation about the ϕ and ψ dihedral angles. PMFs were calculated using the metadynamics [27] routine incorporated into NAMD [28] with the glycosidic linkage torsion angles used as collective variables. For the three-bond (1→6) linkages, we calculated a two-dimensional PMF as a function of ϕ and ψ only, allowing the ω dihedral to rotate freely. All PMF surfaces were calculated in gas-phase, except for the charged αDNeu5NAc(2→3)βDGal$p$ disaccharide, which required simulation in explicit aqueous solution with a neutralizing counter-ion. Gas phase PMFs for uncharged disaccharides have been demonstrated to be a reasonable approximation to solution PMF in a polysaccharide [25,29,30].

2.2. Molecular Dynamics Simulations

All simulations were performed with the NAMD molecular dynamics program [28] version 2.12 (employing NAMD CUDA extensions for calculation of long-range electrostatics and nonbonded forces on graphics processing units [31]). Carbohydrates were modeled with the CHARMM36 additive force field for carbohydrates [19,32] and water was simulated with the TIP3P model [33].

Initial configurations of three-repeat (3 RU) and six-repeat unit (6 RU) oligosaccharides for GBSIII and Pn14 PS were built using our in-house CarbBuilder software [34,35] which employs the psfgen tool to create "protein structure" (psf) files for modeling with the CHARMM force field and the NAMD molecular dynamics program. These initial oligosaccharide structures were optimized through 20,000 steps of standard NAMD minimization in vacuum and then solvated (using the *solvate* plugin to the Visual Molecular Dynamics (VMD) [36] analysis package) in a periodic cubic unit cell with randomly distributed sodium ions to electrostatically neutralize the system.

All MD simulations were preceded by a 30,000 step minimization phase, with a temperature control and equilibration regime involving 10 K temperature reassignments from 10 K culminating in a maximum temperature of 300 K. Equations of motion were integrated using a Leap-Frog Verlet integrator with a step size of 1 fs and periodic boundary conditions. Simulations were performed under isothermal-isobaric (nPT) conditions at 300 K maintained using a Langevin piston barostat [37] and a Nose-Hoover [38,39] thermostat.

Long-range electrostatic interactions were treated using particle mesh Ewald (PME) summation, with $\kappa = 0.20$ Å^{-1} and 1 Å PME grid spacing. Non-bonded interactions were truncated with a switching function applied between 12.0 and 15.0 Å to groups with integer charge. The 1–4 interactions were not scaled, in accordance with the CHARMM force field recommendations.

Each metadynamics simulation comprised a 1500 ns MD simulation, with a Gaussian hill height of 0.5 and width of 2.5 degrees. Structures were collected at intervals of 250 ps for analysis. For the solution simulation, the αDNeu5NAc(2→3)βDGal$p$ disaccharide was placed in the center of a cubic box with sides of 30 Å. The box was filled with approximately 2500 water molecules and a single Na$^+$ counter ion.

The 3RU strands were placed in the center of a cubic water box with sides of 60 Å, while the 6RU strands employed a box of length 80 Å. The Pn14 strands were solvated with 6810 (3RU) and 16,313 (6 RU) water molecules, while the GBSIII strands used 6790 (3 RU) and 16,279 (6 RU) water molecules. The GBSIII systems were neutralized with 3 (3 RU) and 6 (6 RU) Na$^+$ ions. In each case, the system was equilibrated 0.03 ns with a cycled temperature increase from 0 K to 300 K in 10 K increments with each cycle commencing with a 10,000 step energy minimization followed by a 0.001 ns MD simulation at the specified temperature until 300 K. The 3 RU MD simulations ran for 250 ns and the 6 RU simulations ran for 1 µs.

2.3. Data Analysis

In this work, two-bond (1→X) glycosidic linkages are defined by the torsion angles ϕ = H1′–C1′–OX–CX and ψ = C1′–OX–CX–HX. The (2→3) glycosidic linkages use ϕ = C1′–C2′–O3–C3 and ψ = C2′–O3–C3–H3. These definitions for ϕ and ψ are analogous to ϕ_H and ψ_H in IUPAC convention. For the (1→6) glycosidic linkage, the three dihedral angles are defined as ϕ = H1′–C1′–O6–C6, ψ = C1′–O6–C6–C5 and ω = O6–C6–C5–O5.

Analysis of the simulations used time series frames 25 ps apart, discarding the first 100 ns as equilibration. Molecular conformations extracted from the MD simulations were depicted with VMD, where necessary using the PaperChain visualization algorithm for carbohydrates [40] to highlight the hexose rings. Dihedral angles from the simulations and the DP2-Fab complex crystal structure (PDB ID code 5M63) were extracted using VMD's Tcl scripting interface and statistical values calculated with in-house Python scripts. The DP2 fragment comprises RU2 with a terminal 2,5-anhydro-D-Man. The GBSIII 6RU simulation conformations and the DP2-Fab complex crystal structure were aligned for comparison on the ring atoms of the αDNeu5NAc(2→3)βDGal$p$(1→4)βDGlc$p$NAc branch point.

Conformations from both 3RU trajectories were clustered using VMD's internal *measure cluster* command to calculate clusters according to the quality threshold algorithm [41]. Frames were aligned on the GlcNAc residues in RU1 to RU5 of the 6RU chains. Clustering was then performed with a cut-off of 7 Å on an RMSD fit to the atoms in the backbone residues of RU1 to RU5.

2.4. NMR Analysis

The GBSIII polysaccharide sample (10 mg) was lyophilized and exchanged twice with 99.9% D$_2$O (Sigma Aldrich, Pty. Ltd., Johannesburg, South Africa), then dissolved in 600 µL of D$_2$O and introduced into a 5 mm NMR tube for data acquisition. 1D ^{1}H and ^{13}C and 2D, COSY, TOCSY, NOESY, HSQC, HMBC and hybrid HSQC-TOCSY and HSQC-NOESY spectra were obtained using a Bruker Avance III 600 MHz NMR spectrometer (Bruker BioSpin AG, Fällanden, Switzerland) equipped with a BBO Prodigy cryoprobe and processed using standard Bruker software (Topspin 3.2). The probe temperature was set at 343 K. The 2D TOCSY experiment was performed using a mixing time of 180 ms and the 1D variants using a mixing time of 200 ms. The 2D NOESY experiment was performed using a mixing times of 300 and 500 ms and the 1D variants using mixing times of 300, 400 and 500 ms. The ^{1}H-^{13}C HSQC and HMBC experiments were optimized for J = 145 Hz and 8 Hz, and the HSQC-TOCSY and HSQC-NOESY experiments were recorded using mixing times of 120 and 250 ms, respectively. 2D experiments were recorded using non-uniform sampling: 50% for homonuclear and 25% for heteronuclear experiments. Spectra were referenced relative to the H3ax/C3 signal of terminal sialic acid: ^{1}H at 1.79 ppm and ^{13}C at 40.68 ppm [42].

3. Results

Our 1 µs simulations of 6 RU show that polysaccharides with the →6)βDGlcpNAc(1→3)βD Galp(1→4)βDGlcp(1→ backbone are all extremely flexible, with none of the well-defined conformations we have found in other, linear bacterial polysaccharides [24,25]. However, a closer inspection of the range of motion for GBSIII PS, Pn14 PS and the unbranched backbone PS reveal a common dominant conformational habit, as well as significant differences in flexibility.

3.1. PS Chain Conformations

In Figure 2, we quantify range of motion for these very flexible polysaccharides with the simple end-to-end distance, r, measured between the GlcNAc O5 atoms in repeat units RU1 and RU6 (illustrated on a sample conformation in Figure 2a). Comparison of the time series (Figure 2, center column) and distribution (right column) of r shows that GBSIII PS is the most conformationally defined, and the unbranched polysaccharide backbone the most flexible, of the three molecules. Only 12% of the GBSIII PS conformations have $r < 40$ Å, as compared to 25% for Pn14 and 33% for the unbranched backbone. Overall, the unbranched backbone is less extended (more globular) than the branched polysaccharides and shows more rapid conformational transitions (compare time series plots in Figure 2b–d). The corresponding mean squared end-to-end distances for the simulations reflect this trend: 2505 Å (GBSIII), 2157 Å (Pn14) and 1993 Å (backbone).

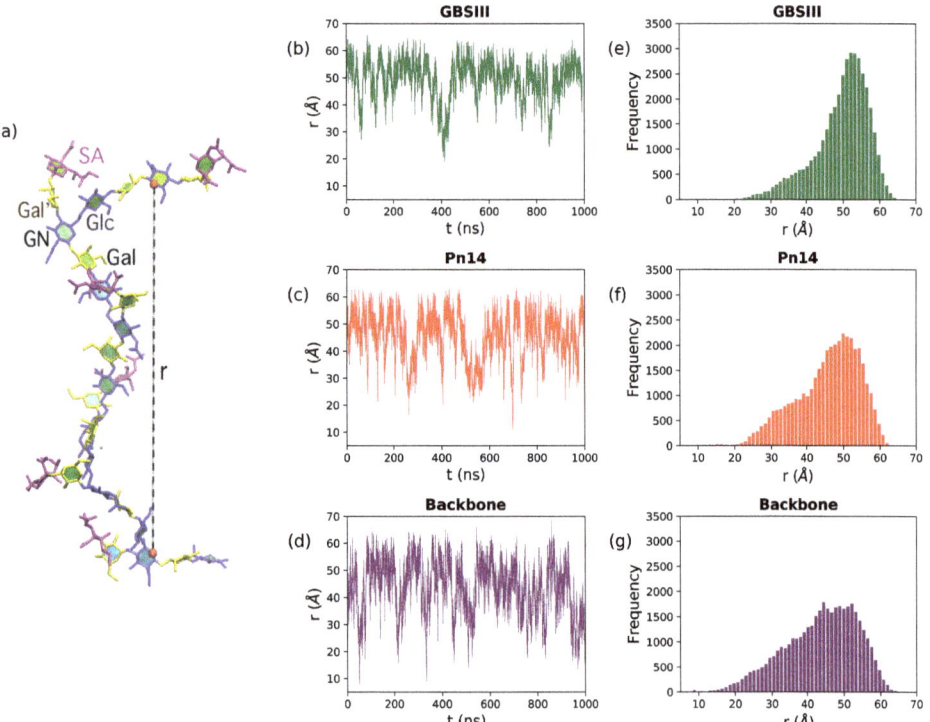

Figure 2. Polysaccharide end-to-end distance distributions for the 6RU PS. (**a**) The molecular end-to-end distance, r, is defined as the distance between O5 atoms in GlcNAc residues in RU1 and RU6, here shown on the GBSIII PS. The center column shows the r time series for (**b**) GBSIII PS, (**c**) Pn14 PS and (**d**) unbranched backbone PS. The corresponding distance distributions are in the rightmost column for (**e**) GBSIII PS, (**f**) Pn14 PS and (**g**) the unbranched backbone PS.

Although flexible, the GBSIII PS and Pn14 PS have a similar dominant overall conformation with $48 < r < 58$ Å. Here the PS backbone has an overall "zig-zag" arrangement, bending at the 1→6 linkage, with the side chains exposed at the branch points, as shown in the GBSIII schematic in Figure 3a and the sample conformation in Figure 3b.

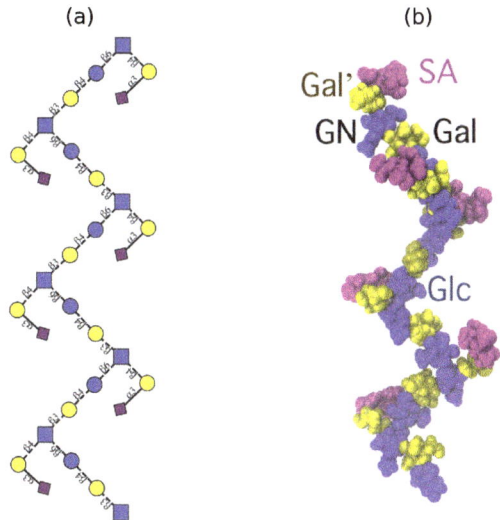

Figure 3. The 'zig-zag' conformational habit of GBSIII and Pn14 PS. (**a**) Schematic representation with the ESN symbol set [16] (yellow circle: Gal, blue circle: Glc, blue square: GlcNAc, purple diamond: Neu5Ac) and (**b**) a representative 6RU GBSIII PS simulation snapshot. Residues are highlighted as follows: Glc and GlcNAc: blue; Gal: yellow; sialic acid: purple.

This conformation is in very good agreement with the new antibody binding model recently proposed for GBSIII PS (see Figure 5 in Carboni et al. [13]). Figure 4 shows the GBSIII PS conformations from our 6RU simulation superimposed on the solved crystal structure for DP2-Fab. The zig-zag conformation of the backbone exposes the sialic acid side chain for binding (Figure 4a) with the flexible backbone held well away from the antibody over the course of the simulation (Figure 4b). Conversely, we find no evidence in our simulations to support the helical model for GBSIII PS previously proposed [10,11]. Further, in the zig-zag conformation, the polysaccharide backbone is relatively inaccessible to antibody binding.

However, although the 6RU backbone shows the same dominant conformation for GBSIII PS, Pn14 PS and the unbranched backbone PS, they have a significant difference in flexibility. Clustering of the simulation conformations shows that, while GBSIII PS is in this general zig-zag conformational family for 85% of the simulation, Pn14 PS is more flexible and is in a zig-zag for 78% of the simulations, moving occasionally into alternative, more bent conformations (with smaller r). The unbranched backbone polysaccharide is the most disorganised, with the zig-zag appearing for 66% of the simulation and showing significant sub-populations of globular conformations (with $r < 25$ Å).

The source of the conformational differences between the polysaccharides is a conformational constraint on the βDGlc(1→6)[βDGal(1→4)]βDGlcNAc linkage in GBSIII PS and, to a lesser extent, in Pn14 PS. The conformation and flexibility of the other backbone linkages (βDGlcpNAc(1→3)βDGalp and βDGalp(1→4)βDGlcp) is very similar in all three polysaccharides—see a detailed analysis in Appendix A, particularly Figure A1. However, for the βDGlcp(1→6)βDGlcpNAc linkage, proximity of the side chains impose a restriction on rotation, as follows.

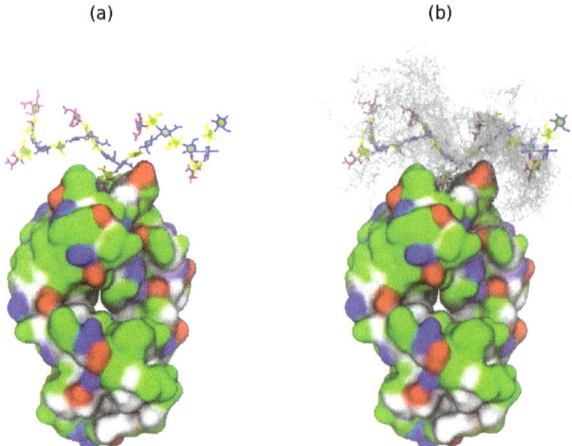

Figure 4. GBSIII 6RU structures superimposed on the bound branch point of the DP2-FAb crystal structure from Carboni et al. [13] (PDB ID code 5M63): (**a**) a single representative structure and (**b**) superimposed conformational snapshots at 12.5 ns intervals (with the first 125 ns discarded as equilibration).

3.2. Conformations of the 1→6 Linkage

Figure 5 provides a comparison of the flexibility of the three-bond glycosidic linkage in a βDGlc$p$(1→6)βDGlc$p$NAc disaccharide and the GBSIII PS, Pn14 PS and unbranched backbone PS. The three dihedral angles describing rotation about the three bonds in the (1→6) glycosidic linkage are here defined as ϕ = H1′–C1′–O6–C6, ψ = C1′–O6–C6–C5 and ω = O6–C6–C5–O5. These dihedrals are labeled on the GBSIII fragment in Figure 5, left. A PMF energy surface for the (1→6) glycosidic linkage has, therefore, three dimensions. However, for ease of visualization and comprehension, we show only 2D projections of the 3D volume: the ϕ, ψ PMF (Figure 5a) and the ϕ, ω PMF surface (Figure 5b) for a βDGlc(1→6)βDGlcNAc disaccharide in the gas phase. These PMF surfaces illustrate the range of motion possible for an unrestrained linkage. The ϕ, ψ PMF in Figure 5a reveals that the central bond in the linkage described by the ψ dihedral is relatively flexible, with multiple minima within the 2 kcal·mol^{-1} contours: a global minimum conformation at ψ = 71°, a secondary *anti* minimum conformation at ψ = −179° and a tertiary minimum in the ψ = −60 region. In contrast, rotation about the ϕ dihedral is much more constrained, with a broad global minimum around 0° < ϕ < 75° and a narrow secondary well at ϕ = 160°. The ϕ, ω PMF surface in Figure 5b confirms these minima for ϕ and shows the expected three minima for the ω dihedral, which are by convention termed *gg* ($\omega \approx -60°$), *gt* ($\omega \approx 60°$) and *tg* $\omega \approx 180°$). Glucopyranosides are expected to be primarily in the *gg* conformation, with the *gg*:*gt*:*tg* population ratios approximately 6:4:0 [43].

As a comparison to the unrestrained disaccharide, the range of motion actually explored during the simulations of the 6RU oligosaccharides is revealed by the corresponding dihedral time series scatter plots superimposed on the disaccharide PMFs. The restriction of the βDGlc(1→6)βDGlcNAc linkage in GBSIII is apparent in the time series scatterplots for the 6RU GBSIII oligosaccharide strand (Figure 5, second column). These confirm a single dominant conformer for GBSIII, with average torsion angle values ϕ, ψ, ω = 51°, −175°, −67° (standard deviations = 10, 11, 8 respectively). These angles are compatible with the GBSIII DP2-Fab complex crystal structure where this linkage has ϕ, ψ, ω = 51°, 140°, −70° (indicated by 'X' on the PMF plots in Figure 5a,b). The central 1→6 linkage in GBSIII PS is in this dominant conformation for 100% of the simulation and the ω dihedrals remain in the low-energy *gg* conformation for the duration.

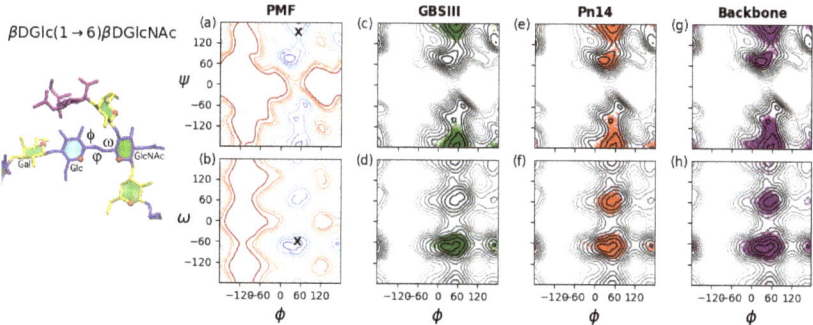

Figure 5. Rotation of the three-bond βDGlc(1→6)βDGlcNAc linkages in GBSIII, Pn14 and the unbranched backbone PS. The ϕ, ψ and ω angles describing the orientation of this linkage are labeled on the GBSIII fragment shown on the left. Contoured 2D (**a**) ϕ, ψ PMF and (**b**) the ϕ, ω PMF surfaces for a βDGlc(1→6)βDGlcNAc disaccharide in the gas phase illustrate the range of motion possible for an unrestrained linkage. Contours are drawn at intervals of 1 kcal·mol^{-1} to a maximum of 12 kcal·mol^{-1} and 'X' markers indicate dihedral angle values from the six-sugar GBSIII epitope identified in the DP2-Fab crystal structure [13]. The range of motion actually explored by the 6RU oligosaccharides is demonstrated with time series scatter plots of the two central βDGlc(1→6)βDGlcNAc linkages in the 6RU strands superimposed on the PMFs as follows: (**c**) GBSIII ϕ, ψ; (**d**) GBSIII ϕ, ω; (**e**) Pn14 ϕ, ψ; (**f**) Pn14 ϕ, ω; (**g**) unbranched backbone ϕ, ψ; and (**f**) unbranched backbone ϕ, ω.

The average torsion angle values for Pn14 PS are ϕ, ψ, ω = 50°, 180°, −62° (standard deviations = 12, 18, 26 respectively). The central βDGlc(1→6)βDGlcNAc linkage is in the dominant conformation (equivalent to the GBSIII PS) for 91% of the simulation. The increase in standard deviation for the ϕ and ω dihedrals relative to GBSIII PS is indicative of increased flexibility and alternative conformations of the ω dihedral, which shows a ratio of approximate 10:1 of *gg* to *gt* conformations, with no *tg* conformations appearing. Therefore, the 1→6 linkage shows a slight increase in flexibility relative to GBSIII PS, which is cumulative with increasing chain length. This reflects the increased constraint on the backbone imposed by the terminal sialic in the GBSIII side chain.

The 1→6 linkage is markedly more flexible in the unbranched backbone saccharide and the zig-zag conformation drops to 86% of the simulation. The average torsion angle values for the unbranched backbone are ϕ, ψ, ω = 50°, −179°, −69° (standard deviations = 15, 22, 30 respectively). In particular, the ω dihedral has an 8% population of *gt* conformations and a small population of *tg* conformations. In addition, both the ϕ and ψ dihedrals show a broader range of rotation.

Interestingly, we saw no effect on conformation and dynamics of increasing chain length. Our simulations of 3RU for GBSIII and Pn14 PS showed the same dihedral populations as the middle linkages in the 6RU simulations (data not shown). Further, we performed a 250 ns simulation of the effective branch epitope previously identified (Figure 1d) [14,15]. This molecule shows the same conformation of the branch point and other dihedrals as Pn14 PS (see Appendix B, Figure A2) and is thus a faithful representation of the branch point in the Pn14 PS.

3.3. Inter-Residue Atomic Contacts in GBSIII

In GBSIII PS, interactions between the side chain and the backbone residues stabilize the conformation of the 1→6 linkage. We compare the simulation data with NMR NOESY experiments on the GBSIII PS, focussing on inter-residue NOEs that are diagnostic for close proximity of the side chain to the backbone.

In GBSIII PS, hydrogen bonding interactions between the side chain sialic acid (SA) and side chain Gal (Gal') and the backbone Glc and Gal stabilize the conformation of the 1→6 linkage, as follows. Transient hydrogen bonds occur between the bound SA O9 and backbone Gal O2 (shown in Figure 6a) as well as SA O9 – Glc O3 and SA O8 – Glc O2 hydrogen bonds (occasionally simultaneous, as in Figure 6b). The crystal structure for the GBSIII PS fragment in DP2-Fab shows a close hydrogen bond between SA O9 and and the Glc O6, with distance of 2.8 Å [13]. We do not find this hydrogen bond in our simulations, although the atoms come within 4 Å of each other. This is due to the fact that the sialic acid is in an alternative (higher energy) conformation in the crystal structure—possibly stabilized by interactions with the antibody. The conformation of this sialyl linkage is known to have no fixed standard conformation and to be heavily dependent on the molecular environment [44]. See Appendix A and Figure A1e for more detailed analysis of the sialic acid conformation. Unfortunately, considerable overlap between the signals of the NAc group of SA and GlcNAc precluded investigation of contact between the sialic acid side chain and the backbone in GBSIII, as previously reported [13].

Additional hydrogen bonds occur between the Gal' O2 and backbone Glc O3 in both the GBSIII PS and Pn14 PS simulations. In this case, NMR signals are better resolved: a series of 1D and 2D NOESY experiments gave key H1 Glc crosspeaks to H4, H5 and both H6s of the neighboring GlcNAc (consistent with the βDGlc(1→6)[βDGal(1→4)]βDGlcNAc linkage) as well as small additional correlations to the main chain repeating unit (Figure 6c(iii)). In particular, peaks for H1 Glc to H1 Gal' as well as H1 Glc to H3 Gal' provide evidence for close proximity of the side chain to the backbone and are consistent with our simulations. This is corroborated by 2D NOESY cross peaks, as well as peaks from the well-resolved H2 of Glc at 3.36 ppm to H1 and H3 of Gal' (Figure 6c(iv)).

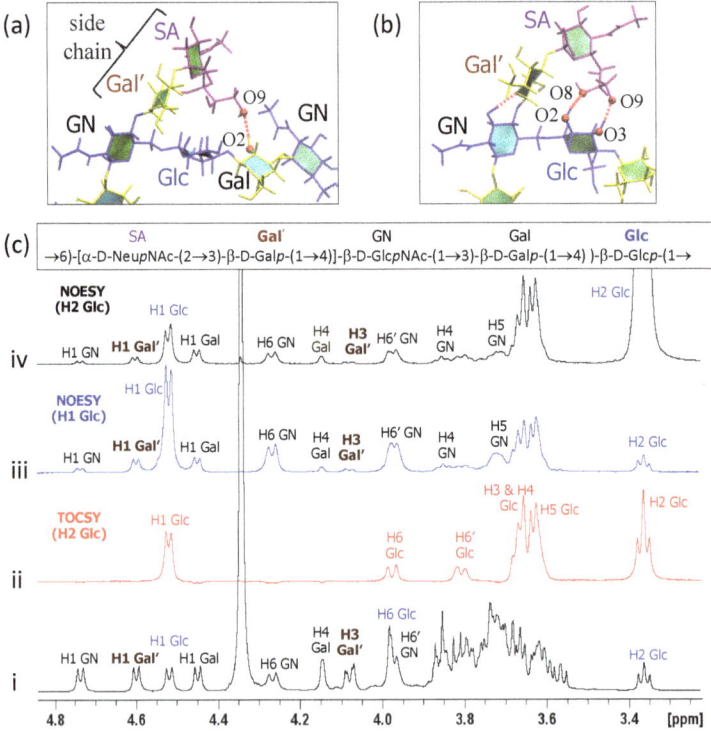

Figure 6. Inter-residue contacts in GBSIII PS. (**a**) Example of SA O9–Gal O2 hydrogen bond between the side chain and the backbone residues. (**b**) Example of simultaneous SA O9–Glc O3 and SA O8–Glc O2 hydrogen bonds. (**c**) Overlay of 1D NMR experiments of GBSIII PS showing (**i**) 1D proton spectrum; (**ii**) 1D TOCSY (200 ms) with irradiation of H2 Glc; (**iii**) 1D NOESY (500 ms) with irradiation of H1 Glc; and (**iv**) 1D NOESY (500 ms) with irradiation of H2 Glc.

4. Discussion

This modeling study shows that the polysaccharide backbone conformation is very similar in the GBSIII and Pn14 polysaccharides, albeit with increased flexibility for Pn14 PS. Both GBSIII and Pn14 PS exhibit a constrained branch epitope and a flexible zig-zag backbone. The zig-zag conformation is in remarkable agreement with the binding model for GBSIII PS proposed by Carboni et al. [13]. The βDGlc(1→6)[βDGal(1→4)]βDGlcNAc branch point is a relatively rigid and exposed component of the flexible backbone, and thus a likely site for antibody binding. This stationary branch point is in agreement with preclinical evidence that has indicated that the Pn14 branching element βDGalp(1→4)]βDGlcpNAc is necessary and sufficient for induction of an effective antibody response [14]. Further, the lack of accessibility of the backbone in GBSIII and Pn14 PS to antibody binding together with increased flexibility and alternative conformations of the unbranched backbone provides a rational for why antibodies to linear oligosaccharide fragments of GBSIII PS (such as Gal-Glc-GlcNAc, Glc-GlcNAc-Gal, and GlcNAc-Gal-Glc) bound neither GBSIII PS nor Pn14 PS [7]. In addition, the lack of extended conformational epitopes supports experimental data that finds short epitopes to be effective for GBSIII and Pn14, epitopes comprising solely their respective branch points and side chain (i.e., βDGlc(1→6)[αDNeu5Ac(2→3)βDGal(1→4)]βDGlcNAc and βDGlc(1→6)[βDGal(1→4)]βDGlcNAc, respectively). This is consistent with the DP2-Fab crystal structure elucidated by Carboni et al.: the binding involves the branch and does not require a conformational epitope [13].

Kurbatova et al. identified a βDGalp(1→4)βDGlcp(1→6)[βDGalp(1→4)]βDGlcpNAc tetrasaccharide as the most effective epitope for Pn14 PS, as compared to hexa- and octasaccharides in a mouse model [15]. Our work provides a possible explanation for this: vaccination with this primary epitope could raise a single class of effective antibody, as opposed to a family of antibodies raised by the more flexible hexa- and octasaccharides, thus making this short chain more protective. In contrast, the hexa- and octasaccharides could potentially present epitopes not present in the polysaccharide, as seen in the unbranched backbone.

The flexible zig-zag conformation and stationary branch point were not identified for the Pn14 PS in the earlier study. In contrast to the small 8% population of the gt conformation in Pn14 that we see in these simulations, in the 5RU simulations with the AMBER force field by González-Outeiriño et al. the Pn14 oligosaccharide showed a nearly 50:50 mixture of the gg to gt rotamers, whereas the GBSIII PS remained almost constantly in the gg conformation. This discrepancy was attributed to an anomaly arising from insufficient equilibration in the 50 ns simulations [10]. Therefore, the extreme flexibility of Pn14 PS and disordered structure as compared to GBSIII PS suggested by this prior work could be a consequence of the increased flexibility of this dihedral in the AMBER force field as compared to the CHARMM force field. In the presence of competing computational models, experimental evidence is key. The DP2-Fab crystal structure provides evidence that a short strand can effectively bind to an antibody and that a helical conformation of the backbone is not necessary for antigen binding. In addition, we observed inter-residue NMR NOEs for the GBSIII PS that are consistent with our simulations.

The branches of the GBSIII and Pn14 PS both present common terminal glycan epitopes: 3-Sialyl-N-acetyllactosamine is present in human biofluids and is a common sequence terminating N- and O-glycans on the surface of all mammalian cells, while the shorter βDGalp(1→4)]βDGlcpNAc constitutes the ubiquitous LacNAc building block in mammalian N-linked protein glycans. In general, mimics of mammalian cell surface residues can subvert the immune system.

This work thus suggests a strategy for bacterial evasion of the host immune system: expression of a very flexible backbone that is shielded from the immune system by both its zig-zag conformation and hyper-mobility, combined with exposed, inflexible branches that present human-mimic epitopes. This strategy should be considered with other polysaccharides with similar backbones and human-like branch epitopes, where it is likely that the branch points will be key to immunogenicity.

In summary, this work demonstrates how small structural features such as side chains can alter the conformation of a polysaccharide by restricting rotation around backbone linkages. It also highlights the explanatory power of simulation for optimal antigen design and the development of effective conjugate vaccines.

Author Contributions: Conceptualization, M.M.K. and N.R.; Funding acquisition, M.M.K. and N.R.; Investigation, M.M.K. and N.R.; Methodology, M.M.K. and N.R.; Project administration, M.M.K.; Resources, N.R.; Software, M.M.K.; Validation, N.R.; Visualization, M.M.K.; Writing—original draft, M.M.K.; Writing—review & editing, M.M.K. and N.R.

Funding: This research was funded by The South African National Research Foundation grant number 103805 and grant number 86038 (NMR equipment).

Acknowledgments: Computations were performed using facilities provided by the University of Cape Town's ICTS High Performance Computing team: http://hpc.uct.ac.za. The authors thank PATH and the Biovac Institute for providing the GBSIII polysaccharide sample.

Conflicts of Interest: The authors declare no conflict of interest. The funders had no role in the design of the study; in the collection, analyses, or interpretation of data; in the writing of the manuscript, or in the decision to publish the results.

Abbreviations

The following abbreviations are used in this manuscript:
NMR   Nuclear Magnetic Resonance
PS   polysaccharide
RU   repeat unit

Appendix A. Analysis of Glycosidic Linkages

The GBSIII glycosidic linkages can be conveniently classified into the three linkages which make up the common polymer backbone and the two glycosidic linkages which comprise the side chains. The contoured disaccharide ϕ, ψ PMF energy surfaces for disaccharides representing all the constituent linkages in GBSIII (Pn14 and the backbone being subsets) are shown in the left column of Figure A1. The three linkages which make up the common polymer backbone are shown in the top three rows and the two glycosidic linkages which comprise the side chains in the bottom two rows.

Appendix A.1. βDGlcNAc(1→3)βDGal

The βDGlcNAc(1→3)βDGal backbone linkage is flexible: the ϕ, ψ PMF (Figure A1a, left) shows a broad, shallow central well, encompassing the global energy minimum at $\phi, \psi = 54°, 16°$, and a secondary syn-syn minimum at $\phi, \psi = 44°, -54°$ with $\Delta G = 1$ kcal·mol^{-1}. This is compatible with the GBSIII DP2-Fab complex crystal structure [13], where this linkage has angles equivalent to $\phi, \psi = 35°, -9°$ (indicated by 'X' on the PMF plot). In addition, the tertiary anti-ψ minimum is also relatively low in energy ($\Delta G = 1.5$ kcal·mol^{-1}), albeit with a high energy barrier to rotation of >6 kcal·mol^{-1}.

The time series scatter plots for this linkage in GBSIII, Pn14 and the unbranched backbone show that all 6RU oligosaccharides explored the full range of linkage conformations in the central well, with the average ϕ,ψ value showing a shift to favor the secondary well in solution (Table A1). This is in agreement with the reported behaviour of this linkage in the sialyl Lewis X pentasaccharide (sLe^X-5) for a 500 ns MD simulation at 37 °C in explicit water [45]. However, transitions to the anti-ψ conformation occurred rarely throughout the duration simulations. This is in contrast to sLe^X-5, where the unconstrained terminal βDGal showed a significant population of the anti-ψ conformation. This difference is likely due to the more constrained environment in the oligosaccharides, as our βDGlcNAc(1→3)βDGal vacuum PMF is very similar to the energy map calculated for this linkage in sLe^X-5. Indeed, the previous 5RU simulations of GBSIII and Pn14 by González-Outeiriño et al. showed an even smaller range of motion for the βDGlcNAc(1→3)βDGal linkage, encompassing only the vacuum global energy minimum (Table A1). This can be attributed to limited conformational sampling in the earlier 50 ns simulations, as transitions between the two minima in the central well occurred on a 20- to 50 ns time scale in our oligosaccharide simulations.

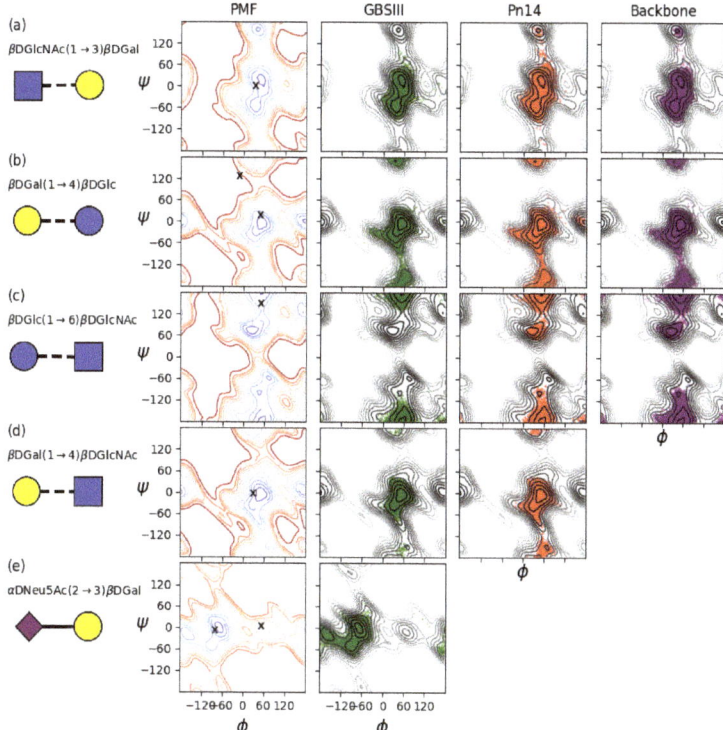

Figure A1. The left column shows contoured disaccharide ϕ, ψ PMF surfaces for (a) βDGlcNAc(1→3)βDGal, (b) βDGal(1→4)βDGlc, (c) βDGlc(1→6)βDGlcNAc, (d) βDGal(1→4)βDGlcNAc and (e) αDNeu5Ac(2→3)βDGal. The PMF for the charged αDNeu5Ac(2→3)βDGal disaccharide is in solution, all others are gas-phase. Contours are drawn at intervals of 1 kcal·mol^{-1} to a maximum of 12 kcal·mol^{-1} and 'X' markers indicate dihedral angle values from the six-sugar GBSIII epitope in complex with Fab crystal structure [13]. Scatter plots of the corresponding two central linkages in the 6RU oligosaccharide strands for the last 900 ns of simulation time are superimposed on the PMFs for 6RU of GBSIII (column 2, green), Pn14 (column 3, red) and the unbranched backbone (right column, purple).

Table A1. Average values of the glycosidic dihedrals in degrees for the two middle repeating units of 6 RU of GBSIII and Pn14 and the unbranched backbone, including comparison with González-Outeiriño et al. [10] (standard deviations in parenthesis). * Note that the 1→6 linkage comprises three diehdrals.

	PMF ϕ, ψ, ω	GBSIII ϕ, ψ, ω	Pn14 ϕ, ψ, ω	Backbone
βDGlcNAc(1→3)βDGal	54, 16	45 (12), −22 (25)	45 (13), −20 (27)	44 (12), −23 (26)
González-Outeiriño et al.		42 (13), 2 (18)	41 (12), 1 (19)	
βDGal(1→4)βDGlc	56, −1	47 (14), −14 (40)	49 (15), −14 (37)	49 (14), −17 (46)
González-Outeiriño et al.		47 (12), 8 (12)	43 (12), −7 (16)	
βDGlc(1→6)βDGlcNAc *	26, 71	51 (10), −175 (11), −67 (8)	50 (12), −180 (18), −62 (26)	50 (15), −179 (22), −69 (30)
González-Outeiriño et al.		41 (10), −159 (22), −67 (9)	40 (14), −167 (31), −65 (10)	
βDGal(1→4)βDGlcNAc	49, 1	50 (10), 0 (14)	50 (11), −2 (18)	
González-Outeiriño et al.		39 (10), 5 (10)	43 (11), 5 (11)	
αDNeu5Ac(2→3)βDGal	−66, 1	−70 (21), −8 (19)	-	
González-Outeiriño et al.		−173 (14), −11 (11)		

Appendix A.1.1. βDGal(1→4)βDGlc

The βDGal(1→4)βDGlc linkage is also flexible. The ϕ, ψ PMF (Figure A1b, right) has a single central syn-syn well with the global energy minimum at $\phi, \psi = 56°, -1°$ and both a narrow anti-ϕ minimum ($\Delta G = 0.5$ kcal·mol^{-1}) and an anti-ψ minimum ($\Delta G = 3.6$ kcal·mol^{-1}). In the crystal structure of the six-sugar GBSIII epitope in complex with Fab, this linkage has angles equivalent to $\phi, \psi = -14°, 6°$ and $\phi, \psi = 45°, -6°$ (indicated by 'X's on the PMF plot). The 6RU simulations of GBSIII and Pn14 show sub-populations of anti-ψ conformations: transitions to this conformation are infrequent and require long simulation times to become apparent. Indeed, anti-ψ conformations of this linkage were not reported for the previous 50 ns simulation, which accounts for the smaller ψ standard deviation in the average value reported by González-Outeiriño et al. (Table A1).

Appendix A.1.2. βDGlc(1→6)βDGlcNAc

This linkage is discussed in detail in the main text.

Appendix A.2. βDGal(1→4)βDGlcNAc

Comparison of the PMF maps reveals that addition of a N-Acetyl group restricts the range of motion of the βDGal(1→4)βDGlcNAc linkage (Figure A1d, left) somewhat as compared to the βDGal(1→4)βDGlc linkage (Figure A1b, left). The energy of the anti-ψ minimum is slightly lowered and the anti-ϕ minimum raised. This is reflected in the narrower range of rotation in the simulations of the GBSIII and Pn14 6RU oligosaccharides (Figure A1d). Rotation to the *anti-ψ* orientation of this linkage is prevented by the proximity of the backbone βDGlc residue. In Pn14, the last RU which is not in contact with a branch has a significant population of the anti-ψ conformer. This is in agreement with simulations of both sLe^X [20] and sLe^X-5 [45], where the same linkage is constrained by the close proximity of the branching αLFuc.

Appendix A.3. αDNeu5Ac(2→3)βDGal

The PMF for the charged αDNeu5Ac(2→3)βDGal disaccharide PMF (Figure A1c, left) was computed in water and shows a very flexible linkage with multiple minima separated by low energy barriers. The conformation of this sialyl linkage is known to have no fixed fixed standard conformation and to be heavily dependent on the molecular environment [44]. Indeed, in contrast to the flexibility of the disaccharide, in our simulation of GBSIII 6RU, a *gauche* conformation predominates for this branching residue, with an average value of $\phi, \psi = -67°, -4°$. The angle distribution for this linkage is consistent with previous MD simulations of sLe^X [20] and sLe^X-5 [45]. In contrast, González-Outeiriño et al. found that the ($\phi \approx -180°$) *anti-phi* conformations predominated with the mean of $\phi, \psi = -173°, -11°$ and a population ratio for the anti/gauche states of approximately 96:4 [10].

In the GBSIII DP2-Fab complex crystal structure [13], the unbound branch has angles equivalent to ϕ, $\psi = -80°, -17°$ (close to our values) the bound branch has $\phi, \psi = 54°, -4°$ (indicated by 'X's on the PMF plot).

Appendix B. Branch Point in Tetrasaccharide

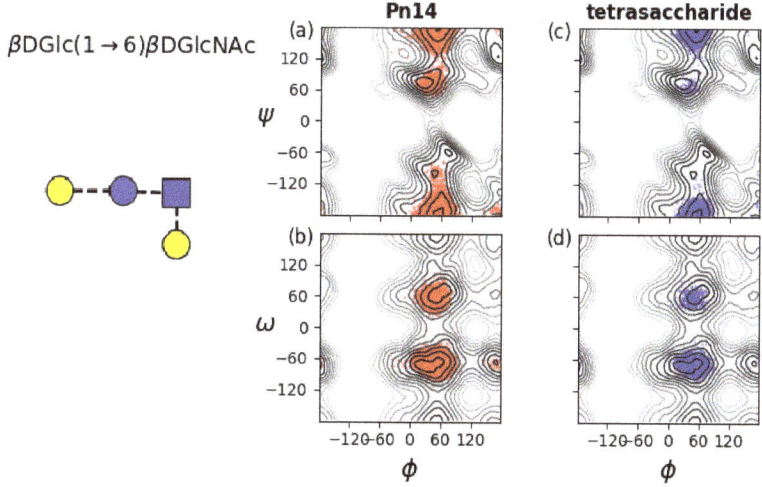

Figure A2. Rotation of the three-bond βDGlc(1→6)βDGlcNAc linkages in Pn14 and the effective tetrasaccharide epitope previously identified (left) [14]. Time series scatter plots are superimposed on the ϕ, ψ PMF (top row) and the ϕ, ω PMF (bottom row) for the two central βDGlc(1→6)βDGlcNAc linkages for: (**a**) Pn14 ϕ, ψ; (**b**) Pn14 ϕ, ω; (**c**) tetrasaccharide ϕ, ψ; and (**d**) tetrasaccharide ϕ, ω.

References

1. Edmond, K.M.; Kortsalioudaki, C.; Scott, S.; Schrag, S.J.; Zaidi, A.K.M.; Cousens, S.; Heath, P.T. Group B streptococcal disease in infants aged younger than 3 months: Systematic review and meta-analysis. *Lancet* **2012**, *379*, 547–556. [CrossRef]
2. Johnson, H.L.; Deloria-Knoll, M.; Levine, O.S.; Stoszek, S.K.; Hance, L.F.; Reithinger, R.; Muenz, L.; O'Brien, K.L. Systematic evaluation of serotypes causing invasive pneumococcal disease among children under five: The pneumococcal global serotype project. *PLoS Med.* **2010**, *7*, e1000348. [CrossRef] [PubMed]
3. Donders, G.; Halperin, S.; Devlieger, R.; Baker, S.; Forte, P.; Wittke, F.; Slobod, K.; Dull, P. Maternal immunization with an investigational trivalent group B Streptococcal vaccine: A randomized controlled trial. *Obstet. Gynecol.* **2016**, *127*, 213–221. [CrossRef] [PubMed]
4. Madhi, S.; Koen, A.; Cutland, C.; Jose, L.; Govender, N.; Wittke, F.; Olugbosi, M.; Sobanjo-ter Meulen, A.; Baker, S.; Dull, P.; Narasimhan, V. Antibody Kinetics and Response to Routine Vaccinations in Infants Born to Women Who Received an Investigational Trivalent Group B Streptococcus Polysaccharide CRM197-Conjugate Vaccine During Pregnancy. *Clin. Infect. Dis.* **2017**, *65*, 1897–1904. [CrossRef] [PubMed]
5. Crumrine, M.; Fischer, G.; Balk, M. Immunochemical cross-reactions between type III group B streptococcus and type 14 *Streptococcus pneumoniae*. *Infect. Immun.* **1979**, *25*, 960–963. [PubMed]
6. Guttormsen, H.K.; Baker, C.J.; Nahm, M.H.; Zughaier, L.C.P.S.M.; Edwards, M.S.; Kasper, D.L. Type III Group B Streptococcal Polysaccharide Induces Antibodies That Cross-React with *Streptococcus pneumoniae* Type 14. *Infect. Immun.* **2002**, *70*, 1724–1738. [CrossRef] [PubMed]
7. Safari, D.; Dekker, H.A.T.; Rijkers, G.T.; van der Ende, A.; Kamerling, J.P.; Snippe, H. The immune response to group B streptococcus type III capsular polysaccharide is directed to the -Glc-GlcNAc-Gal- backbone epitope. *Glycoconj. J.* **2011**, *28*, 557–562. [CrossRef] [PubMed]

8. Kasper, D.L.; Baker, C.; Baltimore, R.; Crabb, J.; Schiffman, G.; Jennings, H. Immunodeterminant specificity of human immunity to type III group B streptococcus. *J. Exp. Med.* **1979**, *149*, 327–339. [CrossRef] [PubMed]
9. Jennings, H.J.; Lugowski, C.; Kasper, D.L. Conformational aspects critical to the immunospecificity of the type III group B streptococcal polysaccharide. *Biochemistry* **1981**, *20*, 4511–4518. [CrossRef] [PubMed]
10. González-Outeiriño, J.; Kadirvelraj, R.; Woods, R.J. Structural elucidation of type III group B Streptococcus capsular polysaccharide using molecular dynamics simulations: The role of sialic acid. *Carbohydr. Res.* **2005**, *340*, 1007–1018. [CrossRef] [PubMed]
11. Kadirvelraj, R.; González-Outeiriño, J.; Foley, L.; Beckham, M.L.; Jennings, H.J.; Foote, S.; Ford, M.G.; Woods, R.J. Understanding the bacterial polysaccharide antigenicity of *Streptococcus agalactiae* versus *Streptococcus pneumoniae*. *Proc. Natl. Acad. Sci. USA* **2006**, *103*, 8149–8154. [CrossRef] [PubMed]
12. Jennings, H.J.; Katzenellenbogen, E.; Lugowski, C.; Michon, F.; Roy, R.; Kasper, L.D. Structure, conformation and immunology of sialic acid containing polysaccharides of human pathogenic bacteria. *Pure Appl. Chem.* **1984**, *56*, 893–905. [CrossRef]
13. Carboni, F.; Adamo, R.; Fabbrini, M.; Ricco, R.D.; Cattaneo, V.; Brogioni, B.; Veggi, D.; Pinto, V.; Passalacqua, I.; Oldrini, D.; Rappuoli, R.; Malito, E.; Margarita, I.R.; Berti, F. Structure of a protective epitope of group B Streptococcus type III capsular polysaccharide. *Proc. Natl. Acad. Sci. USA* **2017**, *114*, 5017–5022. [CrossRef] [PubMed]
14. Safari, D.; Dekker, H.A.T.; Joosten, J.A.; Michalik, D.; de Souza, A.C.; Adamo, R.; Lahmann, M.; Sundgren, A.; Oscarson, S.; Kamerling, J.P.; Snippe, H. Identification of the smallest structure capable of evoking opsonophagocytic antibodies against *Streptococcus pneumoniae* type 14. *Infect. Immun.* **2008**, *76*, 4615–4623. [CrossRef] [PubMed]
15. Kurbatova, E.A.; Akhmatova, N.K.; Akhmatova, E.A.; Egorova, N.B.; Yastrebova, N.E.; Sukhova, E.V.; Yashunsky, D.V.; Tsvetkov, Y.E.; Gening, M.L.; Nifantiev, N.E. Neoglycoconjugate of Tetrasaccharide Representing One Repeating Unit of the *Streptococcus pneumoniae* Type 14 Capsular Polysaccharide Induces the Production of Opsonizing IgG1 Antibodies and Possesses the Highest Protective Activity As Compared to Hexa- and Octasaccharide Conjugates. *Front. Immunol.* **2017**, *8*, 659.
16. Varki, A.; Freeze, H.H.; Manzi, A.E. Overview of Glycoconjugate Analysis. *Curr. Protoc. Protein Sci.* **2009**, *57*, 12.
17. Kuttel, M.M.; Ravenscroft, N. The Role of Molecular Modeling in Predicting Carbohydrate Antigen Conformation and Understanding Vaccine Immunogenicity. In *Carbohydrate-Based Vaccines: From Concept to Clinic*; ACS Symposium Series; American Chemical Society: Washington, DC, USA, 2018; Volume 1290, Chapter 7, pp. 139–173.
18. Kirschner, K.; Yongye, A.; Tschampel, S.; Gonzalez-Outeirino, J.; Daniels, C.; Foley, B.; Woods, R. GLYCAM06: A Generalizable Biomolecular Force Field. Carbohydrates. *J. Comput. Chem.* **2008**, *29*, 622–655. [CrossRef]
19. Guvench, O.; Hatcher, E.; Venable, R.M.; Pastor, R.W.; Alexander, D.; MacKerell, J. CHARMM Additive All-Atom Force Field for Glycosidic Linkages between Hexopyranoses. *J. Chem. Theory Comput.* **2009**, *5*, 2353–2370. [CrossRef]
20. Guvench, O.; Mallajosyula, S.S.; Raman, E.P.; Hatcher, E.; Vanommeslaeghe, K.; Foster, T.J.; Jamison, F.W., II; MacKerell, A.D., Jr. CHARMM Additive All-Atom Force Field for Carbohydrate Derivatives and Its Utility in Polysaccharide and CarbohydrateProtein Modeling. *J. Chem. Theory Comput.* **2011**, *7*, 3162–3180. [CrossRef]
21. Mallajosyula, S.S.; Guvench, O.; Hatcher, E.; MacKerell, A.D., Jr. CHARMM Additive All-Atom Force Field for Phosphate and Sulfate linked to carbohydrates. *J. Chem. Theory Comput.* **2012**, *8*, 759–776. [CrossRef]
22. Lewis, A.L.; Nizet, V.; Varki, A. Discovery and characterization of sialic acid O-acetylation in group B Streptococcus. *Proc. Natl. Acad. Sci. USA* **2004**, *101*, 11123–11128. [CrossRef] [PubMed]
23. Pannaraj, P.S.; Edwards, M.S.; Ewing, K.T.; Lewis, A.L.; Rencha, M.A.; Baker, C.J. Group B streptococcal conjugate vaccines elicit functional antibodies independent of strain O-acetylation. *Vaccine* **2009**, *27*, 4452–4456. [CrossRef] [PubMed]
24. Kuttel, M.M.; Jackson, G.E.; Mafata, M.; Ravenscroft, N. Capsular polysaccharide conformations in pneumococcal serotypes 19F and 19A. *Carbohydr. Res.* **2015**, *406*, 27–33. [CrossRef] [PubMed]
25. Kuttel, M.M.; Timol, Z.; Ravenscroft, N. Cross-protection in *Neisseria meningitidis* serogroups Y and W polysaccharides: A comparative conformational analysis. *Carbohydr. Res.* **2017**, *446–447*, 40–47. [CrossRef] [PubMed]

26. Hlozek, J.; Kuttel, M.M.; Ravenscroft, N. Conformations of *Neisseria meningitidis* serogroup A and X polysaccharides: The effects of chain length and O-acetylation. *Carbohy. Res.* **2018**, *465*, 44–51. [CrossRef] [PubMed]
27. Laio, A.; Parrinello, M. Escaping free energy minima. *Proc. Natl. Acad. Sci. USA* **2002**, *99*, 12562–12565. [CrossRef] [PubMed]
28. Phillips, J.C.; Braun, R.; Wang, W.; Gumbart, J.; Tajkhorshid, E.; Villa, E.; Chipot, C.; Skeel, R.D.; Kale, L.; Schulten, K. Scalable Molecular Dynamics with NAMD. *J. Comput. Chem.* **2005**, *26*, 1781–1802. [CrossRef]
29. Yang, M.; MacKerell, A.D. Conformational Sampling of Oligosaccharides Using Hamiltonian Replica Exchange with Two-Dimensional Dihedral Biasing Potentials and the Weighted Histogram Analysis Method (WHAM). *J. Chem. Theory Comput.* **2015**, *11*, 788–799. [CrossRef]
30. Kuttel, M.M. Conformational free energy maps for globobiose (α-D-Gal-(1-4)-β-D-Gal) in implicit and explict aqueous solution. *Carbohydr. Res.* **2008**, *343*, 1091–1098. [CrossRef]
31. Stone, J.E.; Phillips, J.C.; Freddolino, P.L.; Hardy, J.; Trabuco, L.G.; Schulten, K. Accelerating Molecular Modeling Applications with Graphics Processors. *J. Comput. Chem.* **2007**, *28*, 2618–2639. [CrossRef]
32. Guvench, O.; Greene, S.N.; Kamath, G.; Brady, J.W.; Venable, R.M.; Pastor, R.W.; MacKerell, A.D. Additive Empirical Force Field for Hexopyranose Monosaccharides. *J. Comput. Chem.* **2008**, *29*, 2543–2564. [CrossRef] [PubMed]
33. Jorgensen, W.L.; Chandrasekhar, J.; Madura, J.D.; Impey, R.W.; Klein, M.L. Comparison of simple potential functions for simulations of liquid water. *J. Chem. Phys.* **1983**, *79*, 926–935. [CrossRef]
34. Kuttel, M.; Ravenscroft, N.; Foschiatti, M.; Cescutti, P.; Rizzo, R. Conformational properties of two exopolysaccharides produced by *Inquilinus limosus*, a cystic fibrosis lung pathogen. *Carbohydr. Res.* **2012**, *350*, 40–48. [CrossRef] [PubMed]
35. Kuttel, M.M.; Ståhle, J.; Widmalm, G. CarbBuilder: Software for Building Molecular Models of Complex Oligo- and Polysaccharide Structures. *J. Comput. Chem.* **2016**, *37*, 2098–2105. [CrossRef] [PubMed]
36. Humphrey, W.; Dalke, A.; Schulten, K. VMD—Visual Molecular Dynamics. *J. Mol. Graph.* **1996**, *14*, 33–38. [CrossRef]
37. Feller, S.E.; Zhang, Y.; Pastor, R.W.; Brooks, B.R. Constant pressure molecular dynamics simulation: The Langevin piston method. *J. Chem. Phys.* **1995**, *103*, 4613–4621. [CrossRef]
38. Nose, S.; Lein, M.L. Constant pressure molecular dynamics for molecular systems. *Mol. Phys.* **1983**, *50*, 1055–1076. [CrossRef]
39. Hoover, W.G. Canonical dynamics: Equilibrium phase-space distributions. *Phys. Rev. A* **1985**, *31*. [CrossRef]
40. Cross, S.; Kuttel, M.M.; Stone, J.E.; Gain, J.E. Visualisation of Cyclic and Multi-Branched Molecules with VMD. *J. Mol. Graph. Model.* **2009**, *28*, 131–139. [CrossRef] [PubMed]
41. Heyer, L.J.; Kruglyak, S.; Yooseph, S. Exploring Expression Data: Identification and Analysis of Coexpressed Genes. *Genome Res.* **1999**, *9*, 1106–1115. [CrossRef] [PubMed]
42. Lundborg, M.; Widmalm, G. Structure Analysis of Glycans by NMR Chemical Shift Prediction. *Anal. Chem.* **2011**, *83*, 1514–1517. [CrossRef] [PubMed]
43. Nishida, Y.; Hori, H.; Ohrui, H.; Meguro, H. ^{1}H-NMR analyses of rotameric distributions of C5-C6 bonds of D-glucopyranoses in solution. *J. Carbohydr. Chem.* **1988**, *7*, 239–250. [CrossRef]
44. Miyazaki, T.; Sato, H.; Sakakibara, T.; Kajihara, Y. An Approach to the Precise Chemoenzymatic Synthesis of ^{13}C-Labeled Sialyloligosaccharide on an Intact Glycoprotein: A Novel One-Pot [3-^{13}C]-Labeling Method for Sialic Acid Analogues by Control of the Reversible Aldolase Reaction, Enzymatic Synthesis of [3-^{13}C]-NeuAc-α-(2→3)-[U-^{13}C]-Gal-β-(1→4)-GlcNAc-β- Sequence onto Glycoprotein, and Its Conformational Analysis by Developed NMR Techniques. *J. Am. Chem. Soc.* **2000**, *122*, 5678–5694.
45. Battistel, M.D.; Azurmendi, H.F.; Frank, M.; Freedberg, D.I. Uncovering Nonconventional and Conventional Hydrogen Bonds in Oligosaccharides through NMR Experiments and Molecular Modeling: Application to Sialyl Lewis X. *J. Am. Chem. Soc.* **2015**, *137*, 13444–13447. [CrossRef] [PubMed]

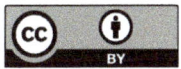

© 2019 by the authors. Licensee MDPI, Basel, Switzerland. This article is an open access article distributed under the terms and conditions of the Creative Commons Attribution (CC BY) license (http://creativecommons.org/licenses/by/4.0/).

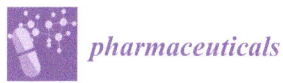

Review

Developments in Carbohydrate-Based Cancer Therapeutics

Farzana Hossain and Peter R. Andreana *

Department of Chemistry and Biochemistry, University of Toledo, Toledo, OH 43606, USA; Farzana.Hossain@rockets.utoledo.edu
* Correspondence: peter.andreana@utoledo.edu

Received: 3 May 2019; Accepted: 29 May 2019; Published: 4 June 2019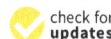

Abstract: Cancer cells of diverse origins express extracellular tumor-specific carbohydrate antigens (TACAs) because of aberrant glycosylation. Overexpressed TACAs on the surface of tumor cells are considered biomarkers for cancer detection and have always been prioritized for the development of novel carbohydrate-based anti-cancer vaccines. In recent years, progress has been made in developing synthetic, carbohydrate-based antitumor vaccines to improve immune responses associated with targeting these specific antigens. Tumor cells also exhaust more energy for proliferation than normal cells, by consuming excessive amounts of glucose via overexpressed sugar binding or transporting receptors located in the cellular membrane. Furthermore, inspired by the Warburg effect, glycoconjugation strategies of anticancer drugs have gained considerable attention from the scientific community. This review highlights a small cohort of recent efforts which have been made in carbohydrate-based cancer treatments, including vaccine design and the development of glycoconjugate prodrugs, glycosidase inhibiting iminosugars, and early cancer diagnosis.

Keywords: cancer treatment; carbohydrate antigens; carbohydrate-based antitumor vaccines; warburg effect; iminosugar; cancer diagnosis

1. Introduction

Carbohydrates are the most abundant complex biomolecules, which play pivotal roles in many cellular interactions, such as signaling to other cellular molecules or cell surface receptors [1]. A wide range of monosaccharide and oligosaccharide residues are connected by glyosidic linkages to form essential glycoconjugates, including glycoproteins, glycolipids, and glycosylated natural products. Furthermore, the biosynthesis of those glycans is controlled by several enzymes, so any deviation in the structure of cell surface glycans enables them to encode information essential for disease progression [2]. Therefore, carbohydrates, which can induce glycan-mediated interactions, are targeted as pharmaceutical therapeutic agents aimed at treating various pathological diseases.

Historically, many naturally isolated carbohydrates were initially used for the development of cancer diagnostic tools. As time elapsed, scientists began to embrace synthesizing carbohydrates for a number of reasons, including the often difficult and lengthy process of obtaining reasonable quantities of pure compound from natural sources. For example, many research groups have relegated to synthesizing tumor-associated carbohydrate antigens (TACAs), which have been noted by the National Institutes of Health as important biomarkers of cancer prognosis, rather than enduring a cumbersome isolation strategy [3]. In many instances, TACAs alone have been found to be poorly immunogenic, unable to induce a T-cell dependent immune response, which has been noted as critical for cancer therapy [3]. At some point in time, scientists began to conjugate TACAs with T-cell stimulating protein carriers, including keyhole limpet haemocyanin (KLH), tetanus toxoid (TT), bovine serum albumin (BSA), and diphtheria toxin (CRM197) [4]. Initially, the responses of those monovalent vaccines were promising, but with further studies, those protein carriers themselves were found to act as self-immunogenic and suppress antigen-specific immunogenicity [5]. Subsequently, TACAs have been coupled with polysaccharides (zwitterionic polysaccharide, PS A1) [6], Toll-like receptor 2 (TLR2) ligand, Pam$_3$CysSerK$_4$ [7], and T-cell peptide epitopes [8], among others, to develop partially to fully synthetic, self-adjuvating, multi-component cancer vaccines. Some of those aforementioned vaccines have been able to reach different phases of clinical trials, e.g., a hexavalent vaccine construct, incorporating GM2, globo H, Le^y, clustered Thomsen nouveau (Tn), clustered Thomsen-Friedenreich (TF), and glycosylated mucin 1 (MUC1) antigens have been used for the treatment of phase II prostate cancer patients [9].

Aside from carbohydrate-based tumor antigens, cancer cells also contain an increased number of glucose transporters (GLUTs) and lectins on their membrane surface, which can transport or bind carbohydrate moieties, respectively. The demand for increased energy in proliferation of cancer cells is met by GLUTs, which allow for an increased uptake of glucose at a higher rate than normal cells—a phenomenon commonly referred to as the "Warburg effect" [10]. This effect has garnered much attention from the community, as many scientists have designed and developed sugar-based targeted drug delivery. Several cytotoxic agents, e.g., glufosfamide, chlorambucil, busulfan, docetaxel, paclitaxel, have been glycoconjugated and found to be less toxic to normal cells than the parent aglycons [11]. Those sugar prodrugs are thought to be cleaved by various intracellular glycosidases. The majority of carbohydrate-based prodrugs are used to improve pharmacokinetic properties, and the site of glycosidase cleavage is typically extracellular, allowing for the release of active drugs. Further research, however, is required to validate the GLUT-mediated cellular entry or GLUT inhibition of those drugs.

The biosynthesis of certain glycans, such as *N*-glycans, by altered glycosylation is also considered a well-known hallmark for cancer progression. Enhanced expression of various glycosyltransferase enzymes, including *N*-acetylglucosaminyltransferase V (e.g., GalNAc-TV, GnT-V, MGAT5), are responsible for an increased number of *N*-glycans in tumor cells [12]. Some imino natural alkaloids (e.g., swainsonine, deoxymannojirimycin, castanospermine) were found to be good inhibitors of specific glycosidases, thereby blocking complete *N*-glycan processing. Numerous iminoalditols and their analogs have been synthesized and inhibitory activity analyzed [13].

Over the past few decades, there have also been enormous strides in development with various sectors of cancer therapeutics, however, patient survival rates are still low when diagnosis is in late stage tumor progression. Only a few plasma tumor markers, such as prostate specific antigen (PSA), cancer antigen 125 (CA125), and alpha-fetoprotein (AFP), have been clinically used for early stage cancer diagnosis in the United States [14]. Most of the plasma tumor antigens are neither sensitive nor specific enough to detect at a very early stage. Recently, some carbohydrate-based non-invasive diagnosis cancer tools, such as metabolic oligosaccharide engineering (MOE) imaging technology, lectin binding, and glycan micro-arrays, have been used to screen tumors [15].

Although a large amount of data is available, this review will mainly focus on glycoconjugate therapeutics, which have been recently used for cancer treatment and prevention. First, we will discuss the recent carbohydrate-based vaccine developments with improved immune responses, glycoconjugated cytotoxic prodrugs for targeted drug delivery, glucosidase inhibiting iminosugars, and finally early cancer detection.

2. Immune Therapy with Carbohydrate-Based Vaccines

2.1. TACAs and Their Immune Response

Oligosaccharides, which coat the plasma membrane, are linked to proteins or lipids through the machinery of glycosyltransferases. Usually, the sugar moieties of glycolipids are attached to a ceramide chain, and for glycoproteins those moieties are linked to the peptide backbone of proteins via an *N*-linkage (linked to NH residue of arginine or lysine or an *O*-linkage (linked to OH residue of serine or threonine. As oligosaccharides are embedded on the cell surface, they become a point of initial contact for many cellular interactions, including the biological transmission of signals, adhesion of lections, release of cytotoxins, and elicitation of antibodies [16]. However, aberrant or modified glycosylation patterns on cancer cell surfaces are typically associated with up- or down-regulation of many glycosyltransferases. For example, in vitro studies reveal that elevations of serum glycosidases, e.g., β-N-acetylglucosaminidase and β-glucuronidase, have been found to occur in different cancer cells [17]. Resultant abnormal glycans are overexpressed on many carcinomas, including those in biopsies of cancer patients.

TACAs are distinctly marked in large number of tumors, but not on normal cells. They promote tumor cell invasion, cause metastasis, and are immunogenic, making them unique targets for cancer vaccine design and development. TACAs are divided into two classes [18]. One is protein linked, including the Tn, Sialyl-Tn (STn) and TF antigens. These antigens are conjugated to the -OH group of serine and threonine residues, and are the result of truncated glycosylation and premature sialylation of protein (e.g., Mucin protein). The mutation in molecular chaperone, Cosmc, is responsible for the lack of cellular β-3-galactosyltransferase (T-synthase), which promotes Tn-antigen (α-GalNAc-Thr/Ser) formation [19,20]. Furthermore, the blood group precursors, Tn, STn, and TF-antigens, contribute to form an array of antigens on heavily glycosylated mucin proteins, such as MUC1. Another classification of TACAs is glycolipid-based. This classification contains the gangliosides GM2, GD2, GD3, fucosyl-GM1, Globo-H, and Lewis^y (Le^y), which all contain a lipidated reducing end [3]. The glycosphingolipids GM2, GD2, and GD3 are involved in human melanomas and Lewis antigens, such as sialyl Lewis (SLe^a), SLe^x, SLe^x-Le^x, are identified human tumor-associated antigens. However, difficulties in the isolation of those antigens from natural sources, due to the heterogeneity of sugars on the cell-surface of tumor cells, complicates vaccine design and development. Therefore, many carbohydrate-based research groups have been resolved to synthesizing homogeneous sugar antigen constructs, and synthetic efforts are underway to facilitate and advance relevant methods, including one-pot synthesis [21] and automated oligosaccharide synthesis [22], to expand the chemists' reagent repertoire for oligomer assembly.

The feature which hampers the development of carbohydrate-based vaccines is their T-cell independent nature. Furthermore, TACAs are considered "self-antigens" and elicit B-cell dependent specific IgM antibodies (possibly IgG3), with no memory T-cell response. The antibodies against carbohydrate antigens are known to exhibit complement-dependent cytotoxicity (CDC), antibody-dependent cellular cytotoxicity (ADCC), and interfere with receptor-mediated signaling to combat tumor cells [23]. After the binding of carbohydrate antigens with the Ig receptors of B-lymphocytes, they can induce cross-linking with Ig proteins, thus activating B-cells and producing low affinity IgM antibodies [24]. However, to get a high-affinity IgG response via class switching, B-cells are required to communicate with T-helper or CD4+ cells. On the other hand, participation of the antigen-presenting cells (APCs) is necessary for activation of the T-cells (Figure 1). APCs can capture, internalize, and proteolytically cleave the protein antigens into peptide fragments (~12–15 amino acids long). Those fragments, containing specific antigens, can be presented on the surface of the APC cells and form a complex with the major histocompatibility complex (MHC) class II molecules. Afterward, APC cells can migrate to lymphoid organs, and MHC class II-peptide complex can interact with T-cell receptors of naïve T-lymphocytes—they then become activated [7]. Furthermore, cluster of differentiation 40 ligand (CD40L) receptors of activated T-helper cells bind with the CD40 on B-cells, resulting in cytokine signaling by the T-cell. The combination of binding to CD40 and cytokine production can stimulate B-cells to proliferate and differentiate into plasma and memory B-cells. The plasma B-cell can secrete antibodies, which can bind with specific surface antigens on cancer cells. Similarly, long-lived memory B-cells rapidly secrete high affinity antibodies (IgG) on subsequent exposure to antigens [18]. Furthermore, CD8+ T-cells are also able to recognize glycoconjugated TACAs (e.g., Tn, TF) with peptides (e.g., MUC1), which have optimal binding affinity for MHC I molecules [25,26].

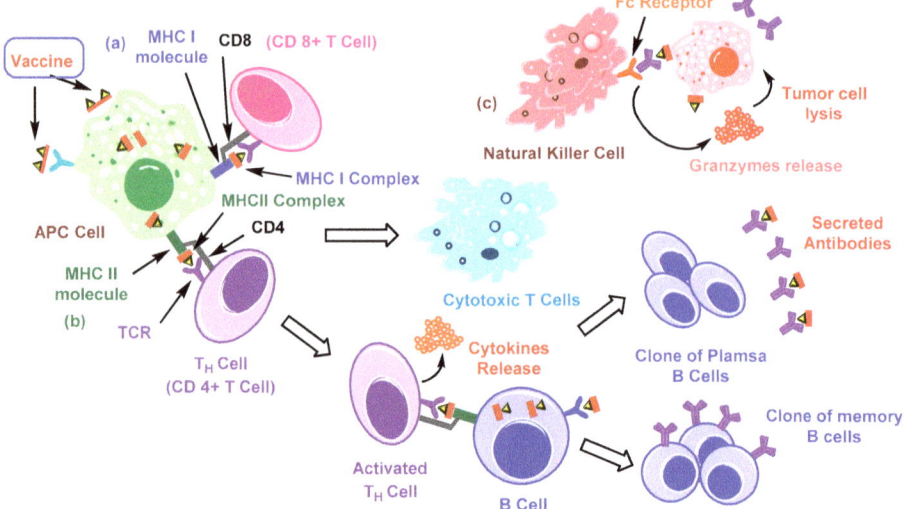

Figure 1. Illustration of immune response to cancer cells. (**a**) Vaccine constructs containing specific antigen(s) get internalized inside antigen-presenting cells (APCs) via endocytosis or binding with specific receptors. While inside APCs, immunogens get proteolyzed by immune proteasomes and divided into several peptide fragments containing antigen(s). If those fragments get loaded onto MHC I then they form MHC I complexes. The resulting complex is transported to the surface so that it can be recognized by CD8+ T-cells. Activated T-cells proliferate to give cytotoxic T-cells [23,27], (**b**) fragments binding with MHC II molecules result in an MHC II complex, which is then transported to the cell surface, activating CD4+ T-cells. Resulting activated cells can further activate B-cells, which present similar antigenic fragments with MHC II. Activated B-cells differentiate into clones of plasma and memory B-cells [23,27], (**c**) antibody-dependent cellular cytotoxicity (ADCC) occurs when IgG antibodies bind with tumor cells, presenting the target specific antigen(s), then Fc receptors of natural killer (NK) cells can recognize them and release granzymes (perforin, proteases, etc.), which causes lysis of tumor cells [28].

2.2. Carrier-Based Carbohydrate Conjugates

To stimulate additional T-cell responses, early attempts to develop carbohydrate–protein conjugate vaccines involved the conjugation of isolated TACAs with a carrier protein, such as keyhole limpet hemocyanin (KLH), bovine serum albumin (BSA), diphtheria toxoid (DT), tetanus toxoid (TT), ovalbumin, human serum albumin (HSA), meningococcal outer membrane protein complex (OMPC), *Hemophilus influenzae* protein D, or *Pseudomonas aeruginosa* exotoxin A (rEPA) [16,18]. Recently, clinical trials of GD3 ganglioside vaccines and anti-idiotypic monoclonal antibodies, which mimics GD3 gangliosides, were carried out on melanoma patients [29]. The patients were sequentially immunized with BEC2, anti-idiotypic monoclonal antibody vaccine mimicking GD3, followed by GD3-lactone-KLH (GD3-L-KLH), or vice versa. Anti-GD3 antibodies were responsive to the GD3-L-KLH vaccine, but there was a noted poor correlation with previous studies and the result was a low survival outcome [29]. Based on previous immune responses, several ganglioside-KLHs have been synthesized and further clinical studies have been carried out [30]. The results obtained led to the synthesis and structural modifications of TACAs to improve immunogenicity. Over the past number of years, Livingston–Danishefsky research teams made enormous contributions to the carbohydrate-based vaccine development field. They reported on the synthesis of a number of oligosaccharides, glycoconjugates, and TACAs, including Globo-H, Lewis^y, Lewis^x, Lewis^b, KH-1, MUC1, GM2, STn, and Tn, and evaluated, preclinically, the first generation monovalent KLH-conjugate vaccines [16]. Later, they developed some multicomponent vaccines by combining different TACAs on a polypeptide backbone and finally linking it to KLH (Figure 2a), and further clinical trials have been carried out with a collaboration at the Memorial Sloan Kettering Cancer Center (MSKCC) [31,32]. Wong et al. also synthesized Globo H vaccines using several protein carriers, such as keyhole limpet hemocyanion, diphtheria toxoid cross-reactive material CRM197 (DT), tetanus toxoid, and BSA [33]. Among them, the Globo H-diphtheria toxoid (GH-DT) vaccine in the presence of α-galactosylceramide C34 adjuvant was able to induce the highest anti-GloboH IgG antibodies for targeting breast cancer cells [33].

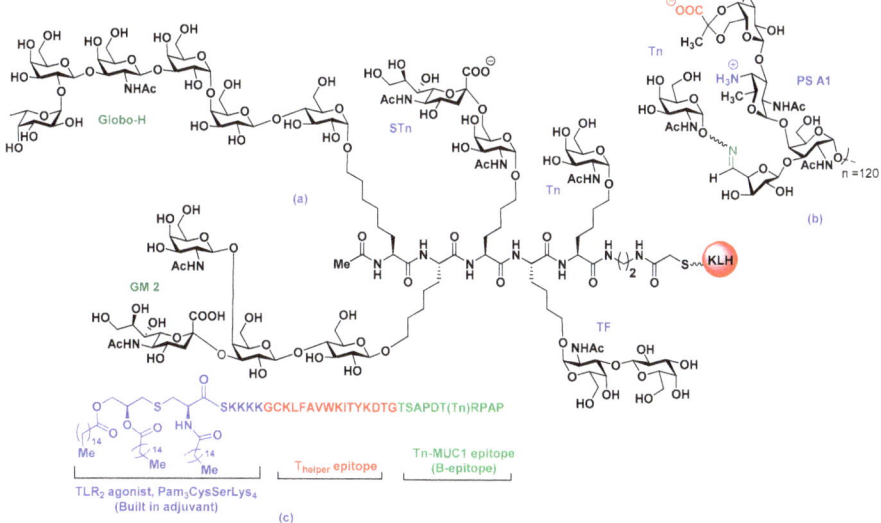

Figure 2. Recent development of tumor-associated carbohydrate antigen (TACA) vaccines. (**a**) Multicomponent vaccine containing different TACAs [23,31], (**b**) entirely carbohydrate-based semi-synthetic vaccine with naturally occurring zwitterionic polysaccharide [34], (**c**) fully synthetic carbohydrate vaccine containing Pam$_3$CysSerLys$_4$, T-helper epitope, and Tn-MUC1 epitope [7,35].

The classical method for conjugating TACAs with a protein involves the utilization of a linker moiety. It has been well documented that linkers themselves can be self-immunogenic or even suppress the antibody production against carbohydrate antigens. For example, in 2004, Boons et al. reported that the immunogenicity of the Le^y conjugate vaccine was suppressed by a rigid bifunctional cross-linker—cyclohexyl maleimide [23]. The linker produced strong IgM and IgG responses, but when a more flexible 3-(bromoacetamido)-propionate linker was used, lower titers of antibody production against the linker was observed [23]. Recently, a number of linkers, including succinimide esters, m-maleimidobenzoyl hydrazide, 4-(4-N-maleimidomethyl)cyclohexane-1-carboxyl hydrazide, squaric acid diesters, and p-nitrophenol esters, have been utilized, depending on the relatively easily accessible functional groups on the carrier protein and carbohydrate antigen [16]. Other concerns regarding linkers are chain length, water solubility, low yield, and first attachment either to a protein or antigen. Even though protein conjugate vaccines contributed to the initial development of tumor therapeutic vaccines, the immunogenicity of the desired TACA or epitope is now known to be suppressed by inherently immunogenic protein carrier.

As an alternative to carrier proteins, our group has isolated several zwitterionic polysaccharides (ZPSs), including PS A1 and PS B from anerobic *Bacteroides fragilis* (ATCC 25285/NCTC 9343) and specific type 1 polysaccharide (Sp1) from *Streptococcus pneumoniae* serotype 1. Like some carrier proteins, ZPSs are also known to elicit a CD4+ T-cell dependent immune response and invoke class switching from IgM to IgG [36]. The co-stimulatory molecules CD40 and CD86 or CD80 on the surface of APCs also can be induced by PS A1 [37]. PS A1 is also known to bind with toll like receptor-2 (TLR-2) of dendritic cells, which plays an active role in releasing IL-12 and IFN-γ [38].

Our group has synthesized aminooxy Tn, TF, STn, and Globo-H antigens and conjugated them to chemically treated, oxidized PS A1, aiming to develop entirely carbohydrate-based cancer vaccines (Figure 2b) [6,34]. The vaccine constructs were injected into C57BL/6J mice, either in the presence or absence of the TiterMax®Gold and Sigma adjuvant system (SAS)®, which generated antigen specific, highly robust immune responses (IgM and IgG) noted in enzyme-linked immunosorbent assay (ELISA) [6,34]. Antibody responses of Tn-PS A1 from adjuvant-free vaccinated mice sera indicate the possibility of a dual role of PS A1 as both carrier and adjuvant. Further flow cytometry (FACS) data, with TF and STn-PS B vaccines, also indicated antibody binding to TF-laced MCF-7 cells. Recently, our group has synthesized a tetrasaccharide repeating unit of PS A1, with alternative charges on adjacent monosaccharides, and experiments are underway to unlock the mystery surrounding unknown aspects of carbohydrate immunity [39].

2.3. Fully Synthetic Carbohydrate Vaccines

To avoid immunosuppressive carrier proteins, many self-adjuvating, multicomponent, fully synthetic vaccines have been proposed by a number of research groups. For example, Boons et al. proposed a multicomponent vaccine to elicit both cytotoxic T lymphocytes (CTLs) and antibody-dependent cellular cytotoxicity (ADCC)-mediated humoral immunity [7]. The tripartite vaccine is comprised of the immunoadjuvant Pam_3CysSK_4, a peptide T-helper epitope, and an aberrantly glycosylated MUC1 peptide (B-epitope) (Figure 2c) [7]. The TLR2 ligand is known to enhance local inflammation and activate the components of the adaptive immune system. The vaccine containing glycosylated MUC1 was more lytic compared to a non-glycosylated counterpart. The mucin 1 (MUC1) is a transmembrane protein overexpressed in various tumors, like lung, breast, pancreas, kidney, ovary, and colon tumors. The extracellular N-terminal domain of MUC1 contains a variable number of 20 amino acid tandem repeat (VNTR) units, like HGVTSAPDTRPAPGSTAPPA. It is aberrantly glycosylated in cancer cells but highly glycosylated in normal cells. Because of this distinguishable characteristic, the National Cancer Institute (NCI) has declared MUC1 as a prioritized cancer antigen among 75 TACAs, therefore many research groups are attempting to develop vaccine constructs utilizing peptide backbones present in VNTR [35].

Mice are usually immunized with vaccines in the presence of adjuvants, which is thought to make the vaccine immunogenic enough to ignore the self-tolerance immunogenicity towards TACAs and boost the immune response [40]. Recently, self-adjuvating vaccines, containing the immunogenic antigens as well as the adjuvants, in a single-entity, have begun to draw much attention in the vaccine arena. For example, in 2017, Yin and co-workers reported a fully synthetic self-adjuvating vaccine candidate [41]. This two-component vaccine contains: (i) an invariant natural killer T (iNKT) cell ligand, α-galactosylceramide (αGalCer), and (ii) a sialyl Tn (STn). This STn-αGalCer vaccine construct showed remarkable efficacy in inducing antibody class switching from IgM to STn-specific IgG (IgG1 and IgG3 subtypes) antibodies [41].

To improve the antigen stability against glycosidases and enhance the in vivo bioavailability, a fully synthetic vaccine has been reported. The vaccine is comprised of four clustered Tn-antigen analogs, an immunostimulant peptide (OvaPADRE), and a cyclopeptide scaffold. This vaccine prototype, thus far, has elicited long-lasting antibodies able to bind Tn expressing MCF-7 human breast cancer cells, and it was observed to produce high titers of IgG1, IgG2a, and IgG3 antibodies [42].

3. Glycosylation for Specific Anticancer Drug Delivery

3.1. Glucose Metabolism in Cancer Cells and Warburg Effects

Unlike normal cells, many cancer cells consume an abundance of glucose, and have a higher rate of aerobic glycolysis to supply the increased energy required for their rapid proliferation [43].

Tumor cells can alter cellular metabolism during the transition from a normal to abnormal state. Normally, during glucose metabolism or glycolysis, one molecule of glucose is converted into two pyruvates, two molecules of ATP, and two reduced nicotinamide adenine dinucleotide (NADH) molecules. In the presence of oxygen, pyruvate undergoes oxidation to CO_2 and H_2O, and generates 36 additional ATPs per glucose (Figure 3), whereas in the absence of oxygen, pyruvate gets reduced to lactic acid [44]. However, in cancer cells, a large amount of glucose can also be converted to lactic acid, regardless of the availability of oxygen. This kind of unusual metabolism opens the windows for many cancer-targeting therapeutics. This tendency of a higher rate of glucose consumption or increased aerobic glycosylation phenomenon, known as the Warburg effect, was first observed by the German scientist Otto Warburg in 1926, and has become an object of significant interest in defeating cancer [10]. The Warburg Effect was later utilized in a clinical study, when the use of a radio labeled glucose-analog, 2-deoxy-2(^{18}F)fluoro-D-glucose (^{18}F-FDG), was consumed by cancer cells observed via positron emission tomography (PET) analysis. This study is now considered one of the hallmarks in the fight against cancer [45]. Based on this effect, many glycosylated prodrugs have been designed over the past few years with the aim of a targeted delivery of respective active anticancer drugs towards cancer cells, and to improve pharmacokinetics, like water solubility and serum stability [46].

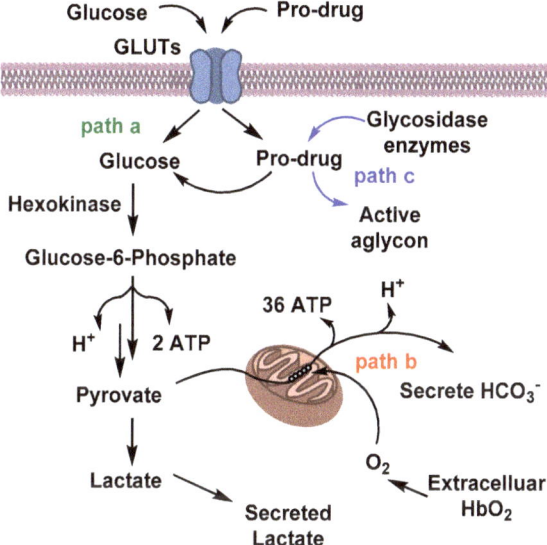

Figure 3. Glucose metabolism and prodrug route inside the cells: Glucose or glyco-conjugated pro drugs get internalized inside the cells via glucose transporters (GLUTs). Glucose metabolism follows either **path a**—anaerobic glycosylation; **path b**—aerobic glycosylation; or **path c**—cleavage of the active drug by a glycosydic enzyme.

For the transportation of polar molecules, especially sugars, inside cells, some carrier proteins are located on the plasma membrane. There are two types of transporter families: one is facilitated glucose transporters (GLUTs), which facilitates glucose transportation between external and internal plasma membrane via concentration gradient [43]. To date, 14 different kinds of GLUTs (GLUT-1–14) have been classified according to their structure and sequence. Among them, GLUT-1 is the most reported facilitative sugar transporter and is known to be overexpressed in cancerous cells [47]. Another kind of transporter is known as sodium-dependent sugar transporter (SGLT), which requires energy for sugar transport [43]. Many cancer cells have overexpressed glucose transporters (GLUTs) to facilitate a higher glucose consumption than that of normal cells. This observation has opened new windows for targeted chemotherapy with fewer side effects. Many groups have conjugated sugars at different positions of cytotoxic agents and analyzed their ability to target glucose transporters, especially GLUT-1. However, to analyze GLUT-1 receptor mediated transportation of glycan-based paclitaxel prodrugs, the receptor was co-treated with GLUT-1 inhibitors, such as phloretin and phlorizin [48]. Due to the similarity in structures among the GLUTs, it is difficult to determine which one gets targeted by glucose-conjugates. No prodrug co-crystalized with human GLUT-1 is known due to rapid interchangeable conformations, which impede crystallization [49]. However, after cellular uptake, the effectiveness of the prodrugs depends on the successful cleavage by the hydrolytic enzymes to release the active drugs for tumor killing.

3.2. Carbohydrate-Based Prodrugs for Specific Targeting

In 1995, Glufosfamide (Figure 4a), the first sugar-conjugated prodrug, was synthesized by Wiessler et al. in an attempt to decrease molecular toxicity and increase the cancer selectivity of a DNA alkylating aglycon ifosfamide mustard [50]. Glufosfamide showed 4.5-fold less toxicity than its active aglycon ifosfamide in rats (in mg kg^{-1}) [50]. The first human clinical trial, with 20 patients, was initiated in Europe by Briasoulis et al. in 1997 [51]. More clinical trials ensued and further patients with various solid tumors were evaluated in Japan and USA; results proved promising [11]. Many anticancer drugs, such as chlorambucil, busulfan, docetaxel, and paclitaxel, were conjugated with several monosaccharides (see Figure 4), utilizing varying linkers, such as esters, amides, ureas, and succinic acids. Several groups reported preliminary biological assessments of the library of glycoconjugated derivatives by comparing the derivatives with their respective aglycons. A recent review by Calvaresi et al. discussed the glycoconjugation of some active cancer therapeutics [11]. Table 1 highlights some recent glycoconjugated anticancer agents, with their biological activity and mode of delivery towards cancer cells via glucose transporters (also see a comprehensive review by Calvaresi) [11].

Carbohydrate-based polymers, such as hydrogels, nanoparticles, micelles, and nanogels, have been shown to be promising delivery vehicles. Hydrophilic or hydrophobic drugs loaded onto hydrogels, through noncovalent interactions, allow in-situ release under specific and well-regulated conditions. Blanchette et al. synthesized P(MAA-g-EG) hydrogel nanoparticles to investigate the oral delivery of hydrophilic anticancer drug bleomycin [52]. This co-polymer solution mixture consists of methacrylic acid (MAA), a hydrophilic monomer, and ethylene glycol (EG) in a 1:1 molar ratio. To allow in situ polymerization, bleomycin was added to the above solution and then treated with UV light to initiate free radical polymerization, forming hydrogel nanospheres P(MAA-g-EG) [52]. For the oral delivery of hydrophobic drugs, Puranik et al. used hydrophobic monomers, such as *tert*-butyl methacrylate (*t*-BMA), *n*-butyl methacrylate (nBMA), *n*-butyl acrylate (nBA), and methyl methacrylate (MMA), along with MAA [53].

To improve the bioactivity and biodegradability of nanoparticles (NPs), and to reduce side effects, scientists are currently trying to find polysaccharide-based NPs (PNPs) for many cancer related treatments. Different polysaccharides, such as chitosan, hyaluronic acid (HA), chondroitin sulfate, heparin, alginate, and pullulan, have been used for the development of various NPs [54]. Furthermore, for specific delivery to the colon, different types of polysaccharides, such as chitosan and cyclodextrin, chitosan and pectin, have been utilized for achieving colon-specific delivery [54]. A number of anti-cancer drugs, such as doxorubicin (DOX), paclitaxel, docetaxel, cisplatin, and 5-fluorouracil, have been conjugated to polysaccharides to achieve their polysaccharide-based delivery to cancer cells [55].

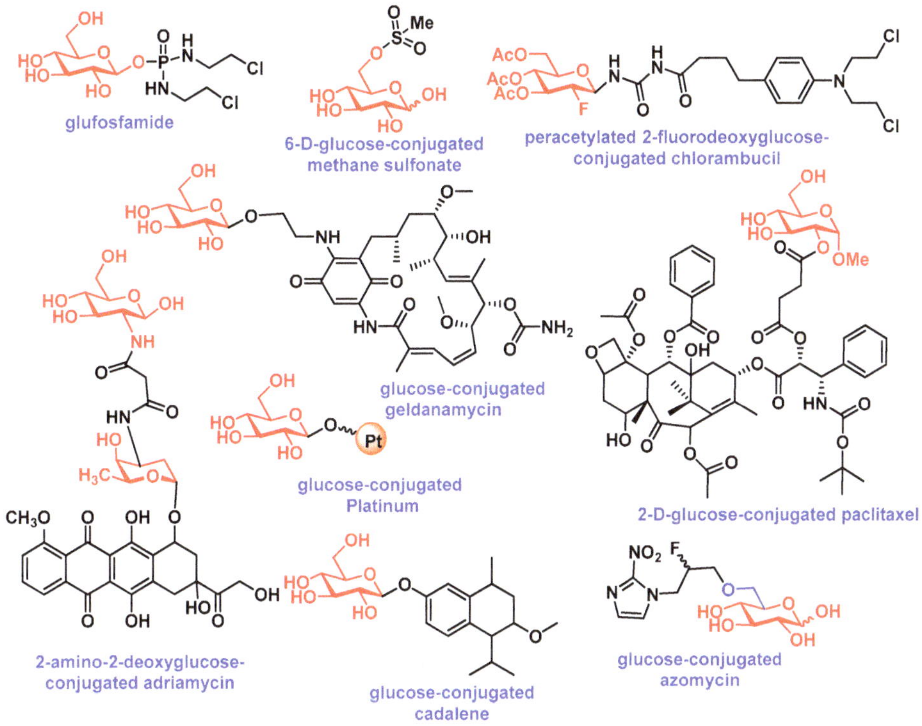

Figure 4. Glycoconjugated prodrugs for targeted delivery via GLUTs.

Recently, a pH sensitive DOX-loaded mesoporous silica nanoparticle (MSN) was conjugated with lectin for the treatment of bone cancer [56]. The building blocks of the multifunctional nanosystem consisted of a polyacrylic acid (PAA) capping layer, which is grafted to MSN, a glycan (sialic acid) targeting ligand, and plant lectin concanavalin A (ConA). This nano-device exhibited 8-fold higher toxicity on tumor cells than free DOX.

Table 1. List of glycoconjugated prodrugs.

Aglycons	Conjugated Sugars	Response of Glycoconjugates Compared to Aglycon in In-Vitro or In-Vivo	Transportation Mode	Ref(s)
Chlorambucil	Peracetylated 2-fluorodeoxyglucose	Human fibroblasts, MCF-7 (25-fold more active) and Mice (Increased in MTD)	-	[57]
Docetaxel	Glucose, galactose, mannose, xylose	B16 murine melanoma cells (3 to 18-fold more active)	-	[58]
Docetaxel	galactose	Syngeneic P388 murine leukemia tumor model (equivalent)	-	[59]
Paclitaxel	Glucose, glucuronic Acid	HUV-EC-C and CHO-K1, NCI-H838, Hep-3B, A498, MES-SA, HCT-116, NPC-TW01, MKN-45 (All less toxic)	Partially GLUT-1, /GLUT-3/GLUT-4 mediated	[48,60]
Chlorambucil	Amino derivatives of glucose, mannose, galactose, xylose, lyxose, D-threoside	NCI-H460, A549, Du145, SKOV3, Hep3b, SF268, MCF7, HT29, HCT15, H1299 (induce decrease in cell growth)	-	[61]
Benzylguanine	Glucose	HeLa S3 and HeLa MR cells (inhibition of O^6-methyl-guanine-DNA methyltransferase, MGMT)	-	[62]
Azomycin	Glucose	Several immortalized murine and human cancer cells (improved selectivity towards hypoxic tumor as radiosensitizer)	GLUTs mediated	[63]
Adriamycin	2-amino-2-deoxy-glucose	MCF-7, Bel-7402, HepG2, MDA-MB-231, U87MG, HELF, SKOV3, and S180, HELF and mice (enhance selectivity towards cancer cells)	GLUTs mediated	[64]
Geldanamycin	Glucose, lactose, galactose	SW620, HT29, MCF7, K562 (one showed 3- to 40-fold enhanced activity with β-galactosidase)	-	[65]
Platinum	Glucose	DU145, RWPE2	GLUTs mediated	[66]
Cadalene	Glucose, lactose, galactose		-	[67]
Ketoprofen	Glucose	In vitro (less toxic) and in vivo (reduced tumor size) Cross blood–brain barrier (BBB)	GLUTs mediated	[68]
Nordihydroguaiaretic acid	Galactose, glucose	NCI/ADR-RES, Hep3B, MCF-7, HT-29	-	[69]

4. Iminosugar Analogs for Cancer Therapy

4.1. Aberrant N-Linked Glycosylation and Inhibition of Glycosidase Enzyme

Cell glycans are synthesized by many glycosyltransferases, and the process generally occurs in the endoplasmic reticulum or Golgi apparatus [70,71]. For example, some enzymes are responsible for the aberrant addition or truncation of the carbohydrate moieties on cell surface lipids, proteins, or peptides, which also play roles in distinguishing tumor cells from normal cells and tumor metastasis [72]. Similar to mutations in genes, due to aberrant O-glycosylation, N-linked oligosaccharides also play a critical role in tumor cell progression and mitosis. The biosynthesis of N-glycoproteins, that normally begins in the endoplasmic reticulum (ER), involves three major sequences. The first phase involves the synthesis of a dolichol-linked precursor oligosaccharide, $GLc_3Man_9GlcNAc_2$-PP-Dol. The lipid molecule, dolichol, is found to be attached to the membrane of ER and contains one phosphate group to add various sugar molecules (two GlcNAc, nine mannose, and three glucose), with a pyrophosphate group. After synthesis of the precursor molecule, it gets transferred to an asparagine (Asn) residue of a protein by oligosaccharyltransferases. The final phase involves modification of the oligosaccharide chain by several trimming reactions, such as the stepwise removal of three glucose molecules and up to six mannose residues by glucosidase I and II. Following the attack by enzymes, the remaining central core undergoes further processing reactions, e.g., the addition of other sugars, such as N-acetylglucosamine, galactose, neuraminic acid, L-fucose, and N-acetylgalactoseamine performed by several glycotransferase enzymes to produce three different types of N-glycans (Figure 5). High mannose-type glycans contain additional mannose units, whereas both hybrid and complex types contain additional monosaccharide units attached to the core. Due to the complex nature of those aglycons, any variation in this biosynthesis may lead to oncogenesis and tumor metastasis. Therefore, the identification of new therapeutic strategies for the inhibition of those glycosidases has captured the attention of scientists to prevent aberrant N-glycosylation, and, hence, halt cancer.

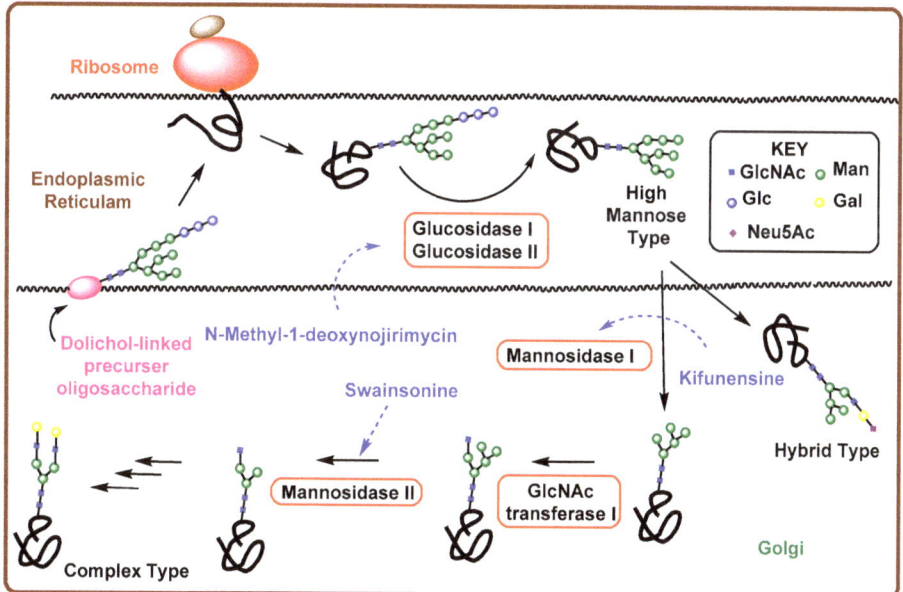

Figure 5. Biosynthetic pathways for N-glycans and iminosugars, inhibiting different glycosidase enzymes.

4.2. Iminosugars as Enzyme Inhibitors

Several naturally-occurring iminosugars have noted anticancer activity through their ability to target the N-glycan biosynthesis pathway. These azo sugars are carbohydrate analogs, in which the oxygen heteroatom position in the ring is replaced by a more basic trivalent nitrogen. This simple substitution makes synthesis challenging and generates opportunities for evaluation of biological activities. The most common naturally occurring rings for this class are pyrrolidine, piperidine, pyrrolizidine, indolizidine, and nor-tropane (Figure 6). Since the first isolation of nojirimycin from *Streptomyces roseochromogenes* R-468, as an antibiotic, approximately 200 naturally occurring azo sugars have been isolated, but still very few are available for pharmaceutical applications [73]. The initial biological evaluations of these sugar analogs indicate their glycosidase and glycosyltransferase inhibitory properties [73]. Recently, these analogs have gained importance in the development of new anticancer drugs. Most of the investigations were, however, carried out on plant glycosidases. Hence, further work is required on mammalian glycosidases to uncover their potential in cancer research.

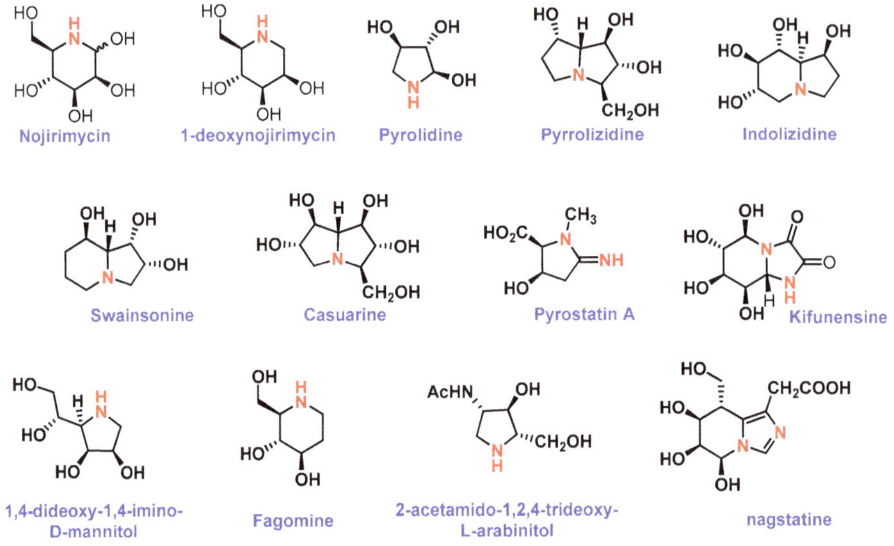

Figure 6. Structures of different iminosugars.

(−)-Swainsonine, (1S,2R,8R,8aR)-1,2,8-trihydroxyindolizidine is the most investigated iminofuranoside that can be found in several natural sources. It is an effective inhibitor of lysosomal α1-3 and α-1-6-mannosidase and Golgi α-manosidase II. The inhibition of Golgi α-manosidase II by (−)-swainsonine can block the expression of the β(1→6)-branched complex type N-glycans in malignant human and rodent cells. With this finding, a phase I study was conducted, in which the potency of glycoprotein processing iminosugars and swainsonine hydrochloride (GD0039) were tested as anti-cancer drugs. Subsequently, clinical phase II trials were conducted in Canada in and around 2002 [13]. The phase II results from 40 patients with advanced renal cell cancer or 5-florouracil (5-FU) resistant advanced colorectal cancer were deemed auspicious. Unfortunately, during the pharmacokinetics and pharmacodynamics investigations of oral GD0039, all the cancer patients at an advanced stage discontinued treatment due to disease progression or toxicity. However, GD0039 was shown to prevent metastasis, inhibit the growth of tumor cells, activate lymphocyte proliferation, and enhance T-cell stimulation. Inspired by biological interactions, various derivatives have been synthesized and anti-cancer activities evaluated, however none of them were observed to be as potent as their predecessor. On the other hand, casuarine, a pentahydroxylated pyrrolizidine, was found to be a good glucosidase inhibitor, showing immune responses such as increasing levels of cytokines IL-2, IL-12, and IFN-γ. Interestingly, those immunological responses do not necessarily depend on glucosidase inhibition. Other iminoalditols and their specific glycosidase inhibitory activities are listed in Table 2.

Table 2. List of iminosugars and their inhibitory effects.

Amino Sugars	Glucosidase Inhibition	Other Anti-Tumor Activities	Ref (s)
Swainsonine	Lysosomal α-1-3- (IC$_{50}$ 0.70 nM) and α-1-6-mannosidase (K$_i$ 40 nM) and Golgi α-mannosidase	Inhibits growth of tumor cells	[13]
1,4-Dideoxy-1,4-imino-D-mannitol	α-mannosidase, Lysosomal Golgi α-mannosidase II, glycogen phosphorylase	Human Glioblastoma and Melanoma Cells	[74]
1-Deoxymannojirimycin	α-1-2-mannosidase (IC$_{50}$ 0.02 mM), Golgi α-mannosidase II (IC$_{50}$ 400 µM)	Interact with recombinant tumor necrosis factor (rTNF) and recombinant interleukin 1 (rIL-1)	[75]
2-aminomethyl-5-(hydroxymethyl) pyrrolidine3,4-diol derivative	Jack bean α-Mannosidase (IC$_{50}$ 55 µM)	Inhibits growth of human glioblastoma cells and melanoma cells, DNA, synthesis of proteins	[74,76]
Castanospermine	α- and β-glucosidases	Inhibitor of breast cancer	[77]
1-deoxynojirimycin	Glucosidase I and II	Anti-metastatic activity, reduce adhesion of tumor cells to vascular endothelium, inhibit cellular transformation, prevent morphological differentiation of endothelial cells	[13]
(+)-Lentiginosine	amyloglucosidases	Inhibits ATPase and Chaperone Activity of Hsp90	[78]
Siastatin B	β-glucuronidase, NAG-ase	Antimetastatic activity	[13]

5. Carbohydrate-Based Diagnosis

Some serum glycoprotein biomarkers, such as carcino-embryonic antigen (CEA), carbohydrate antigens 19-9 (CA19-9) and 125 (CA125), alpha-fetoprotein (AFP), and prostate-specific antigen (PSA) have been found to be useful in the initial detection of colon, ovarian, and prostate cancers [79]. Alternatively, early detection is possible in positron emission tomography (PET), based on an increased concentration of 2-flurodeoxy-D-glucose (^{18}FDG) in tumor cells. As cancer cells are more metabolically active, another imaging probe strategy, named metabolic oligosaccharide engineering (MOE) technology, has recently opened a new era in cancer diagnosis. In this strategy, non-natural derivatives of sialic acid, GalNAc, and fucose are supplied exogenously and get incorporated, using biosynthetic machinery, within the cellular glycans chains (Figure 7a). Those glycans get tagged with chemical imaging probes using biorthogonal reactions, and then are monitored with magnetic resonance imaging (MRI) [80].

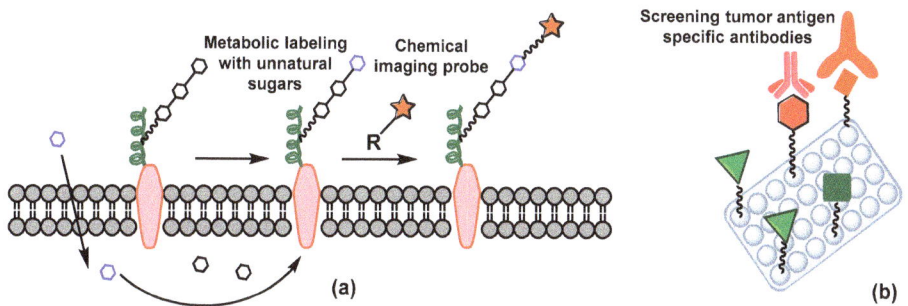

Figure 7. Early detection of cancer (**a**) metabolic oligosaccharide engineering (MOE) technology, (**b**) glycan micro array strategies.

The use of specific lectins to screen potential carbohydrate tumor biomarkers has gained traction in the diagnosis of cancer types with a lack of serum biomarkers. Lectins can bind with selective carbohydrates, are able to distinguish abnormal glycosylation, and trigger the mechanism required for tumor cell apoptosis [81]. A group of lectin proteins, such as *Amaranthus caudatus* agglutinin (ACA), *Artocarpus integrifolia* agglutinin (AIA), *Arachis hypogea* agglutinin (AHA), *Vicia villosa* lectin (VVL), *Griffonia simplicifolia* agglutinin I (GSA I), and *Ulex europaeus* agglutinin I (UEA I) can recognize the Tn, TF, and STn alteration of CA125 and human epididymis secretory protein 4 (HE4) antigens (Figure 7b) [82]. Similarly, glycan microarray strategies have been utilized to detect the presence of antibodies against specific antigens (e.g., Globo H) in cancer patients' serum [15]. The array is composed of various carbohydrates on a solid support and provides high-throughput cancer related glycan–protein interactions (Figure 7b).

6. Conclusion

Due to their ubiquitous nature, carbohydrates have long-been used as a means for cancer diagnosis and for the development of safe, small molecule therapeutics. Although several carbohydrate agents have successfully been synthesized and processed for clinical trials, the therapeutic responses have not lived up to their promise in treating cancer. Results from the use of commercially available carbohydrate-based therapeutic agents has also not been shown to be highly significant. Therefore, more exhaustive studies are required to explore potent therapeutic agents able to combat cancer. One approach might be the development of vaccines with non-natural synthetic antigens, which may overcome the immunosuppressive nature of carrier proteins. Another strategy might be an expansion on the co-administration of a vaccine and glycoconjugated prodrug, which can promote specific drug delivery as well as perturb cancer. Although iminosugars have proven to be glycosidase inhibiting agents for *N*-glycan biosynthesis, further evaluations are required for extended development toward novel drugs.

Funding: NIH U01 GM125271.

Conflicts of Interest: The authors declare no conflicts of interest.

References

1. Brandley, B.K.; Schnaar, R.L. Cell-Surface Carbohydrates in Cell Recognition and Response. *J. Leukocyte Biol.* **1986**, *40*, 97–111. [CrossRef] [PubMed]
2. Fernandez-Tejada, A.; Canada, F.J.; Jimenez-Barbero, J. Glycans in Medicinal Chemistry: An Underexploited Resource. *Chem. Med. Chem.* **2015**, *10*, 1291–1295. [CrossRef] [PubMed]
3. Feng, D.; Shaikh, A.S.; Wang, F. Recent Advance in Tumor-Associated Carbohydrate Antigens (TACAs)-based Antitumor Vaccines. *ACS Chem. Biol.* **2016**, *11*, 850–863. [CrossRef] [PubMed]
4. Guo, Z.; Wang, Q. Recent Development in Carbohydrate-Based Cancer Vaccines. *Curr. Opin. Chem. Biol.* **2009**, *13*, 608–617. [CrossRef] [PubMed]
5. Nativi, C.; Renaudet, O. Recent Progress in Antitumoral Synthetic Vaccines. *ACS Med. Chem. Lett.* **2014**, *5*, 1176–1178. [CrossRef] [PubMed]
6. Shi, M.; Kleski, K.A.; Trabbic, K.R.; Bourgault, J.-P.; Andreana, P.R. Sialyl-Tn Polysaccharide A1 as an Entirely Carbohydrate Immunogen: Synthesis and Immunological Evaluation. *J. Am. Chem. Soc.* **2016**, *138*, 14264–14272. [CrossRef] [PubMed]
7. Lakshminarayanan, V.; Thompson, P.; Wolfert, M.A.; Buskas, T.; Bradley, J.M.; Pathangey, L.B.; Madsen, C.S.; Cohen, P.A.; Gendler, S.J.; Boons, G.-J. Immune Recognition of Tumor-Associated Mucin MUC1 is Achieved by a Fully Synthetic Aberrantly Glycosylated MUC1 Tripartite Vaccine. *Proc. Natl. Acad. Sci. USA* **2012**, *109*, 261–266. [CrossRef] [PubMed]
8. Patronov, A.; Doytchinova, I. T-cell Epitope Vaccine Design by Immunoinformatics. *Open Biol.* **2013**, *3*, 120139. [CrossRef]

9. Slovin, S.F.; Ragupathi, G.; Fernandez, C.; Diani, M.; Jefferson, M.P.; Wilton, A.; Kelly, W.K.; Morris, M.; Solit, D.; Clausen, H.; et al. A Polyvalent Vaccine for High-risk Prostate Patients: "Are More Antigens Better?". *Cancer Immunol. Immunother.* **2007**, *56*, 1921–1930. [CrossRef]
10. Warburg, O. On the Origin of Cancer Cells. *Science* **1956**, *123*, 309–314. [CrossRef]
11. Calvaresi, E.C.; Hergenrother, P.J. Glucose Conjugation for the Specific Targeting and Treatment of Cancer. *Chem. Sci.* **2013**, *4*, 2319–2333. [CrossRef] [PubMed]
12. De Freitas Junior, J.C.; Morgado-Diaz, J.A. The Role of N-glycans in Colorectal Cancer Progression: Potential Biomarkers and Therapeutic Applications. *Oncotarget* **2016**, *7*, 19395–19413. [PubMed]
13. Wrodnigg, T.M.; Steiner, A.J.; Ueberbacher, B.J. Natural and Synthetic Iminosugars as Carbohydrate Processing Enzyme Inhibitors for Cancer Therapy. *Anticancer Agents Med. Chem.* **2008**, *8*, 77–85. [CrossRef] [PubMed]
14. Meany, D.L.; Sokoll, L.J.; Chan, D.W. Early Detection of Cancer: Immunoassays for Plasma Tumor Markers. *Expert Opin. Med. Diagn.* **2009**, *3*, 597–605. [CrossRef]
15. Wang, C.-C.; Huang, Y.-L.; Ren, C.-T.; Lin, C.-W.; Hung, J.-T.; Yu, J.-C.; Yu, A.L.; Wu, C.-Y.; Wong, C.-H. Glycan Microarray of Globo H and Related Structures for Quantitative Analysis of Breast Cancer. *Proc. Natl. Acad. Sci. USA* **2008**, *105*, 11661. [CrossRef]
16. Hevey, R.; Ling, C.C. Recent Advances in Developing Synthetic Carbohydrate-based Vaccines for Cancer Immunotherapies. *Future Med. Chem.* **2012**, *4*, 545–584. [CrossRef]
17. Zhou, X.; Huang, Z.; Yang, H.; Jiang, Y.; Wei, W.; Li, Q.; Mo, Q.; Liu, J. Beta-Glucosidase Inhibition Sensitizes Breast Cancer to Chemotherapy. *Biomed. Pharmacother.* **2017**, *91*, 504–509. [CrossRef]
18. Nishat, S.; Andreana, P. Entirely Carbohydrate-Based Vaccines: An Emerging Field for Specific and Selective Immune Responses. *Vaccines* **2016**, *4*, 19. [CrossRef]
19. Ju, T.; Lanneau, G.S.; Gautam, T.; Wang, Y.; Xia, B.; Stowell, S.R.; Willard, M.T.; Wang, W.; Xia, J.Y.; Zuna, R.E.; et al. Human Tumor Antigens Tn and Sialyl Tn Arise from Mutations in Cosmc. *Cancer Res.* **2008**, *68*, 1636–1646. [CrossRef]
20. Ju, T.; Aryal, R.P.; Stowell, C.J.; Cummings, R.D. Regulation of Protein O-Glycosylation by the Endoplasmic Reticulum-Localized Molecular Chaperone Cosmc. *J. Cell Biol.* **2008**, *182*, 531–542. [CrossRef]
21. Mong, T.K.; Lee, H.K.; Duron, S.G.; Wong, C.H. Reactivity-Based One-Pot Total Synthesis of Fucose GM1 Oligosaccharide: a Sialylated Antigenic Epitope of Small-Cell Lung Cancer. *Proc. Natl. Acad. Sci. USA* **2003**, *100*, 797–802. [CrossRef] [PubMed]
22. Seeberger, P.H. Automated Oligosaccharide Synthesis. *Chem. Soc. Rev.* **2008**, *37*, 19–28. [CrossRef] [PubMed]
23. Buskas, T.; Thompson, P.; Boons, G.J. Immunotherapy for Cancer: Synthetic Carbohydrate-Based Vaccines. *Chem. Commun.* **2009**, 5335–5349. [CrossRef] [PubMed]
24. Maddaly, R.; Pai, G.; Balaji, S.; Sivaramakrishnan, P.; Srinivasan, L.; Sunder, S.S.; Paul, S.F.D. Receptors and Signaling Mechanisms for B-lymphocyte Activation, Proliferation and Differentiation—Insights from Both in vivo and in vitro Approaches. *FEBS Lett.* **2010**, *584*, 4883–4894. [CrossRef] [PubMed]
25. Xu, Y.; Sette, A.; Sidney, J.; Gendler, S.J.; Franco, A. Tumor-Associated Carbohydrate Antigens: A Possible Avenue for Cancer Prevention. *Immunol. Cell Biol.* **2005**, *83*, 440–448. [CrossRef] [PubMed]
26. Xu, Y.; Gendler, S.J.; Franco, A. Designer Glycopeptides for Cytotoxic T cell-Based Elimination of Carcinomas. *J. Exp. Med.* **2004**, *199*, 707–716. [CrossRef] [PubMed]
27. Smyth, M.J.; Cretney, E.; Kelly, J.M.; Westwood, J.A.; Street, S.E.; Yagita, H.; Takeda, K.; van Dommelen, S.L.; Degli-Esposti, M.A.; Hayakawa, Y. Activation of NK Cell Cytotoxicity. *Mol. Immunol.* **2005**, *42*, 501–510. [CrossRef]
28. Wang, W.; Erbe, A.K.; Hank, J.A.; Morris, Z.S.; Sondel, P.M. NK Cell-Mediated Antibody-Dependent Cellular Cytotoxicity in Cancer Immunotherapy. *Front. Immunol.* **2015**, *6*, 368. [CrossRef] [PubMed]
29. Chapman, P.B.; Wu, D.; Ragupathi, G.; Lu, S.; Williams, L.; Hwu, W.-J.; Johnson, D.; Livingston, P.O. Sequential Immunization of Melanoma Patients with GD3 Ganglioside Vaccine and Anti-Idiotypic Monoclonal Antibody That Mimics GD3 Ganglioside. *Clin. Cancer. Res.* **2004**, *10*, 4717. [CrossRef]
30. Chapman, P.B.; Morrisey, D.; Panageas, K.S.; Williams, L.; Lewis, J.J.; Israel, R.J.; Hamilton, W.B.; Livingston, P.O. Vaccination with a Bivalent GM2 and GD2 Ganglioside Conjugate Vaccine: A Trial Comparing Doses of GD2-Keyhole Limpet Hemocyanin. *Clin. Cancer. Res.* **2000**, *6*, 4658.

31. Ragupathi, G.; Koide, F.; Livingston, P.O.; Cho, Y.S.; Endo, A.; Wan, Q.; Spassova, M.K.; Keding, S.J.; Allen, J.; Ouerfelli, O.; et al. Preparation and Evaluation of Unimolecular Pentavalent and Hexavalent Antigenic Constructs Targeting Prostate and Breast Cancer: A Synthetic Route to Anticancer Vaccine Candidates. *J. Am. Chem. Soc.* **2006**, *128*, 2715–2725. [CrossRef] [PubMed]
32. Danishefsky, S.J.; Allen, J.R. From the Laboratory to the Clinic: A Retrospective on Fully Synthetic Carbohydrate-Based Anticancer Vaccines Frequently used Abbreviations are Listed in the Appendix. *Angew. Chem. Int. Ed. Engl.* **2000**, *39*, 836–863. [CrossRef]
33. Huang, Y.L.; Hung, J.T.; Cheung, S.K.; Lee, H.Y.; Chu, K.C.; Li, S.T.; Lin, Y.C.; Ren, C.T.; Cheng, T.J.; Hsu, T.L.; et al. Carbohydrate-Based Vaccines with a Glycolipid Adjuvant for Breast Cancer. *Proc. Natl. Acad. Sci. USA* **2013**, *110*, 2517–2522. [CrossRef] [PubMed]
34. De Silva, R.A.; Wang, Q.; Chidley, T.; Appulage, D.K.; Andreana, P.R. Immunological response from An Entirely Carbohydrate Antigen: Design of Synthetic Vaccines Based on Tn-PS A1 Conjugates. *J. Am. Chem. Soc.* **2009**, *131*, 9622–9623. [CrossRef] [PubMed]
35. Hossain, M.K.; Wall, K.A. Immunological Evaluation of Recent MUC1 Glycopeptide Cancer Vaccines. *Vaccines* **2016**, *4*, 25. [CrossRef] [PubMed]
36. Duke, J.A.; Avci, F.Y. Immunological Mechanisms of Glycoconjugate Vaccines. In *Carbohydrate-Based Vaccines: From Concept to Clinic*; ACS Symposium Series: Columbus, OH, USA, 2018; pp. 61–74.
37. Mazmanian, S.K.; Liu, C.H.; Tzianabos, A.O.; Kasper, D.L. An Immunomodulatory Molecule of Symbiotic Bacteria Directs Maturation of the Host Immune System. *Cell* **2005**, *122*, 107–118. [CrossRef]
38. Wang, Q.; McLoughlin, R.M.; Cobb, B.A.; Charrel-Dennis, M.; Zaleski, K.J.; Golenbock, D.; Tzianabos, A.O.; Kasper, D.L. A Bacterial Carbohydrate Links Innate and Adaptive Responses through Toll-Like Receptor 2. *J. Exp. Med.* **2006**, *203*, 2853–2863. [CrossRef]
39. Eradi, P.; Ghosh, S.; Andreana, P.R. Total Synthesis of Zwitterionic Tetrasaccharide Repeating Unit from Bacteroides fragilis ATCC 25285/NCTC 9343 Capsular Polysaccharide PS A1 with Alternating Charges on Adjacent Monosaccharides. *Org. Lett.* **2018**, *20*, 4526–4530. [CrossRef]
40. Mesa, C.; Fernandez, L.E. Challenges Facing Adjuvants for Cancer Immunotherapy. *Immunol. Cell Biol.* **2004**, *82*, 644–650. [CrossRef]
41. Yin, X.-G.; Chen, X.-Z.; Sun, W.-M.; Geng, X.-S.; Zhang, X.-K.; Wang, J.; Ji, P.-P.; Zhou, Z.-Y.; Baek, D.J.; Yang, G.-F.; et al. IgG Antibody Response Elicited by a Fully Synthetic Two-Component Carbohydrate-Based Cancer Vaccine Candidate with α-Galactosylceramide as Built-in Adjuvant. *Org. Lett.* **2017**, *19*, 456–459. [CrossRef]
42. Richichi, B.; Thomas, B.; Fiore, M.; Bosco, R.; Qureshi, H.; Nativi, C.; Renaudet, O.; BenMohamed, L. A Cancer Therapeutic Vaccine based on Clustered Tn-Antigen Mimetics Induces Strong Antibody-Mediated Protective Immunit. *Angew. Chem. Int. Ed.* **2014**, *53*, 11917–11920. [CrossRef]
43. Calvo, M.B.; Figueroa, A.; Pulido, E.G.; Campelo, R.G.; Aparicio, L.A. Potential Role of Sugar Transporters in Cancer and Their Relationship with Anticancer Therapy. *Int. J. Endocrinol.* **2010**, *2010*, 14. [CrossRef]
44. Annibaldi, A.; Widmann, C. Glucose Metabolism in Cancer Cells. *Curr. Opin. Clin. Nutr. Metab. Care* **2010**, *13*, 466–470. [CrossRef]
45. Herrmann, K.; Benz, M.R.; Krause, B.J.; Pomykala, K.L.; Buck, A.K.; Czernin, J. (18)F-FDG-PET/CT in Evaluating Response to Therapy in Solid Tumors: Where We are and Where We Can Go. *Q. J. Nucl. Med. Mol. Imaging* **2011**, *55*, 620–632.
46. Mahato, R.; Tai, W.; Cheng, K. Prodrugs for Improving Tumor Targetability and Efficiency. *Adv. Drug Deliv. Rev.* **2011**, *63*, 659–670. [CrossRef]
47. Carvalho, K.C.; Cunha, I.W.; Rocha, R.M.; Ayala, F.R.; Cajaiba, M.M.; Begnami, M.D.; Vilela, R.S.; Paiva, G.R.; Andrade, R.G.; Soares, F.A. GLUT1 Expression in Malignant Tumors and its Use as an Immunodiagnostic Marker. *Clinics* **2011**, *66*, 965–972. [CrossRef] [PubMed]
48. Lin, Y.S.; Tungpradit, R.; Sinchaikul, S.; An, F.M.; Liu, D.Z.; Phutrakul, S.; Chen, S.T. Targeting the Delivery of Glycan-Based Paclitaxel Prodrugs to Cancer Cells via Glucose Transporters. *J. Med. Chem.* **2008**, *51*, 7428–7441. [CrossRef]
49. Deng, D.; Xu, C.; Sun, P.; Wu, J.; Yan, C.; Hu, M.; Yan, N. Crystal Structure of the Human Glucose Transporter GLUT1. *Nature* **2014**, *510*, 121–125. [CrossRef]

50. Pohl, J.; Bertram, B.; Hilgard, P.; Nowrousian, M.R.; Stuben, J.; Wiessler, M. D-19575–a Sugar-Linked Isophosphoramide Mustard Derivative Exploiting Transmembrane Glucose Transport. *Cancer Chemother. Pharmacol.* **1995**, *35*, 364–370. [CrossRef]
51. Briasoulis, E.; Judson, I.; Pavlidis, N.; Beale, P.; Wanders, J.; Groot, Y.; Veerman, G.; Schuessler, M.; Niebch, G.; Siamopoulos, K.; et al. Phase I trial of 6-hour Infusion of Glufosfamide, a New Alkylating Agent with Potentially Enhanced Selectivity for Tumors that Overexpress Transmembrane Glucose Transporters: a Study of the European Organization for Research and Treatment of Cancer Early Clinical Studies Group. *J. Clin. Oncol.* **2000**, *18*, 3535–3544.
52. Blanchette, J.; Peppas, N.A. Oral Chemotherapeutic Delivery: Design and Cellular Response. *Ann. Biomed. Eng.* **2005**, *33*, 142–149. [CrossRef]
53. Puranik, A.S.; Pao, L.P.; White, V.M.; Peppas, N.A. Synthesis and Characterization of pH-Responsive Nanoscale Hydrogels for Oral Delivery of Hydrophobic Therapeutics. *Eur. J. Pharm. Biopharm.* **2016**, *108*, 196–213. [CrossRef]
54. Ranjbari, J.; Mokhtarzadeh, A.; Alibakhshi, A.; Tabarzad, M.; Hejazi, M.; Ramezani, M. Anti-Cancer Drug Delivery Using Carbohydrate-Based Polymers. *Curr. Pharm. Des.* **2018**, *23*, 6019–6032. [CrossRef]
55. Posocco, B.; Dreussi, E.; De Santa, J.; Toffoli, G.; Abrami, M.; Musiani, F.; Grassi, M.; Farra, R.; Tonon, F.; Grassi, G.; et al. Polysaccharides for the Delivery of Antitumor Drugs. *Materials* **2015**, *8*, 2569–2615. [CrossRef]
56. Martínez-Carmona, M.; Lozano, D.; Colilla, M.; Vallet-Regí, M. Lectin-Conjugated pH-Responsive Mesoporous Silica Nanoparticles for Targeted Bone Cancer Treatment. *Acta Biomater.* **2018**, *65*, 393–404. [CrossRef] [PubMed]
57. Miot-Noirault, E.; Reux, B.; Debiton, E.; Madelmont, J.C.; Chezal, J.M.; Coudert, P.; Weber, V. Preclinical Investigation of Tolerance and Antitumour Activity of New Fluorodeoxyglucose-Coupled Chlorambucil Alkylating Agents. *Invest. New Drug.* **2011**, *29*, 424–433. [CrossRef]
58. Mandai, T.; Okumoto, H.; Oshitari, T.; Nakanishi, K.; Mikuni, K.; Hara, K.; Hara, K.; Iwatani, W.; Amano, T.; Nakamura, K.; et al. Synthesis and Biological Evaluation of Water Soluble Taxoids Bearing Sugar Moieties. *Heterocycles* **2001**, *54*, 561–566. [CrossRef]
59. Mikuni, K.; Nakanishi, K.; Hara, K.; Hara, K.; Iwatani, W.; Amano, T.; Nakamura, K.; Tsuchiya, Y.; Okumoto, H.; Mandai, T. In vivo Antitumor Activity of Novel Water-Soluble Taxoids. *Biol. Pharm. Bull.* **2008**, *31*, 1155–1158. [CrossRef]
60. Fu, Y.; Li, S.; Zu, Y.; Yang, G.; Yang, Z.; Luo, M.; Jiang, S.; Wink, M.; Efferth, T. Medicinal Chemistry of Paclitaxel and its Analogues. *Curr. Med. Chem.* **2009**, *16*, 3966–3985. [CrossRef]
61. Goff, R.D.; Thorson, J.S. Assessment of Chemoselective Neoglycosylation Methods Using Chlorambucil as a Model. *J. Med. Chem.* **2010**, *53*, 8129–8139. [CrossRef]
62. Reinhard, J.; Eichhorn, U.; Wiessler, M.; Kaina, B. Inactivation of O(6)-methylguanine-DNA methyltransferase by glucose-conjugated inhibitors. *Int. J. Cancer* **2001**, *93*, 373–379. [CrossRef] [PubMed]
63. Kumar, P.; Shustov, G.; Liang, H.; Khlebnikov, V.; Zheng, W.; Yang, X.-H.; Cheeseman, C.; Wiebe, L.I. Design, Synthesis, and Preliminary Biological Evaluation of 6-O-Glucose–Azomycin Adducts for Diagnosis and Therapy of Hypoxic Tumors. *J. Med. Chem.* **2012**, *55*, 6033–6046. [CrossRef] [PubMed]
64. Cao, J.; Cui, S.; Li, S.; Du, C.; Tian, J.; Wan, S.; Qian, Z.; Gu, Y.; Chen, W.R.; Wang, G. Targeted Cancer Therapy with a 2-Deoxyglucose–Based Adriamycin Complex. *Cancer Res.* **2013**, *73*, 1362. [CrossRef]
65. Cheng, H.; Cao, X.; Xian, M.; Fang, L.; Cai, T.B.; Ji, J.J.; Tunac, J.B.; Sun, D.; Wang, P.G. Synthesis and Enzyme-Specific Activation of Carbohydrate–Geldanamycin Conjugates with Potent Anticancer Activity. *J. Med. Chem.* **2005**, *48*, 645–652. [CrossRef] [PubMed]
66. Patra, M.; Awuah, S.G.; Lippard, S.J. Chemical Approach to Positional Isomers of Glucose–Platinum Conjugates Reveals Specific Cancer Targeting through Glucose-Transporter-Mediated Uptake in Vitro and in Vivo. *J. Am. Chem. Soc.* **2016**, *138*, 12541–12551. [CrossRef] [PubMed]
67. Lee, H.Y.; Kwon, J.-T.; Koh, M.; Cho, M.-H.; Park, S.B. Enhanced Efficacy of 7-hydroxy-3-methoxycadalene *via* Glycosylation in In vivo Xenograft Study. *Bioorg. Med. Chem. Lett.* **2007**, *17*, 6335–6339. [CrossRef] [PubMed]
68. Gynther, M.; Ropponen, J.; Laine, K.; Leppänen, J.; Haapakoski, P.; Peura, L.; Järvinen, T.; Rautio, J. Glucose Promoiety Enables Glucose Transporter Mediated Brain Uptake of Ketoprofen and Indomethacin Prodrugs in Rats. *J. Med. Chem.* **2009**, *52*, 3348–3353. [CrossRef] [PubMed]

69. Hwu, J.R.; Hsu, C.-I.; Hsu, M.-H.; Liang, Y.-C.; Huang, R.C.C.; Lee, Y.C. Glycosylated Nordihydroguaiaretic Acids as Anti-Cancer Agents. *Bioorg. Med. Chem. Lett.* **2011**, *21*, 380–382. [CrossRef]
70. Ohtsubo, K.; Marth, J.D. Glycosylation in Cellular Mechanisms of Health and Disease. *Cell* **2006**, *126*, 855–867. [CrossRef]
71. Stanley, P. Golgi Glycosylation. *Cold Spring Harb Perspect Biol.* **2011**, *3*, 1–13. [CrossRef]
72. Ho, W.-L.; Hsu, W.-M.; Huang, M.-C.; Kadomatsu, K.; Nakagawara, A. Protein Glycosylation in Cancers and its Potential Therapeutic Applications in Neuroblastoma. *J. Hematol. Oncol.* **2016**, *9*, 100. [CrossRef] [PubMed]
73. Nash, R.J.; Kato, A.; Yu, C.Y.; Fleet, G.W. Iminosugars as Therapeutic Agents: Recent Advances and Promising Trends. *Future Med. Chem.* **2011**, *3*, 1513–1521. [CrossRef] [PubMed]
74. Fiaux, H.; Popowycz, F.; Favre, S.; Schütz, C.; Vogel, P.; Gerber-Lemaire, S.; Juillerat-Jeanneret, L. Functionalized Pyrrolidines Inhibit α-Mannosidase Activity and Growth of Human Glioblastoma and Melanoma Cells. *J. Med. Chem.* **2005**, *48*, 4237–4246. [CrossRef] [PubMed]
75. Vallee, F.; Karaveg, K.; Herscovics, A.; Moremen, K.W.; Howell, P.L. Structural Basis for Catalysis and Inhibition of N-glycan Processing Class I alpha 1,2-mannosidases. *J. Biol. Chem.* **2000**, *275*, 41287–41298. [CrossRef] [PubMed]
76. Popowycz, F.; Gerber-Lemaire, S.; Schütz, C.; Vogel, P. Syntheses and Glycosidase Inhibitory Activities of 2-(Aminomethyl)-5-(hydroxymethyl)pyrrolidine-3,4-diol Derivatives. *Helv. Chim. Acta* **2004**, *87*, 800–810. [CrossRef]
77. Allan, G.; Ouadid-Ahidouch, H.; Sanchez-Fernandez, E.M.; Risquez-Cuadro, R.; Fernandez, J.M.; Ortiz-Mellet, C.; Ahidouch, A. New Castanospermine Glycoside Analogues Inhibit Breast Cancer Cell Proliferation and Induce Apoptosis Without Affecting Normal Cells. *PLoS One* **2013**, *8*, e76411. [CrossRef] [PubMed]
78. Dal Piaz, F.; Vassallo, A.; Chini, M.G.; Cordero, F.M.; Cardona, F.; Pisano, C.; Bifulco, G.; De Tommasi, N.; Brandi, A. Natural Iminosugar (+)-Lentiginosine Inhibits ATPase and Chaperone Activity of Hsp90. *PLOS ONE* **2012**, *7*, e43316. [CrossRef]
79. Namikawa, T.; Kawanishi, Y.; Fujisawa, K.; Munekage, E.; Iwabu, J.; Munekage, M.; Maeda, H.; Kitagawa, H.; Kobayashi, M.; Hanazaki, K. Serum Carbohydrate Antigen 125 is a Significant Prognostic Marker in Patients with Unresectable Advanced or Recurrent Gastric Cancer. *Surg. Today* **2018**, *48*, 388–394. [CrossRef]
80. Dube, D.H.; Bertozzi, C.R. Metabolic Oligosaccharide Engineering as a Tool for Glycobiology. *Curr. Opin. Chem. Biol.* **2003**, *7*, 616–625. [CrossRef]
81. Evellyne de Oliveira, F.; Cassia Regina Albuquerque da, C.; Priscilla, B.S.A.; Raiana Apolinario de, P.; Mary Angela, A.-S.; Matheus Silva, A.; Adrielle, Z.; Maria, G.C.-d.-C.; Luis Claudio Nascimento da, S.; Maria Tereza dos Santos, C. Lectin-Carbohydrate Interactions: Implications for the Development of New Anticancer Agents. *Curr. Med. Chem.* **2017**, *24*, 3667–3680.
82. Coulibaly, F.C.; Youan, B.-B. Current Status of Lectin-Based Cancer Diagnosis and Therapy. *AIMS Mol. Sci.* **2017**, *4*, 1–27.

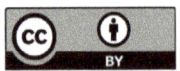

© 2019 by the authors. Licensee MDPI, Basel, Switzerland. This article is an open access article distributed under the terms and conditions of the Creative Commons Attribution (CC BY) license (http://creativecommons.org/licenses/by/4.0/).

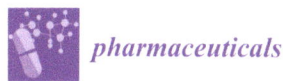

Review

Strategies for the Development of Glycomimetic Drug Candidates

Rachel Hevey

Molecular Pharmacy, Dept. Pharmaceutical Sciences, University of Basel, Klingelbergstr. 50, 4056 Basel, Switzerland; rachel.hevey@unibas.ch

Received: 15 March 2019; Accepted: 9 April 2019; Published: 11 April 2019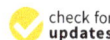

Abstract: Carbohydrates are a structurally-diverse group of natural products which play an important role in numerous biological processes, including immune regulation, infection, and cancer metastasis. Many diseases have been correlated with changes in the composition of cell-surface glycans, highlighting their potential as a therapeutic target. Unfortunately, native carbohydrates suffer from inherently weak binding affinities and poor pharmacokinetic properties. To enhance their usefulness as drug candidates, 'glycomimetics' have been developed: more drug-like compounds which mimic the structure and function of native carbohydrates. Approaches to improve binding affinities (e.g., deoxygenation, pre-organization) and pharmacokinetic properties (e.g., limiting metabolic degradation, improving permeability) have been highlighted in this review, accompanied by relevant examples. By utilizing these strategies, high-affinity ligands with optimized properties can be rationally designed and used to address therapies for novel carbohydrate-binding targets.

Keywords: carbohydrate; glycomimetic; drug development; lectin; lead optimization; binding affinity

1. Introduction

As one of the most abundant natural products, carbohydrates play many integral roles throughout our environment, for example as a metabolic energy source, a structural component of cell walls, and cellular recognition. They are present as various biological conjugates, including glycoproteins, proteoglycans, and glycolipids, and typically form a thick layer at the cell surface of approximately 10–100 Å which is referred to as the 'glycocalyx' [1,2]. This expression at the extracellular surface makes them ideally suited for interactions with neighboring cells and biomolecules.

In mammals, oligosaccharides are comprised of unique combinations of a defined group of monosaccharide residues which exhibit impressive structural complexity [3]. In contrast to amino acids and nucleotides which are typically assembled in a linear fashion, carbohydrates can form both linear and branched structures with contiguous stereocenters, affording a diverse array of structures. In addition to varying stereochemistry and regiochemistry of their glycosidic linkages, the monosaccharides forming these complex structures can also vary in their ring size (e.g., furanose, pyranose) and are often further modified (e.g., acetylation, sulfation, methylation) (Figure 1). The syntheses of oligosaccharides in vivo are accomplished by carbohydrate-processing enzymes: (i) glycosylases, which hydrolyze terminal residues; (ii) glycosyltransferases, which add residues to an existing structure; and (iii) other glycan-processing enzymes, such as sulfotransferases, which structurally fine tune individual functional groups.

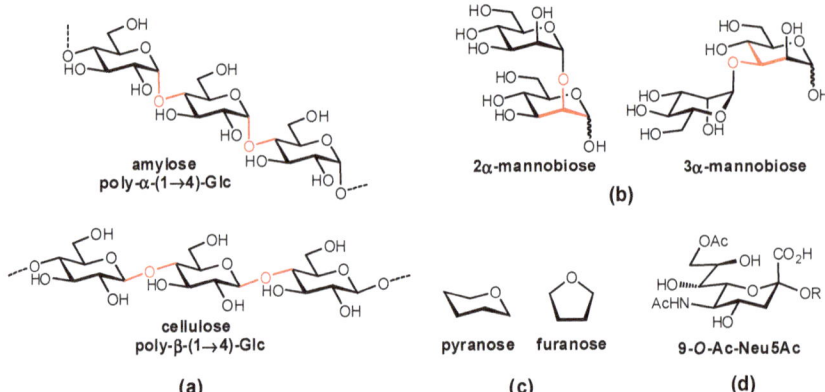

Figure 1. Structural variation in glycans arises from differences in: (**a**) anomeric stereochemistry; (**b**) regiochemistry of linkages; (**c**) ring size; and (**d**) further covalent modifications.

Carbohydrate structures attached to proteins are commonly classified as either O-linked (e.g., to serine or threonine amino acid side chains) or N-linked (e.g., to asparagine side chains). The biosyntheses of these two groups occur via two distinct mechanisms. O-Linked glycans are synthesized in a much more straightforward fashion: a monosaccharide is first transferred to the Ser/Thr sidechain and then other glycosyltransferases subsequently add to the structure, making it increasingly complex. In contrast, the formation of N-linked glycans involves the initial assembly of a complex oligosaccharide onto a phospholipid scaffold (dolichyl pyrophosphate), which then gets transferred within the endoplasmic reticulum to a protein asparagine residue; the glycan is then further elaborated through a combination of glycosidases which can partially deconstruct the original glycan construct, and glycosyltransferases which add additional sugar residues. Further functionalization of the glycan can then occur via the addition of acetate, sulfate, phosphate, or other groups to various positions of the oligosaccharide.

Proteins which bind to carbohydrate ligands can be broadly classified into enzymatic proteins (e.g., glycosidases, glycosyltransferases), lectins (non-enzymatic, signaling proteins), or glycosaminoglycan-binding proteins. Lectins play a prominent role in host recognition processes, and are primarily located at the cell surface but can also be found as soluble proteins. Lectins can be further classified into various sub-groups, such as the C-type lectins (e.g., selectins) which require Ca^{2+} ions for protein binding and play an integral role in intercellular adhesion and pathogen recognition, or I-type lectins (e.g., Siglecs) which are part of the immunoglobulin superfamily and are important for immune regulation. The affinities of carbohydrate-protein interactions are characteristically very weak, with dissociation constants (K_d) in the range of micromolar to millimolar, which has typically been attributed to several factors. Firstly, they lack hydrophobic functional groups and are therefore unable to form hydrophobic interactions with the protein surface; hydrophobic interactions are typically a feature of high affinity interactions. Secondly, their affinity often relies on hydrogen-bonding (H-bonding) interactions with the protein surface and they have a difficult time competing with H-bonding from bulk solvent. Thirdly, since the relatively shallow, solvent-accessible protein binding site and polar surface area of the ligands both form extensive H-bonding networks with bulk solvent, this needs to be removed prior to ligand-protein association and results in large enthalpic penalties for desolvation. Finally, flexibility in their structures can result in high entropic penalties for protein binding.

1.1. Carbohydrates in Disease

Carbohydrates play an important role in a number of biological processes, such as cell adhesion, inflammatory migration, host-pathogen recognition, immune activation, and cancer metastasis [4–6]. Many diseases have been correlated with changes in the composition of cell-surface glycans, a direct result of the differential expression of glycosidases and glycosyltransferases in the diseased state. These altered protein expression levels cause a unique surface glycan composition (for example, hypersialylated or truncated structures) which potentially generates novel targets for disease therapies. Aberrant carbohydrate expression has been linked to various diseases such as cancer, infection (viral, bacterial, and parasitic), and immune dysregulation, among others. Modified glycan expression is not necessarily associated with disease, as it also occurs during different stages of tissue development, cellular differentiation, or inflammatory response.

In addition to aberrant carbohydrate expression, 'normal' glycans also play an important role in disease progression as they are often a target of invading pathogens and their associated toxins. For example, influenza uses haemagglutinin, one of its viral coat proteins, to bind cell-surface sialic acids on human cells, an essential process for facilitating entry of the virus into host cells [7]. Many bacterial toxins also target surface carbohydrates, such as the toxins from botulism, cholera, tetanus, and diphtheria, as well as plant toxins such as abrin and ricin [8].

1.2. Native Carbohydrates as Pharmaceutical Agents

Due to their extensive structural diversity, carbohydrates are excellent as recognition molecules and are a desirable target for drug development, but unfortunately suffer from a number of drawbacks when being considered as therapeutic ligands [9–11].

Since carbohydrates engage proteins through only low energy interactions (H-bonding, metal chelation, salt bridges, and weak hydrophobic interactions), the K_d values of lectins are typically in the high micromolar to millimolar range except for a few examples (e.g., cholera toxin binds its GM_1 ligand with approximately 1 µM affinity, and arabinose-binding protein binds arabinose with approximately 100 µM affinity) [12–14]. The weak interactions formed through protein binding are often unable to compensate for the steep enthalpic penalties required for desolvation of the polar substrate and shallow protein binding site, and therefore, lectins often also rely on multivalent interactions to improve binding affinities.

Native carbohydrate ligands have limited use as orally-administered therapies, since they are unable to passively cross the intestinal enterocyte layer. This passive permeation typically requires molecules of a low molecular mass, with limited polar surface area, and low numbers of H-bond donors and acceptors (in line with the Lipinski and Veber rules) [15,16]; the hydrophilicity of poly-hydroxylated carbohydrates (potentially with additional carboxylates, sulfates, etc.) prohibits this passive permeation.

Due to the ease at which bulk solvent can displace native ligands within the shallow binding sites, the k_{off} rates of lectin interactions are characteristically very high, contributing to very short residence times (often in the range of seconds) which contributes to their unsuitability as drug candidates. Once in the bloodstream, carbohydrates very quickly undergo renal excretion and clearance from the body, contributing to their extremely poor pharmacokinetic properties.

1.3. Development of Glycomimetic Drug Candidates

Glycomimetics are 'drug-like' compounds which mimic the structure and function of native carbohydrates, and have been thoroughly studied in the development of therapeutic candidates for both lectins and enzymatic carbohydrate-processing proteins [11,17]. Well-designed glycomimetics can impart enhanced affinities, increased bioavailabilities, and longer serum half-lives. Glycomimetic compounds can be designed to take advantage of additional interactions which are not present in the native counterpart, offering enhancements in both affinity and selectivity.

Several strategies have been used to overcome the poor drug-like character of carbohydrates, which are described within this review and accompanied by relevant examples. Strategies such as reducing ligand polarity, increasing affinity through the optimization of entropic and enthalpic binding components, ligand pre-organization, and improving pharmacokinetic parameters have all been examined.

In order to rationally design glycomimetics, as much information as possible about the ligand-protein binding event should be collected [11]. To date, the most informative and utilized approaches rely on X-ray crystal structures, nuclear magnetic resonance (NMR) experimentation, and molecular modeling. Crystal structures provide information about the mode of ligand binding, and can convey which functional groups are essential for binding and which should be tolerant to modification. In cases where a crystal structure is not available, computational homology models can be developed to obtain further information. Saturation transfer difference (STD) NMR and transfer Nuclear Overhauser Effect (NOE) NMR have both been used to obtain key information on ligand binding. STD NMR provides insights into which functional groups are in direct contact with the protein, while transfer NOE NMR experiments provide important information on the precise binding conformation that the ligand adopts while bound to the protein, which can be used for ligand pre-organization strategies to reduce entropic binding penalties. By combining information from multiple approaches one can establish which functional groups are most important for target binding, thereby suggesting which groups can be further tuned and modified, for example through bioisostere replacement, derivatization, or deoxygenation. Protein crystal structures can also be used to identify amino acid residues in the vicinity of the binding site which can be targeted for forming additional interactions, such as aromatic residues or hydrophobic pockets.

In silico approaches, useful for generating homology models, have also been developed to predict via molecular dynamics simulations which are the most relevant functional groups for ligand-protein binding; a recent publication by Sood et al. successfully ranked ligand functional groups as either 'critical', 'enhances binding', or 'not important', which could then be used to generate a pharmacophore and design appropriate glycomimetics [18]. Subsequent improvements in computational methods will prove very beneficial for aiding in glycomimetic design.

Apart from direct interactions between the ligand and protein surface, it is also important to consider the impact of structural waters on ligand binding. For highly constrained water molecules, often characterized by their presence in both liganded and unliganded crystal structures, they can typically be regarded as an extension of the binding site and therefore, interactions with these highly ordered waters can afford favorable enthalpic gains [19,20]. In contrast, H-bonding of the ligand to more mobile water molecules in the binding site can create significant entropic penalties by restricting the movement of the water molecule in the bound state. Several computational methods are in development to help with more accurately predicting structural water molecules and the strength of their interactions. Highly conserved water molecules have been important for considerations in developing glycomimetics against several carbohydrate-binding proteins, for example FimH and L-arabinose binding protein [19,21].

The development of glycomimetics has already proven successful in several cases, with multiple candidates reaching the clinic. These successes mostly target the enzymatic carbohydrate-processing proteins and have typically been based on transition state mimetics. Arguably the most widely known example, oseltamivir (Tamiflu®) is a glycomimetic inhibitor of influenza neuraminidase and is used in the treatment of influenza infection (Figure 2) [22,23]. Zanamivir (Relenza®) is another established neuraminidase inhibitor for influenza treatment [24]; both oseltamivir and zanamivir inhibit the cleavage of terminal sialic acid (Neu5Ac) residues on host cells, which is an essential process for viral propagation and thereby limits disease progression. Miglustat is an inhibitor of glucosylceramide synthase which has been used in the treatment of type I Gaucher disease to prevent the harmful accumulation of glucosylceramide [25]. Another successful family of therapeutic glycomimetics is the α-glucosidase inhibitors (miglitol, voglibose, acarbose) which have been used in the treatment of diabetes and lysosomal storage disorders [26–28]. These glycomimetics are again transition state mimics, and as the target protein α-glucosidase is present in the brush border of the small intestine, passive permeation of the drug through the gastrointestinal membrane is not required for drug activity. As can be seen for miglustat, miglitol, and other transition state glycomimetics which directly inhibit enzymatic processes, ionizable groups are an important chemical feature for mimicking the charged oxocarbenium transition state.

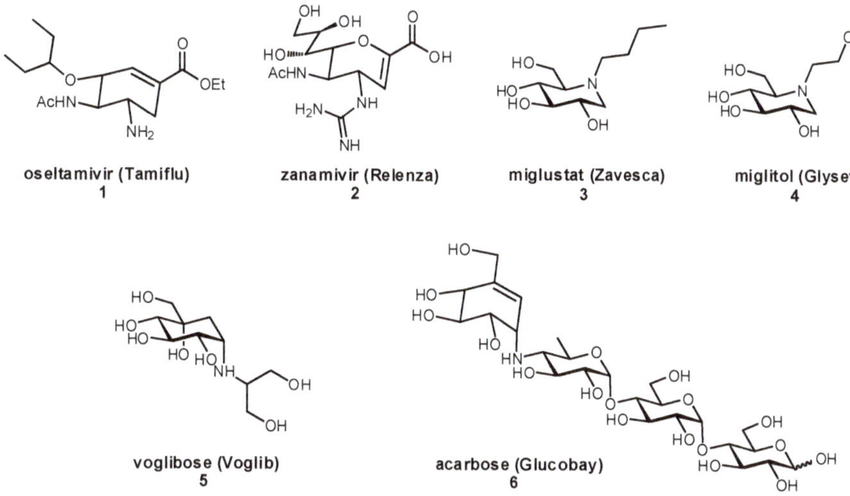

Figure 2. Examples of glycomimetic inhibitors that have successfully reached the market.

For diseases with an unmet clinical option, carbohydrates provide a promising target. In a time of increasing concern over antibiotic resistance, the emergence of anti-adhesive therapies offers a promising alternative [29,30]. Carbohydrates play an imperative role in the adherence of many pathogens to host cells, contributing to both infectivity and pathogen-avoidance of host clearance. Glycomimetic inhibitors, intelligently designed to have enhanced affinities over host cell-surface ligands, can be developed to prevent the adhesion of pathogens to host cells thereby facilitating clearance from the host; as adhesion does not affect overall survival of the pathogen, this approach is also at a considerably lower risk for developing resistance mechanisms. Since it is possible for bacterial and viral pathogens to express multiple types of adhesin proteins simultaneously, co-therapy including antibiotics and other anti-adhesives may ultimately be necessary for treatment success using this approach [31].

Interestingly, glycomimetics have also been used as antigens in carbohydrate-conjugate vaccines [32–37]. The non-native, glycomimetic structures have been observed to enhance immunogenicity, and if designed properly can elicit the production of antibodies that are cross-reactive with native glycans. Approaches to obtain glycomimetics with bioisosteric functional groups and glycosidic linkages have both been used in efforts toward vaccine development.

2. Glycomimetic Design – Strategies to Improve Binding Affinities

2.1. Deoxygenation

Several examples of glycomimetics have illustrated that a reduction in ligand polar surface area can enhance binding affinities by both generating new hydrophobic contacts with the protein, as well as reducing the enthalpic cost of ligand desolvation. Therefore, the removal of polar functional groups uninvolved in protein binding, most commonly the hydroxy moieties, has been well demonstrated to enhance binding affinities.

The thermodynamics of ligand-protein binding can be quantified by calculating the Gibbs free energy of an interaction, ΔG (Equation (1)), from its individual enthalpic (ΔH) and entropic (TΔS) terms, where a negative free energy is essential for productive binding events:

$$\Delta G = \Delta H - T\Delta S \tag{1}$$

To better understand the high enthalpic cost of desolvation, one can compare the thermodynamic quantities calculated by Cabani et al. [19,38]. The enthalpic penalty of desolvating a single hydroxy group, ΔH = 35 kJ/mol, is only partially offset by the favorable entropy term that results from the release of structured water molecules into bulk solvent, ΔS = 10 kJ/mol. This results in a net free energy of +25 kJ/mol, which cannot be compensated for by the energy gain afforded by a single H-bond (approx. ΔG = −18 kJ/mol). Although vicinal hydroxy groups experience a somewhat reduced desolvation penalty in comparison to individual hydroxy moieties (approx. ΔG = 34 kJ/mol for two vicinal hydroxy groups), the high enthalpic penalty of desolvation is still unfavorable for a binding event. This suggests that a minimum of two H-bonds should form between a ligand hydroxy group and the protein in order for the free energy of binding to be considered favorable. As exemplified in the literature, the removal of hydroxy groups forming only a single H-bond with the protein binding site typically enhances binding affinity. In order to optimize affinities in the design of glycomimetic ligands, the aim should be to form a larger number of high-quality H-bonds between each of the ligand's polar groups and the protein surface.

Although the desolvation penalty is often very high for carbohydrate-binding proteins, resulting in part from shallow and solvent-exposed binding sites, proteins with deeper binding pockets are inherently more hydrophobic, less solvated, and therefore often display enhanced affinities. In these hydrophobic binding cavities, the H-bonds between ligand and protein are considerably stronger (approx. 10-fold), experience less competition from bulk solvent, and also have improved residence times (reduced k_{off} rates) [19,39–42]. In these particular cases, where a lower desolvation penalty exists in combination with a higher enthalpic gain per H-bond, the requirement for generating such extensive H-bonding networks is reduced.

Alternative strategies have been used to reduce ligand solvation and thereby minimize the desolvation penalty: although not exemplified with a glycomimetic, Gao et al. nicely illustrated that the addition of a hydrophobic group in a non-binding, non-relevant position of a ligand was successful in disrupting water structure around the ligand and, therefore, reduced the enthalpic cost of desolvation [43]. Even though this portion of the molecule displayed no interactions with the protein surface, it was successful in enhancing the free energy of binding.

Deoxygenation can also provide other beneficial effects. By reducing overall polarity of the molecule, this can increase the electron density on the pyranose ring and thereby enhance nucleophilicity of its remaining hydroxy groups. This enhanced nucleophilicity can strengthen interactions involving complexation of metal ions or salt bridges. Alternatively, deoxygenation of 6-OH groups removes a rotational degree of freedom yet still leaves the C-6 methyl group intact for influencing $^4C_1/^1C_4$ pyranose conformational preference, which can further reduce the entropic costs associated with ligand binding.

Replacement of a hydroxy group with a fluorine atom has been used to experimentally probe the necessity of individual hydroxy moieties for H-bonding. This same strategy of OH → F substitution can also be applied in computational modelling. The fluorine atom is useful as a bioisosteric mimic of the hydroxy group, yet is also more hydrophobic and therefore, can retain important characteristics of the hydroxy moiety yet reduce polar surface area of the ligand [44]. Several studies have revealed that upon fluorine substitution, recognition of the mimetic by its native receptor is still possible; for example, in studying the transport of D-glucose across the endothelial membrane of red blood cells, 2-deoxy-2-fluoroglucose and 3-deoxy-3-fluoroglucose afforded very similar transport rates as compared to the native ligand [45]. In another study, fluorinated mimetics of MUC1-based glycopeptides were observed to be cross-reactive with serum antibodies from mice that had been vaccinated with native antigen (compound 7; Figure 3) [46]. This widespread recognition of fluorinated glyco-analogues has been a contributing factor to the success of ^{18}F-2-deoxy-2-fluoro-D-glucose (8) as a radiotracer for diagnosing neoplasia through positron emission tomography (PET) scans) [47,48].

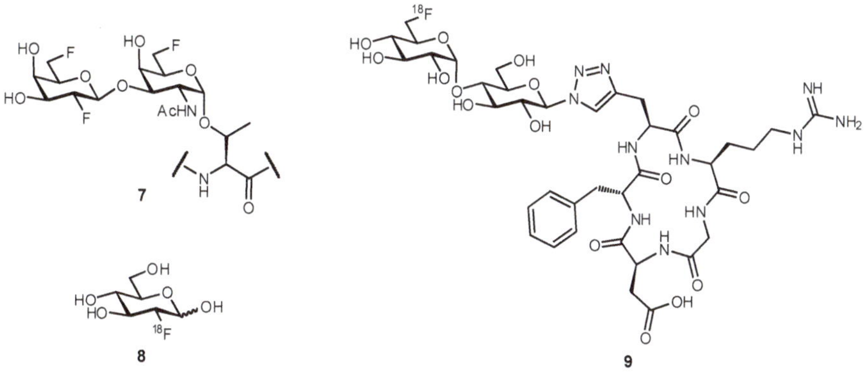

Figure 3. The bioisosteric replacement of hydroxy substituents with one or more fluorine atoms has proven successful in generating glycomimetics [46,48].

2.2. Biomimetic Replacement of Functional Groups

Biomimetic functional groups, i.e., those with comparable electronic and steric properties, can sometimes be used to replace existing functional groups to improve properties of a drug candidate. Bioisosteric replacement is a common practice in medicinal chemistry, with many families of bioisosteres having been reported and evaluated (Table 1). Given the specific requirements for a functional group in a particular binding event (e.g., steric restrictions, H-bond donor/acceptor properties), different bioisosteres can be considered as suitable replacements in different situations.

Table 1. Examples of bioisosteric groups.

Original Group	Potential Replacements
–H	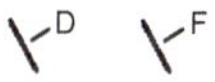 –D, –F
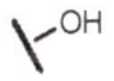 –OH	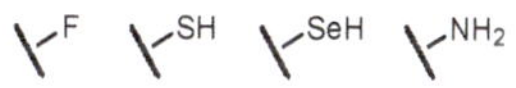 –F, –SH, –SeH, –NH$_2$
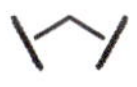 –CH=CH–	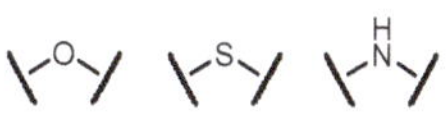 –O–, –S–, –NH–
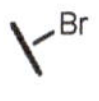 –Br	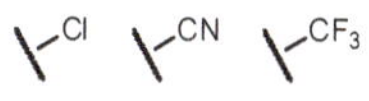 –Cl, –CN, –CF$_3$
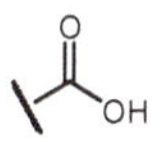 –C(O)OH	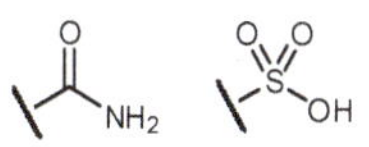 –C(O)NH$_2$, –S(O)$_2$OH

Bioisosteric replacement can afford enhanced affinities in a number of ways; for example, in the previously described OH → F substitutions [45,46,49], the fluorine atom can still facilitate polar interactions with the protein surface yet reduces overall hydrophilicity of the ligand. The fluorine atom can also be used as a suitable replacement for hydrogen, owing to its small size and relative hydrophobicity; replacement of the axial C-3 proton of sialic acid (Neu5Ac), to afford the glycomimetic 10 was successful in generating an inhibitor of sialyltransferase (Figure 4) [50,51]. Substitution with the fluorine atom afforded a ligand which was sterically compatible with the binding site, yet the unique electronic properties of fluorine generated a much more electrophilic anomeric carbon (C-2), improving antagonist ability. To overcome the negligible oral availability associated with such a polar substrate, the drug candidate was peracetylated; treatment in mice successfully impaired the progression of murine melanoma by inhibiting the attachment of metastatic cancer cells to the extracellular matrix and was also observed to slow down tumor growth in vivo.

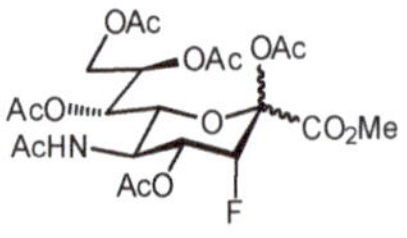

Figure 4. A Neu5Ac-based glycomimetic **10** was successful in preventing tumor metastasis in a mouse model [50].

In alternative biomimetic approaches, hydroxy groups binding to an active-site metal ion can be replaced with improved metal ligands, assuming that this modification is well tolerated by the binding site. Non-covalent interactions between sulfur and π-systems are typically stronger than those with oxygen atoms, suggesting a suitable route for further enhancing binding enthalpies. Aside from enhancing the enthalpic and entropic contributions of binding, bioisosteric replacement can also be useful for the removal of groups prone to metabolic degradation, or those that facilitate rapid excretion; these effects on the pharmacokinetic properties of a drug candidate will be discussed in more detail later.

2.3. Targeting Neighboring Regions of the Binding Site

For lectins with a well-structured binding pocket (which facilitates reduced entropic penalties upon generating additional interactions), it can be beneficial to look for new, enthalpically-favorable binding opportunities. The most promising approaches have targeted nearby aromatic or aliphatic residues and hydrophobic pockets, since ligand modification with hydrophobic groups has the added advantage of reducing the overall polar surface area of the ligand. Although, in general, hydrophobicity is preferred, additional interactions with neighboring ionic groups can also be realized, either through salt bridges or cation-π interactions. The overall approach for developing high-affinity glycomimetics is to optimize the individual entropic and enthalpic binding contributions; the majority of efforts in developing carbohydrate derivatives have focused on targeting surrounding protein sites that can both positively enhance binding contributions and also improve ligand selectivity against a particular target, with some examples highlighted below.

A large body of work has been focused on developing FimH antagonists, as an anti-adhesive approach to treating urinary tract infections (UTIs). UTIs are one of the most common causes of infection in developed countries, typically caused by uropathogenic *Escherichia coli* bacteria [52,53]. Antibiotic resistance has been of increasing concern for treating these infections, and therefore, the possibility of anti-adhesive treatment offers a promising alternative. Type 1-fimbriae on *E. coli* facilitate bacterial adherence to the bladder epithelium and enable the pathogen to avoid clearance during micturition; the FimH protein is located at the tip of the fimbriae, and binds to the highly mannosylated glycoprotein uroplakin 1a present at the epithelial surface [54,55]. Examination of the FimH crystal structure was very beneficial for glycomimetic development, as it provided pertinent information on the ligand binding mode and also suggested further modifications to improve ligand affinity [55]. It was observed that the 2-, 3-, 4-, and 6-OH groups of the D-mannose residue form an important H-bond network in the buried ligand cavity with amino acid side chains Asp54, Gln133, Asn135, and Asp140, and backbone atoms from Phe1 and Asp47. Not unexpectedly, attempts to modify these positions have generally proven unsuccessful. Alternatively, the region surrounding the binding site entrance contains two tyrosine residues and one isoleucine residue (Tyr48, Ile52, and Tyr137), often referred to as the 'tyrosine gate', which can form hydrophobic contacts with glycomimetics and have been a major target for improving the affinities of FimH antagonists. First developed were aryl and n-alkyl mannosides, which displayed increased affinities due to interactions with a hydrophobic rim surrounding the deep binding pocket and the aforementioned tyrosine gate. The groups of Janetka and Hultgren improved affinities by using 4′-biaryl mannosides with a meta substituent that could act as an H-bond acceptor (**11** and **12**), in which the aromatic extension formed an optimal π-π interaction with Tyr48 and a new H-bonding electrostatic interaction with Arg98/Glu50, resulting in nanomolar binding affinities (Figure 5) [56]. Contributions from many groups in the development of α-mannosides and oligomannosides have improved FimH antagonists even further [57–62].

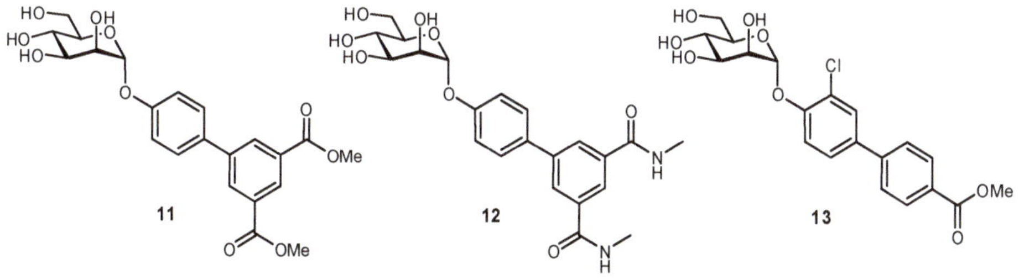

Figure 5. Biaryl mannosides have been successfully developed as nanomolar antagonists of the bacterial protein FimH [56,60].

The targeting of neighboring residues has also been used in the development of antagonists for FimH-like adhesin (FmlH) [31]. FmlH is a pilus adhesin which binds galactosides and N-acetyl-galactosaminosides presented on bladder and kidney tissue, facilitating the adhesion of *E. coli* to these surfaces. In efforts to inhibit this interaction, aryl galactosides and N-acetyl-galactosaminosides were designed which facilitated several key protein interactions: a π-π interaction with Tyr46, a salt bridge between the carboxylate and Arg142, and a H_2O-mediated H-bond between the N-acetyl group and Lys132. The best inhibitor (**14**) displayed a K_i of approximately 90 nM and upon administration in a mouse model was able to reduce the bacterial load in both the kidney and bladder (Figure 6). Co-treatment with a FimH antagonist further improved bacterial elimination.

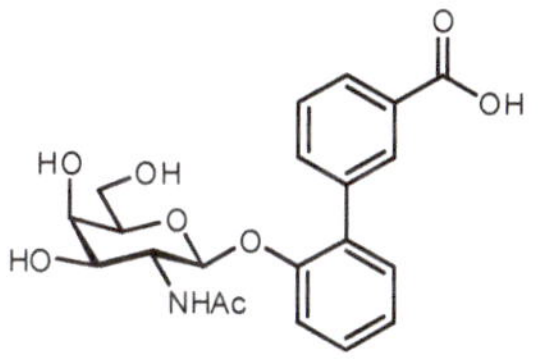

Figure 6. Biaryl glycosides have also been developed as antagonists of the adhesin FmlH; co-treatment with FmlH and FimH antagonists in a mouse model of urinary tract infection significantly facilitated bacterial clearance [31].

In addition to the aforementioned glucosylceramide synthase inhibitor miglustat, iminosugars have also been developed as protein chaperones with picomolar affinities for the treatment of Gaucher disease, the most prevalent lysosomal storage disease (LSD) [63]. LSDs ultimately result from a glycosidase deficiency, as glycosidases are important for the break-down of lysosomal glycosphingolipids. In LSDs such as Gaucher disease and Fabry disease, genetic mutations result in the misfolding of proteins, which are then targeted for degradation in the endoplasmic reticulum instead of being trafficked to the lysosome, resulting in significantly reduced lysosomal concentrations of protein. In pharmacological chaperone therapy, sub-inhibitory concentrations of a protein ligand can be used to stabilize the protein conformation, enabling successful trafficking of the protein to the lysosome; if designed appropriately, upon reaching the lysosome the protein should bind with higher affinity to its native ligand (also present in larger excess), thereby still retaining its native activity. In order to be effective as molecular chaperones, these glycomimetics should both be selective for their target, as well as reach the endoplasmic reticulum. This approach has previously been demonstrated for the glycomimetic 1-deoxygalactonojirimycin (Migalastat®; Figure 7), an inhibitor of α-galactosidase in vitro, which has been successfully used as a pharmacological chaperone in the treatment of Fabry disease [64,65]. Alternatively, glycomimetic inhibitors based on 1-deoxynojirimycin (DNJ) have been developed by Mena-Barragán et al. and García-Moreno et al. in the development of a therapy against Gaucher disease (Figure 7), which results from a β-glucocerebrosidase deficiency [63,66]. Modification of DNJ to form sp^2-iminosugars significantly enhanced targeting to the endoplasmic reticulum, and even more fortunately the ligands were found to have enhanced binding at neutral pH over acidic pH, which suggests that their affinity will decrease after entering the lysosome which should aid in protein dissociation and reduce competition with its native substrates. The iminosugars were found to successfully act as molecular chaperones for proteins expressed in mutated G188S/G183W fibroblasts (a disease-associated genetic mutation); for example, structure **20** afforded a more than 70% increase in protein activity at only 20 pM concentration, and a 300% improvement at a 2 nM concentration.

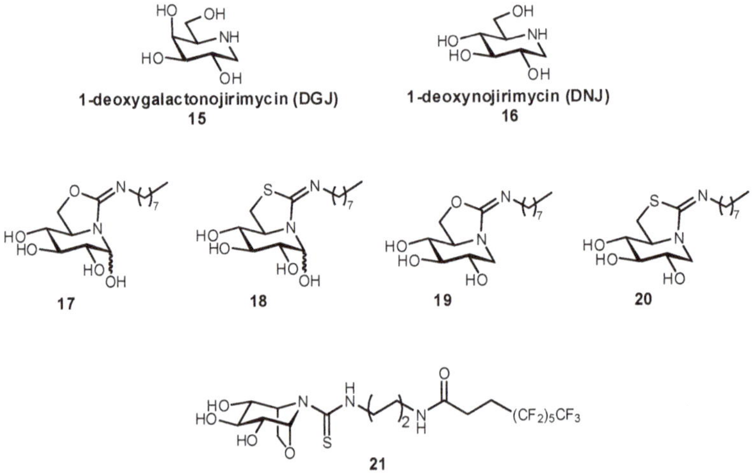

Figure 7. Iminosugars have been used as pharmacological chaperones, in efforts to treat lysosomal storage diseases [63,66].

Several other successful examples of ligand modification have been used to enhance the affinities of glycomimetics for their protein target. For example, Siglec-7 inhibitors have been synthesized which contain C-9 aromatic modifications (also targeting a 'hydrophobic gate' observed in the crystal structure) and/or triazole-containing hydrophobic groups at C-2 of Neu5Ac, in an effort to develop inhibitors which could prevent immune evasion by cancer cells (Figure 8) [67,68]. Similar in structure, Siglec-2 (also known as CD22) Neu5Ac glycomimetics containing a C-9 N-aromatic moiety, C-4 N-acyl derivative, and C-2 n-alkyl group have been used as inhibitors and towards drug conjugates to specifically target uptake into specific subsets of immune cells via Siglec-2-binding clathrin-mediated endocytosis (Figure 9) [69–71]. *Pseudomonas aeruginosa* lectin B (LecB) inhibitors have been developed in an effort to tackle biofilm formation: low molecular weight, nanomolar affinity ligands with good kinetic and thermodynamic properties were developed by targeting a hydrophobic patch on the protein [72]. Additionally, much work has been focused on DC-SIGN antagonists as anti-adhesives, by targeting a hydrophobic groove on the protein [73].

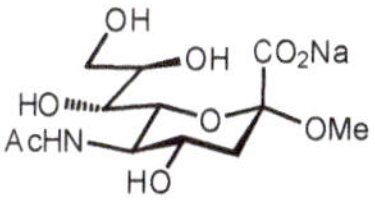

22
IC$_{50}$ 8000 µM

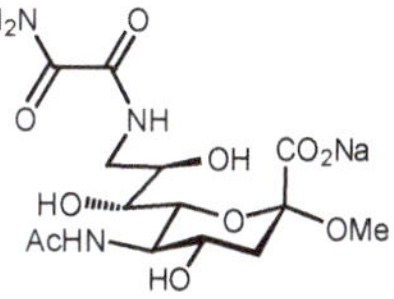

23
IC$_{50}$ 1642 µM

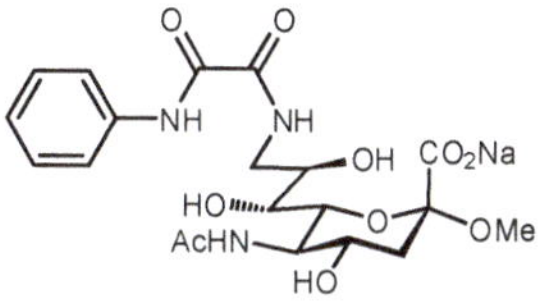

24
rIP 58 (based on 22)

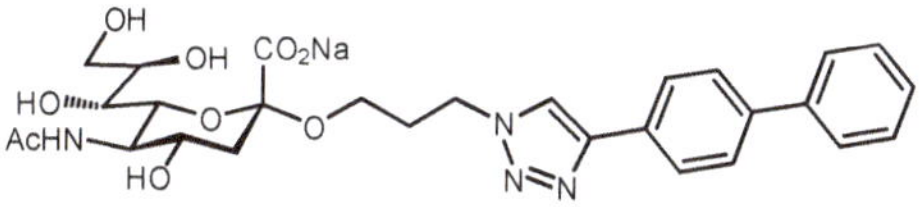

25
IC$_{50}$ 53 µM

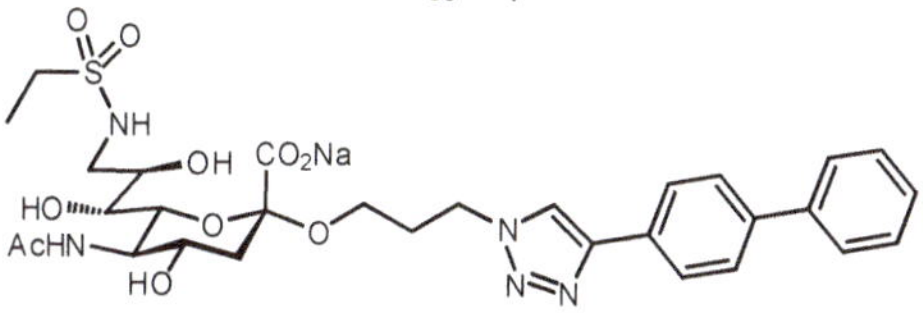

26
IC$_{50}$ 1.6 µM

Figure 8. Inhibitors of Siglec-7 which target additional protein interactions through modification at C-2 and C-9 positions (rIP = relative inhibitory potency) [67,68].

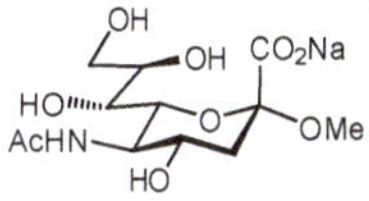

22
IC$_{50}$ 1475 µM

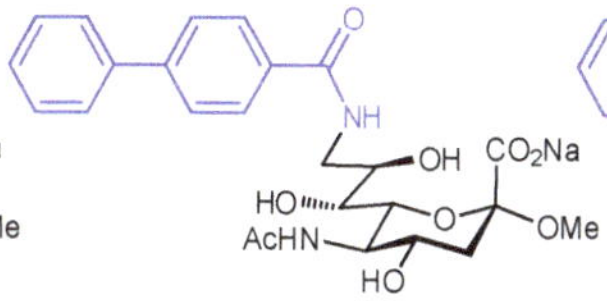

27
IC$_{50}$ 6 µM

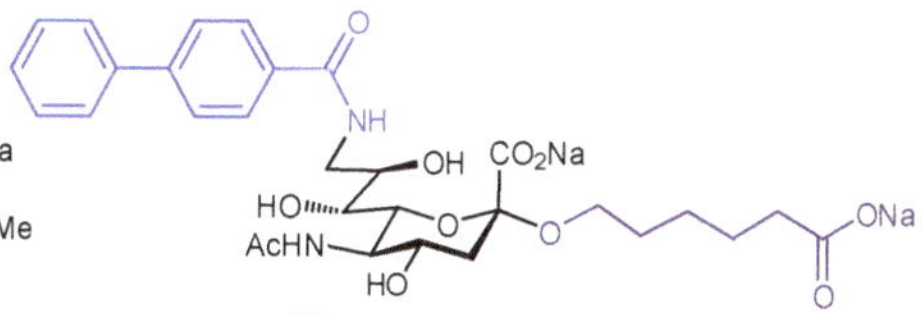

28
IC$_{50}$ 0.048 µM

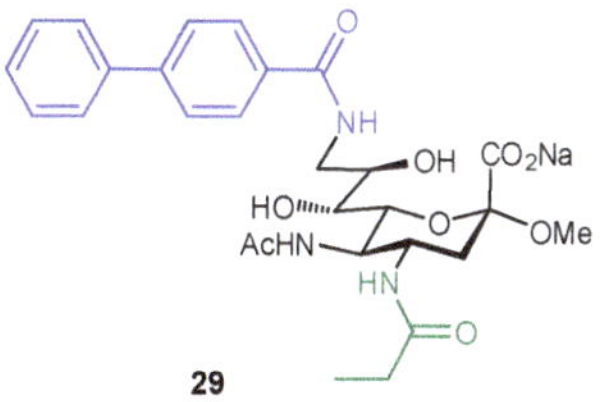

29
IC$_{50}$ 0.18 µM

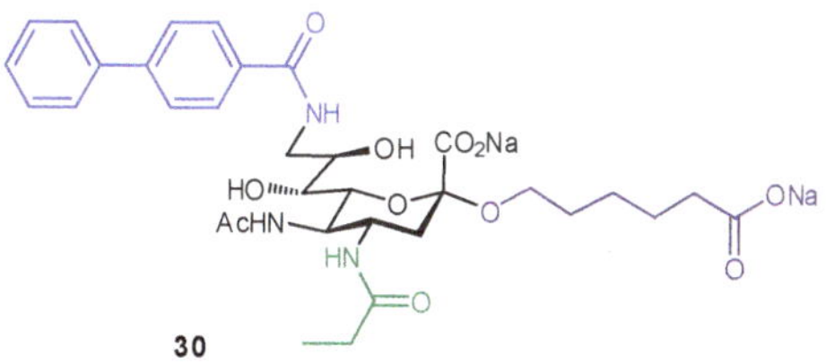

30
IC$_{50}$ 0.012 µM

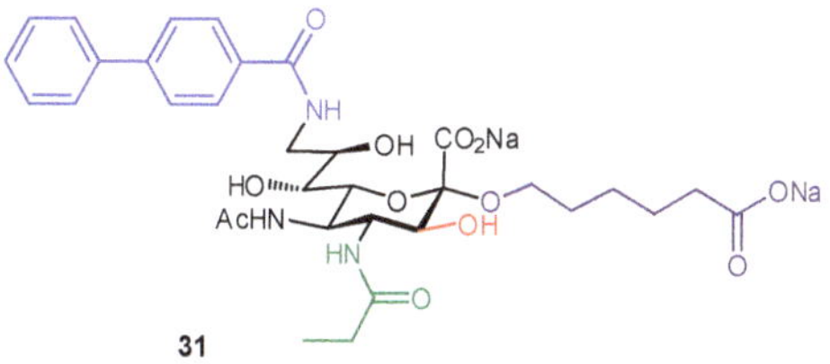

31
IC$_{50}$ 0.006 µM

Figure 9. High-affinity inhibitors of Siglec-2 generated through C-2, C-4, and C-9 modification of sialic acid [70].

A novel approach which also targets neighboring residues of a lectin binding site has been the development of a covalent lectin inhibitor against LecA of *Pseudomonas aeruginosa* [74]. Both LecA and LecB virulence factors have been associated with biofilm formation; although high affinity inhibitors against LecB have been developed, LecA has proven a more challenging target. In order to overcome the large k_{off} associated with LecA-ligand interactions, thereby enhancing affinity, a covalent inhibitor was developed which targets a nearby cysteine (Cys62) residue (Figure 10). This use of a covalent inhibitor attempts to circumvent the inherently weak affinities which arise from the short lifetimes of lectin-ligand complexes by permanently appending the ligand to the protein.

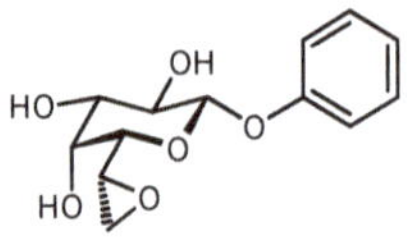

32
IC$_{50}$ 64 µM

Figure 10. The first reported covalent lectin inhibitor, targeting *Pseudomonas aeruginosa* LecA [74].

2.4. Conformational Pre-organization

Improvements in binding affinity through pre-organization have been successful in a number of glycomimetics [75,76]. Pre-organization reduces the entropic penalties associated with binding and additionally tends to reduce polar surface area since internal polar groups interact amongst each other, effectively shielding them from bulk solvent. Molecules have inherent entropy when free in solution, related to both translation and rotation (including internal rotation at single bonds). Entropic costs are associated with the binding of ligands, since a restriction of motion occurs through both a loss of rotational and translational entropy (for both ligand and protein); the greater the rigidity of the formed complex, the higher the entropic penalty of binding [77,78].

As mentioned previously, productive binding can only occur with a negative free energy; this requires that the unfavorable entropic costs from restriction of the binding site be offset by favorable intermolecular interactions of ligand binding, considering both enthalpic contributions (e.g., H-bonding, van der Waals, etc.) and entropic contributions (e.g., release of water molecules from the binding site). Flexible receptors which require an 'induced fit' binding mode suffer from even greater entropic binding penalties, since the protein loses much of its conformational flexibility, therefore requiring even greater enthalpic compensatory interactions to enable productive binding events.

Pre-organization has been shown to play an important role in the development of glycomimetic inhibitors. In the amino-glycosides, distortion of the pyranose ring has been used in efforts to mimic the flattened shape of the enzymatic transition state. This conformational distortion can be accomplished using a variety of approaches, such as the introduction of an sp^2-hybridized center, modification of the ring size, or by generating bicylic or bridged systems [13].

The importance of conformational pre-organization has also been observed in the generation of LecB inhibitors. Glycan screening indicated that the Lewis A (Le^a) trisaccharide, β-D-Gal-(1→3)-[α-L-Fuc-(1→4)]-D-GlcNAc, bound LecB with a K_d of 220 nM [79]. Attempts to simplify the structure eliminated the D-galactose moiety entirely to afford the disaccharide α-L-Fuc-(1→4)-D-GlcNAc, but unfortunately isothermal titration calorimetry (ITC) experiments indicated a significantly reduced binding affinity resulting from an increased entropic penalty [80]. To further simplify the construct and reduce flexibility, α-L-fucosides were modified with heterocyclic aglycone substituents to afford substrates which, in some cases, could bind with affinities similar to those of Le^a [81].

Another successful example of pre-organization was illustrated in the development of an E-selectin antagonist. The native ligand of E-selectin, sialyl Lewis X (sLe^x), binds with six solvent-exposed H-bonds and a salt bridge [11,82,83]. In efforts to improve the affinity of sLe^x, a glycomimetic antagonist was developed which could be pre-organized into the binding-site conformation, minimizing the entropic penalties associated with binding. Based on the crystal structure, it was observed that the N-acetyl-D-galactosamine moiety does not form direct contacts with the protein, but instead only acts as a linker between the other residues; therefore, it was replaced by a non-carbohydrate moiety that linked the D-galactose and L-fucose residues in a correct spatial orientation [84]. By strategically placing substituents on the linker, the structure could be even more rigidified to further improve pre-organization and thereby also antagonist affinity [85]. With later iterations, the Neu5Ac moiety was replaced by (S)-cyclohexyl lactic acid which even further rigidified the glycomimetic conformation [84].

The importance of pre-organization has also been demonstrated in the development of FimH antagonists, upon comparing septanose versus pyranose glycomimetic scaffolds (Figure 11) [86]. In an examination of binding to the conformationally rigid FimH lectin domain, the highly flexible septanose derivative resulted in a 10-fold affinity loss. NMR, X-ray crystal structure, and molecular modeling all indicated that the related septanose and pyranose derivatives formed a superimposable network of H-bonds, yet the septanose displayed lower affinities; ITC confirmed that this loss of affinity resulted from an entropic penalty arising from flexibility of the septanose core.

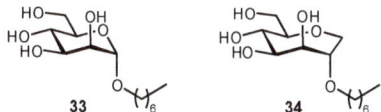

Figure 11. *n*-Heptyl pyranose and septanose FimH ligands have been used to study the effects of pre-organization on binding thermodynamics [86].

2.5. Multivalency

Numerous glycomimetics have incorporated multivalency in order to better mimic the multivalent presentation of native ligands [81,87–91]. Multivalency can improve binding affinities in several ways: (i) chelation; (ii) statistical rebinding effects; or (iii) clustering of soluble binding partners [92,93]. The design of multivalent scaffolds must be carefully considered in order to incorporate proper spacing and flexibility, enabling a correct fit of the ligand into the binding site, yet concomitantly minimizing the entropic costs of binding. In general, flexible scaffolds are often more forgiving if poorly designed, but suffer from much greater entropic penalties upon binding. A recent study from the Hartmann and Lindhorst groups has also nicely demonstrated that tuning scaffold hydrophobicity can also play a significant role in the affinity of multivalent constructs [94].

In an elegant study, DC-SIGN glycomimetic antagonists were conjugated to oligovalent molecular rods and used to study multivalency effects of binding, affording nanomolar antagonists (Figure 12) [93,95]. The constructs contained a rigidified core based on phenylene-ethynylene units (previously used in the generation of *P. aeruginosa* LecA inhibitors), and were designed to be an ideal length (approx. 4 nm) for chelation to bridge carbohydrate recognition domains on neighboring DC-SIGN subunits. The length of the rigid core could be controlled, with the rigidity effectively reducing entropic binding penalties, while the ends of the rods contained trivalent constructs which had been assembled using short, more flexible linkers. The incorporated trivalent groups were intended to address favorable statistical rebinding, with the flexible linkers aimed at facilitating a better fit of ligand into the binding site (at a minor entropic cost). This intelligent design (with appropriate control compounds) was able to probe the different effects of ligand, rigid rod, and proximity effects individually.

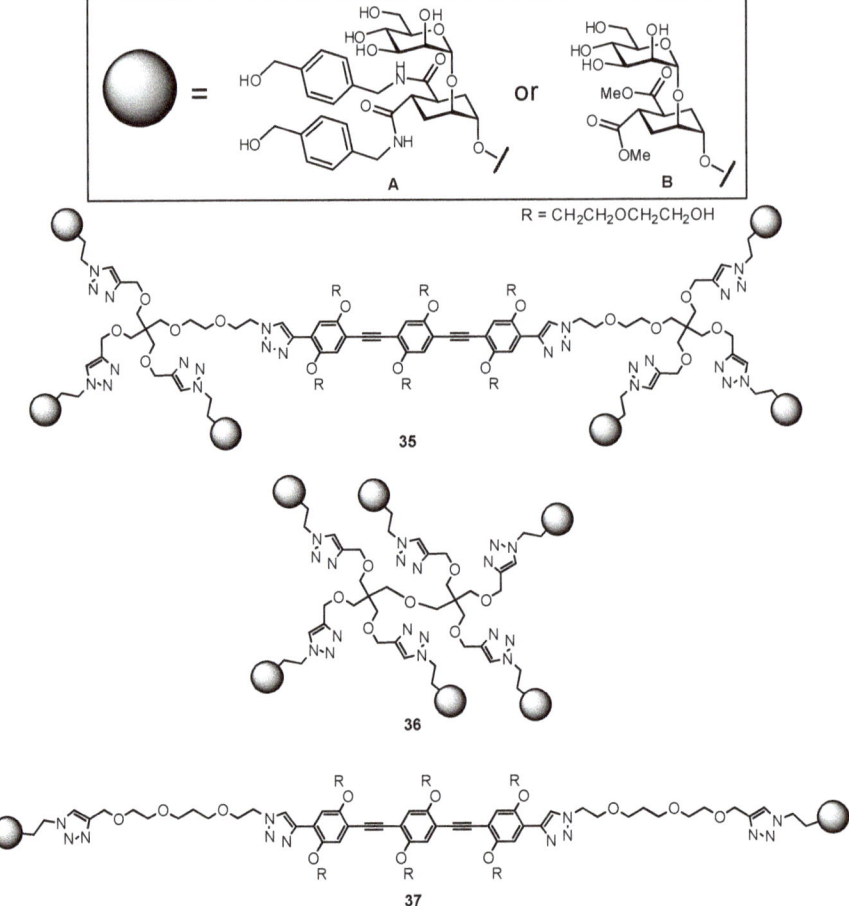

Figure 12. Multivalent constructs based on a DC-SIGN glycomimetic antagonist, used to probe the effects of chelation versus statistical rebinding multivalency effects [93].

Various other multivalent constructs have been generated in the development of carbohydrate-based pharmaceuticals, often with a lead monovalent glycomimetic being incorporated into a polyvalent construct at a later stage of project development. Multivalent constructs have targeted fucose-binding pathogenic soluble receptors, in efforts to improve the outcome of patients with cystic fibrosis, or alternatively to generate simplified mimetics of sLe^x that can mimic its native structure yet are easier to access synthetically [87].

3. Glycomimetic Design—Strategies to Improve Pharmacokinetic Properties

It has been well established that native carbohydrates display inherently poor pharmacokinetic properties [11,17]. They are sensitive to hydrolysis both in the gut and by endogenous proteins, they are not orally available, are rapidly excreted upon entering the bloodstream, and have very short receptor residence times. Many strategies have been used to improve these properties, with some overlap from the approaches used for affinity enhancement, and have been briefly outlined below.

3.1. Preventing Glycosidic Hydrolysis

Several approaches have been used in an effort to slow down the metabolic degradation of oligosaccharides, which are prone to hydrolysis both in the acidic environment of the gastrointestinal tract, as well as through endogenous enzymes (digestive, plasma, and cellular glycosidases). A major focus has been on generating O-glycoside mimetics, most commonly by replacing the bridging glycosidic oxygen atom with a more stable carbon atom, or alternatively by adding electron-withdrawing groups to the pyranose core to destabilize the oxocarbenium intermediate required for degradation. The metabolic stability of glycomimetics can be evaluated by examining the rate of degradation with serum or liver microsomes.

C-Glycosides can be used to improve the hydrolytic stability of oligosaccharides, but can also introduce new challenges due to an enhanced conformational flexibility, primarily resulting from a loss of the *exo*-anomeric effect [96]. Although the *exo*-anomeric effect cannot control the aglycone conformation in C-glycosides, in a number of examples steric bulk has been used to better restrict the aglycone unit in a gauche conformation, similar to that observed in O-glycosides [97–99]. There is indeed greater conformational flexibility observed, but it is evidently not as detrimental to binding as would be expected. Modification of the linked carbon atom with one or two fluorine atoms has also been used to enhance the electronegativity of the bridging unit and further limit its conformational flexibility, yet retain the benefit of the metabolically stable C-glycoside [100–102]. C-Glycosides have been used in the glycomimetic design of numerous inhibitors, including sLe^x [96], GM$_4$ ganglioside [103], galactopyranosides [104,105], mannopyranosides [105–107], fucopyranosides [105,108,109], and pseudoglycopeptides [106], among others.

In addition to the C-glycosides, other atoms or groups have been used to substitute the glycosidic linkage, aiming for an ideal balance between hydrolytic stability and conformational pre-organization. These include various N-linked glycosides, as well as selenium, sulfur, and even dithioacetal analogues (Figure 13) [32,110–114].

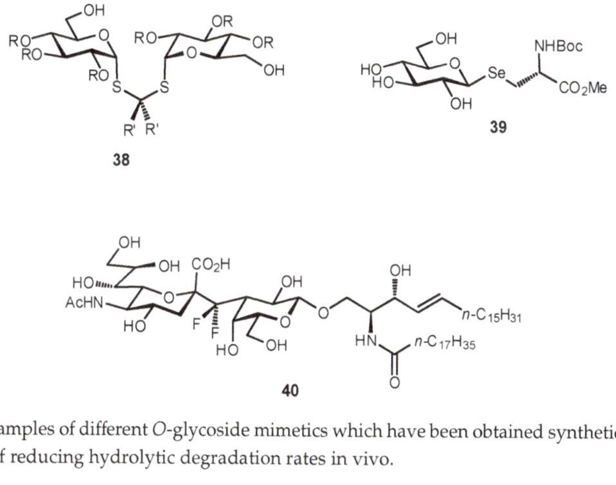

Figure 13. Examples of different O-glycoside mimetics which have been obtained synthetically, with the general aim of reducing hydrolytic degradation rates in vivo.

The biaryl mannoside antagonists of FimH for UTI therapy discussed previously were observed to suffer from very low bioavailability and rapid degradation in vivo, presumably due to metabolic instability of the O-glycosidic linkage in the acidic milieu of the stomach and intestinal tract, as well as to enzymatic mannosidases [115]. In order to improve pharmacokinetic parameters, C-glycoside derivatives were synthesized which indeed displayed enhanced stability and, in some cases, even improved inhibition (Figure 14); this improvement resulted in better efficacy in mouse models of both acute and chronic urinary tract infection. Replacement of the glycosidic linkage was also used for FimH antagonists developed as a potential therapy for patients affected with Crohn's disease, in an effort to reduce the bacterial load of adherent-invasive *E. coli* in the ileal mucosa [116]. Thiazolylaminomannosides were synthesized with an anomeric *N*-linked aryl moiety that could form a favorable interaction with Tyr48 as well as improve hydrolytic stability and solubility of the compound (Figure 15). Unfortunately, the high affinity *N*-linked glycans were observed to anomerize from the active α-mannoside to the inactive β-mannoside in the acidic environment of the stomach [117,118]. To circumvent this anomerization, the amino group was replaced by various linkages (-OCH_2-, -SCH_2-, -CH_2S-, -CH_2CH_2-, -OCH_2CH_2-, -CH_2NH-), which had been slightly extended compared to the first generation in order to improve π-π stacking with Tyr48; this strategy afforded optimized substrate **49** [117,119].

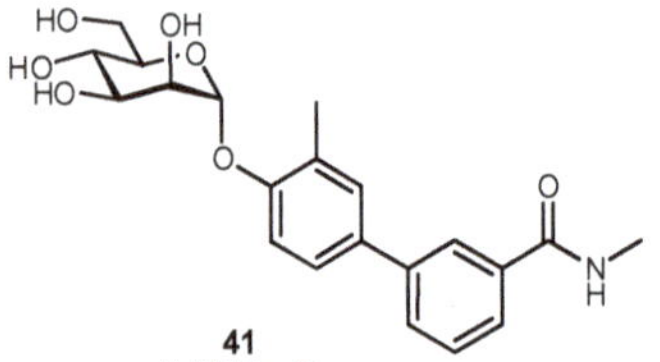

41
HAI 62 nM

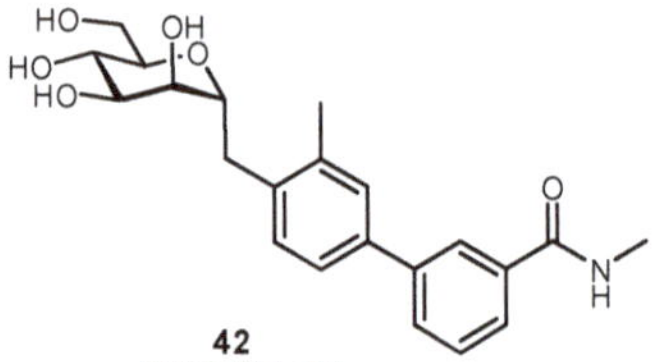

42
HAI 2000 nM

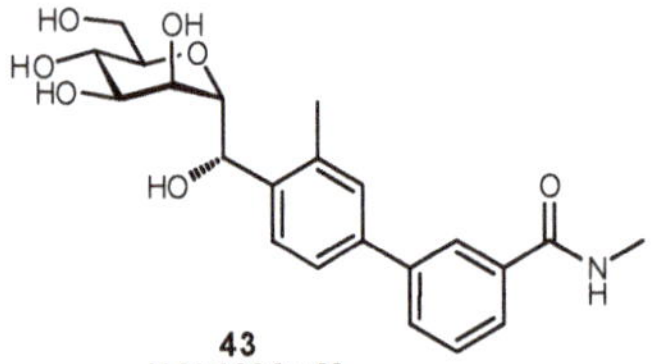

43
HAI 6000 nM

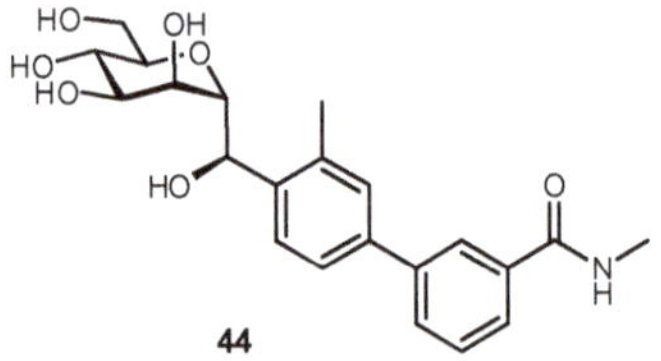

44
HAI 31 nM

Figure 14. The development of *C*-glycosides for treatment of UTIs has been used to improve the metabolic stability of biaryl FimH antagonists (HAI = hemagglutination inhibition assay) [115].

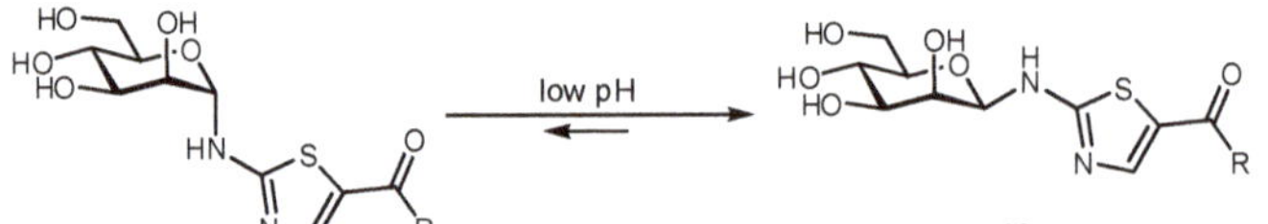

45
(active)

46
(inactive)

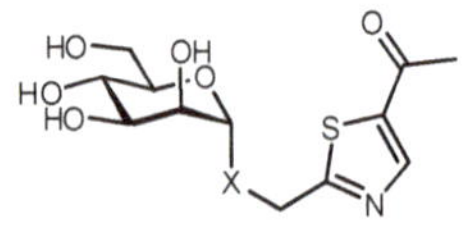

47
(X=O,S,CH_2)

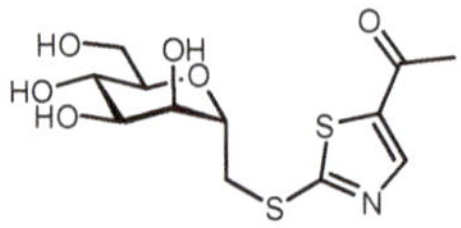

48

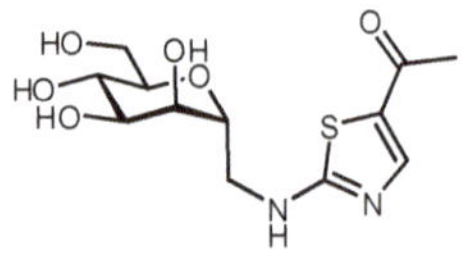

49

Figure 15. A comparison of *O*-, *N*-, *S*-, and *C*-glycosides as FimH antagonists for therapy in Crohn's disease [116,117,119].

Fluorination is well established to be an effective method for modulating the pK_a and pK_b properties of neighboring functional groups, thereby influencing the net charge of a molecule at physiological pH, the strength of ionic interactions, etc. In addition, it has been shown to enhance lipophilicity, and is often used in medicinal chemistry to block sites of undesired metabolism [100,120]. Although not widely used, potentially owing to its synthetic challenges, the fluorination of pyranose structures has been used to destabilize the oxocarbenium intermediate required for glycoside hydrolysis, thereby reducing the rate of metabolic degradation of glycomimetics.

3.2. Improving Oral Bioavailability

Native carbohydrates are not orally available due to their high hydrophilicity which prevents passive permeation across the intestinal membrane, but this can be improved by modifying carbohydrates to reduce their polar surface area. This can be achieved by using some of the techniques already discussed, such as deoxygenation of hydroxy groups or the addition of hydrophobic substituents. Appending a moiety which is known to undergo active transport into the bloodstream can also facilitate improved oral bioavailability. For example, specific amino acid sequences known to target peptide transporters (e.g., PEPT1, PEPT2) have been used; valacyclovir (Valtrex®), an antiviral drug targeting herpes simplex, contains the active component acyclovir (Zovirax®) conjugated to a valine which affords a five-fold increase in oral bioavailability [121,122].

Interestingly, pre-organization can also improve oral bioavailability, as it reduces the polar surface area and thereby substrates can more effectively permeate the membrane. This concept was nicely demonstrated in a study of peptides, where rigidified cyclic peptides were confirmed to have less exposed polar surface area when compared to more flexible cyclic peptides [123]. The rigidified peptides, with their buried polar groups, had better membrane permeability and metabolic stability.

An alternative to improving oral bioavailability is to use the prodrug approach [124]. By modifying a polar substrate with a hydrophobic moiety (e.g., through ester formation), the hydrophilicity becomes temporarily reduced enabling passive permeation through the membrane. Upon entry into the bloodstream, ubiquitous endogenous esterases can cleave the pro-moiety, unmasking the active component. With the condition that the esters are not cleaved prematurely by gastrointestinal esterases, this approach has been very important for improving the absorption of glycomimetic compounds, such as oseltamivir (Tamiflu®; Figure 16) [22,23,125]. Alternatively, for glycomimetics which have been modified with aromatic substituents to engage new protein interactions, they are often membrane permeable but suffer instead from poor aqueous solubility. In these instances, the prodrug approach can also be used to append a polar moiety which temporarily improves solubility. For example, phosphorylated prodrugs have been used in the development of FimH antagonists; this has proven a useful strategy for phosphorylated derivatives which undergo slower hydrolysis, as rapid hydrolysis can cause undesirable precipitation of the substrate (Figure 16) [24,126].

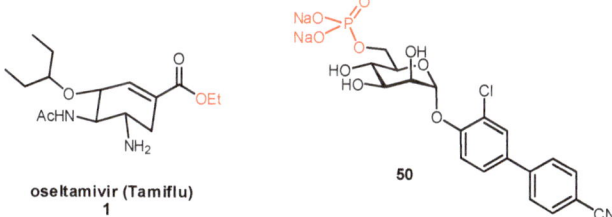

Figure 16. Prodrugs can be used to improve oral bioavailability, by improving factors such as intestinal epithelial membrane permeability (**1**, ester prodrug) or solubility (**50**, phosphate prodrug) [125,126].

3.3. Improving Residence Times and Plasma Half-lives

The residence times of lectins with their physiological ligands is typically in the range of a few seconds. In order for carbohydrate-based molecules to be suitable as therapeutics, it is necessary to extend both the residence time and circulation times (from minutes to hours) [127]. Several strategies have been utilized to improve the plasma half-lives of glycomimetics and to reduce their rate of clearance from the bloodstream. For example, the FimH antagonist **51** displayed high affinity but poor therapeutic potential as it was rapidly eliminated by the kidneys and had low reabsorption by renal tubules [128]. These poor pharmacokinetic properties were attributed to the carboxylate moiety which had been introduced for enhancing π-π interactions between FimH and the biaryl aglycone. To improve therapeutic usefulness, bioisosteres of the carboxylate were generated to afford FimH antagonists with optimized pharmacokinetic profiles (Figure 17). In comparison to the original substrate, some bioisosteres with greater hydrophobicity (reduced desolvation penalty) and conformational rigidity (reduced entropic cost of binding) even displayed enhanced affinities.

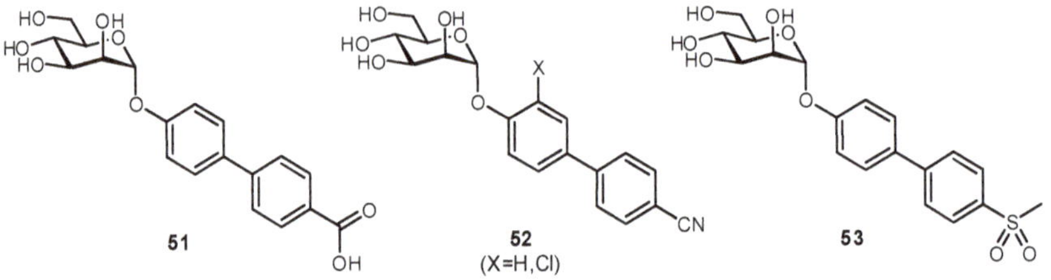

Figure 17. Bioisosteric replacement of a carboxylate moiety was used to optimize FimH antagonist **51** which suffered from rapid renal clearance and low tubular reabsorption in vivo [128].

Another approach involves removing functional groups from glycomimetics which enable active transport or are prone to metabolic degradation. For example, organic anion and cation transporters (OATs and OCTs, respectively) in the liver and kidneys can actively excrete certain glycoconjugates, and are often responsible for their very short half-lives [129]. OAT1 to OAT5 can recognize various anions connected to a hydrophobic ring. It has been demonstrated that the active oseltamivir metabolite is recognized by OAT transporters, and co-therapy with an OAT1 competitive inhibitor (probenecid) considerably improved serum half-life [130]. By elucidating which functional groups are responsible for active transport and/or metabolic degradation, these groups can be replaced by similar bioisosteres and/or modified by fluorination, an approach commonly used to block sites of cytochrome oxidation and other metabolic processes.

An alternative approach to increasing serum half-life is to append a moiety which is known to bind serum proteins, thereby increasing circulation time in the bloodstream. Plasma half-lives can be significantly extended when the carbohydrate ligand interacts with blood plasma components; for example, the heparins naturally bind to plasma proteins and display improved half-lives which make them more suitable for therapeutic use as anti-coagulants [131,132].

A somewhat drastic approach to glycomimetics is to completely replace the carbohydrate with a non-carbohydrate-based scaffold, and then to build in the essential functional groups while retaining their same spatial orientation as compared to the binding mode of the native ligand. Additional hydrophobic or charged moieties can also be appended to the scaffold to facilitate secondary interactions. A number of different scaffolds have been utilized in this approach to mimic either pyranoses or their enzymatic transition states, ranging from peptides to four-membered rings (such as oxetanes, azetidines, thietanes, and cyclobutanes; recently reviewed by Hazelard and Compain) [13,133–138]. Although potentially more difficult to design rationally, these scaffolds can offer additional advantages in terms of stability and more constrained structures (reducing entropic binding penalties). To identify novel scaffolds, the screening of molecule libraries has been utilized to identify potential new substrates which mimic the original glycan; these often rely on the generation of an antibody against the native glycan, with the antibody then used for screening to identify lead structures which can be further evaluated as competitive inhibitors. Although arguably less elegant, this strategy has been successful in identifying a mimic of Le^x which could elicit improvements in neuronal survival and neurite outgrowth [139], or mimetics of heparins which have been used to protect endothelial colony forming progenitor cells in diabetic patients [140], potentially leading to a solution for improved vascular endothelial repair and wound healing for foot ulcers. This approach has also been used in a glycomimetic-containing carbohydrate-based vaccine, where cross-reactive antibodies identified potential peptides through library screening, which were then more immunogenic, cross-reactive with the native substrate, and more easily obtainable through synthesis [141–143].

3.4. Other Considerations

Although methods to improve pharmacokinetic parameters have just been discussed, some of the approaches described may not be desirable for particular therapeutic targets. For example, in some glycomimetics, oral bioavailability is not required: the α-glucosidase inhibitors used to treat diabetes target proteins in the brush border of the small intestine, and therefore do not need to be passively transported across the intestinal membrane. This is also the case for neuraminidase inhibitors such as zanamivir (Relenza®) which can be used to target viral infections in the pharyngeal mucosa.

Similarly, for some glycomimetic therapeutics it could be desirable to have shorter serum half-lives; for example, the FimH antagonists discussed previously rely on renal excretion to reach their desired protein targets in the urinary tract. Although a faster renal clearance is desirable in the treatment of urinary tract infections, glycomimetics that are cleared too quickly would require too frequent dosing; therefore, some hydrophobicity is still desirable to facilitate renal tubular reabsorption and somewhat prolong circulation times.

4. Conclusions

Although historically carbohydrate-based therapeutics have not been overly successful in the drug development pipeline, there have been numerous successful approaches recently developed which can be used to circumvent the weak affinities and poor pharmacokinetic properties typically attributed to glycans. Given their extensive structural diversity and involvement in a broad range of diseases, carbohydrates and their associated glycomimetics have recently come back into focus as a very promising therapeutic option. By identifying an appropriate target and applying several of the strategies discussed in the context of this review, high affinity glycomimetics with favorable pharmacokinetic profiles can be developed, and eventually carried forward into the clinic.

Funding: This research received no external funding.

Acknowledgments: A very grateful acknowledgement goes to Dr. Jacqueline Bezençon for her time and helpful feedback in preparing this manuscript.

Conflicts of Interest: The authors declare no conflict of interest.

References

1. Nieuwdorp, M.; Meuwese, M.C.; Mooij, H.L.; Ince, C.; Broekhuizen, L.N.; Kastelein, J.J.P.; Stroes, E.S.G.; Vink, H. Measuring endothelial glycocalyx dimensions in humans: A potential novel tool to monitor vascular vulnerability. *J. Appl. Physiol.* **2008**, *104*, 845–852. [CrossRef]
2. Van Teeffelen, J.W.; Brands, J.; Stroes, E.S.; Vink, H. Endothelial glycocalyx: Sweet shield of blood vessels. *Trends Cardiovasc. Med.* **2007**, *17*, 101–105. [CrossRef]
3. Varki, A.; Cummings, R.D.; Esko, J.D.; Stanley, P.; Hart, G.W.; Aebi, M.; Darvill, A.G.; Kinoshita, T.; Packer, N.H.; Prestegard, J.H.; et al. (Eds.) *Essentials of Glycobiology*, 3rd ed.; Cold Spring Harbor: New York, NY, USA, 2017.
4. Taylor, S.L.; McGuckin, M.A.; Wesselingh, S.; Rogers, G.B. Infection's sweet tooth: How glycans mediate infection and disease susceptibility. *Trends Microbiol.* **2018**, *26*, 92–101. [CrossRef]
5. Fuster, M.M.; Esko, J.D. The sweet and sour of cancer: Glycans as novel therapeutic targets. *Nat. Rev. Cancer* **2005**, *5*, 526–542. [CrossRef] [PubMed]
6. Dube, D.H.; Bertozzi, C.R. Glycans in cancer and inflammation—Potential for therapeutics and diagnostics. *Nat. Rev. Drug Discov.* **2005**, *4*, 477–488. [CrossRef] [PubMed]
7. Gamblin, S.J.; Skehel, J.J. Influenza hemagglutinin and neuraminidase membrane glycoproteins. *J. Biol. Chem.* **2010**, *285*, 28403–28409. [CrossRef] [PubMed]
8. Smith, D.C.; Lord, J.M.; Roberts, L.M.; Johannes, L. Glycosphingolipids as toxin receptors. *Semin. Cell Dev. Biol.* **2004**, *15*, 397–408. [CrossRef] [PubMed]

9. Seeberger, P.H.; Rademacher, C. (Eds.) *Carbohydrates as Drugs*; Springer: Berlin, Germany, 2014.
10. Zhang, Y.; Wang, F. Carbohydrate drugs: Current status and development prospect. *Drug Discov. Ther.* **2015**, *9*, 79–87. [CrossRef] [PubMed]
11. Ernst, B.; Magnani, J.L. From carbohydrate leads to glycomimetic drugs. *Nat. Rev. Drug Discov.* **2009**, *8*, 661–677. [CrossRef]
12. Quiocho, F.A. Probing the atomic interactions between proteins and carbohydrates. *Biochem. Soc. Trans.* **1993**, *21*, 442–448. [CrossRef]
13. Sears, P.; Wong, C.-H. Carbohydrate mimetics: A new strategy for tackling the problem of carbohydrate-mediated biological recognition. *Angew. Chem. Int. Ed.* **1999**, *38*, 2300–2324. [CrossRef]
14. Schön, A.; Freire, E. Thermodynamics of intersubunit interactions in cholera toxin upon binding to the oligosaccharide portion of its cell surface receptor, ganglioside GM1. *Biochemistry* **1989**, *28*, 5019–5024. [CrossRef] [PubMed]
15. Lipinski, C.A.; Lombardo, F.; Dominy, B.W.; Feeney, P.J. Experimental and computational approaches to estimate solubility and permeability in drug discovery and development settings. *Adv. Drug Deliv. Rev.* **1997**, *23*, 3–25. [CrossRef]
16. Veber, D.F.; Johnson, S.R.; Cheng, H.-Y.; Smith, B.R.; Ward, K.W.; Kopple, K.D. Molecular properties that influence the oral bioavailability of drug candidates. *J. Med. Chem.* **2002**, *45*, 2615–2623. [CrossRef] [PubMed]
17. Magnani, J.L.; Ernst, B. Glycomimetic drugs—A new source of therapeutic opportunities. *Discov. Med.* **2009**, *8*, 247–252.
18. Sood, A.; Gerlits, O.O.; Ji, Y.; Bovin, N.V.; Coates, L.; Woods, R.J. Defining the specificity of carbohydrate-protein interactions by quantifying functional group contributions. *J. Chem. Inf. Model.* **2018**, *58*, 1889–1901. [CrossRef]
19. Sager, C.P.; Eriş, D.; Smieško, M.; Hevey, R.; Ernst, B. What contributes to an effective mannose recognition domain? *Beilstein J. Org. Chem.* **2017**, *13*, 2584–2595. [CrossRef]
20. Modenutti, C.; Gauto, D.; Radusky, L.; Blanco, J.; Turjanski, A.; Hajos, S.; Marti, M.A. Using crystallographic water properties for the analysis and prediction of lectin-carbohydrate complex structures. *Glycobiology* **2015**, *25*, 181–196. [CrossRef]
21. Quiocho, F.A.; Wilson, D.K.; Vyas, N.K. Substrate specificity and affinity of a protein modulated by bound water molecules. *Nature* **1989**, *340*, 404–407. [CrossRef]
22. Kim, C.U.; Lew, W.; Williams, M.A.; Liu, H.; Zhang, L.; Swaminathan, S.; Bischofberger, N.; Chen, M.S.; Mendel, D.B.; Tai, C.Y.; et al. Influenza neuraminidase inhibitors possessing a novel hydrophobic interaction in the enzyme active site: Design, synthesis, and structural analysis of carbocyclic sialic acid analogues with potent anti-influenza activity. *J. Am. Chem. Soc.* **1997**, *119*, 681–690. [CrossRef] [PubMed]
23. McClellan, K.; Perry, C.M. Oseltamivir—A review of its use in influenza. *Drugs* **2001**, *61*, 263–283. [CrossRef]
24. Von Itzstein, M.; Wu, W.-Y.; Kok, G.B.; Pegg, M.S.; Dyason, J.C.; Jin, B.; Phan, T.V.; Smythe, M.L.; White, H.F.; Oliver, S.W.; et al. Rational design of potent sialidase-based inhibitors of influenza virus replication. *Nature* **1993**, *363*, 418–423. [CrossRef]
25. Cox, T.; Lachmann, R.; Hollak, C.; Aerts, J.; van Weely, S.; Hrebícek, M.; Platt, F.; Butters, T.; Dwek, R.; Moyses, C.; et al. Novel oral treatment of Gaucher's disease with N-butyldeoxynojirimycin (OGT 918) to decrease substrate biosynthesis. *Lancet* **2000**, *355*, 1481–1485. [CrossRef]
26. Campbell, L.K.; Baker, D.E.; Campbell, R.K. Miglitol: Assessment of its role in the treatment of patients with diabetes mellitus. *Ann. Pharmacother.* **2000**, *34*, 1291–1301. [CrossRef]
27. Chen, X.; Zheng, Y.; Shen, Y. Voglibose (Basen, AO-128), one of the most important α-glucosidase inhibitors. *Curr. Med. Chem.* **2006**, *13*, 109–116. [CrossRef]
28. Truscheit, E.; Frommer, W.; Junge, B.; Müller, L.; Schmidt, D.D.; Wingender, W. Chemistry and biochemistry of microbial α-glucosidase inhibitors. *Angew. Chem. Int. Ed. Engl.* **1981**, *20*, 744–761. [CrossRef]
29. Sharon, N. Carbohydrates as future anti-adhesion drugs for infectious diseases. *Biochim. Biophys. Acta* **2006**, *1760*, 527–537. [CrossRef]
30. Ofek, I.; Hasty, D.L.; Sharon, N. Anti-adhesion therapy of bacterial diseases: Prospects and problems. *FEMS Immunol. Med. Microbiol.* **2003**, *38*, 181–191. [CrossRef]
31. Kalas, V.; Hibbing, M.E.; Maddirala, A.R.; Chugani, R.; Pinkner, J.S.; Mydock-McGrane, L.K.; Conover, M.S.; Janetka, J.W.; Hultgren, S.J. Structure-based discovery of glycomimetic FmlH ligands as inhibitors of bacterial adhesion during urinary tract infection. *Proc. Natl. Acad. Sci. USA* **2018**, *115*, E2819–E2828. [CrossRef]

32. Hevey, R.; Ling, C.-C. Conjugation strategies used for the preparation of carbohydrate-conjugate vaccines. In *Chemistry of Bioconjugates: Synthesis, Characterization, and Biomedical Applications*; Narain, R., Ed.; John Wiley & Sons, Inc.: Hoboken, NJ, USA, 2013.
33. Hevey, R.; Ling, C.-C. Recent advances in developing synthetic carbohydrate-based vaccines for cancer immunotherapies. *Future Med. Chem.* **2012**, *4*, 545–584. [CrossRef]
34. Krug, L.M.; Ragupathi, G.; Ng, K.K.; Hood, C.; Jennings, H.J.; Guo, Z.; Kris, M.G.; Miller, V.; Pizzo, B.; Tyson, L.; et al. Vaccination of small cell lung cancer patients with polysialic acid or N-propionylated polysialic acid conjugated to keyhole limpet hemocyanin. *Clin. Cancer Res.* **2004**, *10*, 916–923. [CrossRef] [PubMed]
35. Liao, L.; Auzanneau, F.-A. Synthesis of Lewis A trisaccharide analogues in which D-glucose and L-rhamnose replace D-galactose and L-fucose, respectively. *Carbohydr. Res.* **2006**, *341*, 2426–2433. [CrossRef] [PubMed]
36. Wang, J.-W.; Asnani, A.; Auzanneau, F.-A. Synthesis of a BSA-LeX glycoconjugate and recognition of LeX analogues by the anti-LeX monoclonal antibody SH1: The identification of a non-cross reactive analogue. *Bioorg. Med. Chem.* **2010**, *18*, 7174–7185. [CrossRef] [PubMed]
37. Sahabuddin, S.; Chang, T.-C.; Lin, C.-C.; Jan, F.-D.; Hsiao, H.-Y.; Huang, K.-T.; Chen, J.-H.; Horng, J.-C.; Ho, J.A.; Lin, C.-C. Synthesis of N-modified sTn analogs and evaluation of their immunogenicities by microarray-based immunoassay. *Tetrahedron* **2010**, *66*, 7510–7519. [CrossRef]
38. Cabani, S.; Gianni, P.; Mollica, V.; Lepori, L. Group contributions to the thermodynamic properties of non-ionic organic solutes in dilute aqueous solution. *J. Solut. Chem.* **1981**, *10*, 563–595. [CrossRef]
39. Fitch, C.A.; Karp, D.A.; Lee, K.K.; Stites, W.E.; Lattman, E.E.; García-Moreno, B.E. Experimental pKa values of buried residues: Analysis with continuum methods and role of water penetration. *Biophys. J.* **2002**, *82*, 3289–3304. [CrossRef]
40. Levitt, M.; Park, B.H. Water: Now you see it, now you don't. *Curr. Biol.* **1993**, *1*, 223–226. [CrossRef]
41. Pan, A.C.; Borhani, D.W.; Dror, R.O.; Shaw, D.E. Molecular determinants of drug-receptor binding kinetics. *Drug Discov. Today* **2013**, *18*, 667–673. [CrossRef]
42. Schmidtke, P.; Luque, F.J.; Murray, J.B.; Barril, X. Shielded hydrogen bonds as structural determinants of binding kinetics: Application in drug design. *J. Am. Chem. Soc.* **2011**, *133*, 18903–18910. [CrossRef]
43. Gao, J.; Qiao, S.; Whitesides, G.M. Increasing binding constants of ligands to carbonic anhydrase by using "greasy tails". *J. Med. Chem.* **1995**, *38*, 2292–2301. [CrossRef]
44. Biffinger, J.C.; Kim, H.W.; DiMagno, S.G. The polar hydrophobicity of fluorinated compounds. *ChemBioChem* **2004**, *5*, 622–627. [CrossRef]
45. London, R.E.; Gabel, S.A. Fluorine-19 NMR studies of glucosyl fluoride transport in human erythrocytes. *Biophys. J.* **1995**, *69*, 1814–1818. [CrossRef]
46. Oberbillig, T.; Mersch, C.; Wagner, S.; Hoffmann-Röder, A. Antibody recognition of fluorinated MUC1 glycopeptide antigens. *Chem. Commun.* **2012**, *48*, 1487–1489. [CrossRef]
47. Sprinz, C.; Zanon, M.; Altmayer, S.; Watte, G.; Irion, K.; Marchiori, E.; Hochhegger, B. Effects of blood glucose level on 18F fluorodeoxyglucose (18F-FDG) uptake for PET/CT in normal organs: An analysis on 5623 patients. *Sci. Rep.* **2018**, *8*, 2126. [CrossRef]
48. Maschauer, S.; Haubner, R.; Kuwert, T.; Prante, O. 18F-Glyco-RGD peptides for PET imaging of integrin expression: Efficient radiosynthesis by click chemistry and modulation of biodistribution by glycosylation. *Mol. Pharm.* **2014**, *11*, 505–515. [CrossRef] [PubMed]
49. Sadurní, A.; Gilmour, R. Stereocontrolled synthesis of 2-fluorinated C-glycosides. *Eur. J. Org. Chem.* **2018**, *2018*, 3684–3687. [CrossRef] [PubMed]
50. Büll, C.; Boltje, T.J.; van Dinther, E.A.W.; Peters, T.; de Graaf, A.M.A.; Leusen, J.H.W.; Kreutz, M.; Figdor, C.G.; den Brok, M.H.; Adema, G.J. Targeted delivery of a sialic acid-blocking glycomimetic to cancer cells inhibits metastatic spread. *ACS Nano* **2015**, *9*, 733–745. [CrossRef]
51. Büll, C.; Boltje, T.J.; Wassink, M.; de Graaf, A.M.A.; van Delft, F.L.; den Brok, M.H.; Adema, G.J. Targeting aberrant sialylation in cancer cells using a fluorinated sialic acid analog impairs adhesion, migration, and in vivo tumor growth. *Mol. Cancer Ther.* **2016**, *12*, 1935–1946. [CrossRef]
52. Foxman, B. Epidemiology of urinary tract infections: Incidence, morbidity, and economic costs. *Am. J. Med.* **2002**, *113*, 5S–13S. [CrossRef]
53. Mak, R.H.; Kuo, H.-J. Pathogenesis of urinary tract infection: An update. *Curr. Opin. Pediatr.* **2006**, *18*, 148–152. [CrossRef]

54. Firon, N.; Ofek, I.; Sharon, N. Interaction of mannose-containing oligosaccharides with the fimbrial lectin of *Escherichia coli*. *Biochem. Biophys. Res. Commun.* **1982**, *105*, 1426–1432. [CrossRef]
55. Wellens, A.; Garofalo, C.; Nguyen, H.; Van Gerven, N.; Slättegård, R.; Hernalsteens, J.-P.; Wyns, L.; Oscarson, S.; De Greve, H.; Hultgren, S.; et al. Intervening with urinary tract infections using anti-adhesives based on the crystal structure of the FimH-oligomannose-3 complex. *PLoS ONE* **2008**, *3*, e2040. [CrossRef]
56. Han, Z.; Pinkner, J.S.; Ford, B.; Obermann, R.; Nolan, W.; Wildman, S.A.; Hobbs, D.; Ellenberger, T.; Cusumano, C.K.; Hultgren, S.J.; et al. Structure-based drug design and optimization of mannose bacterial FimH antagonists. *J. Med. Chem.* **2010**, *53*, 4779–4792. [CrossRef] [PubMed]
57. Firon, N.; Ashkenazi, S.; Mirelman, D.; Ofek, I.; Sharon, N. Aromatic alpha-glycosides of mannose are powerful inhibitors of the adherence of type 1 fimbriated *Escherichia coli* to yeast and intestinal epithelial cells. *Infect. Immun.* **1987**, *55*, 472–476. [PubMed]
58. Bouckaert, J.; Berglund, J.; Schembri, M.; De Genst, E.; Cools, L.; Wuhrer, M.; Hung, C.-S.; Pinkner, J.; Slättegård, R.; Zavialov, A.; et al. Receptor binding studies disclose a novel class of high-affinity inhibitors of the *Escherichia coli* FimH adhesin. *Mol. Microbiol.* **2005**, *55*, 441–455. [CrossRef]
59. Sperling, O.; Fuchs, A.; Lindhorst, T.K. Evaluation of the carbohydrate recognition domain of the bacterial adhesin FimH: Design, synthesis and binding properties of mannoside ligands. *Org. Biomol. Chem.* **2006**, *4*, 3913–3922. [CrossRef] [PubMed]
60. Klein, T.; Abgottspon, D.; Wittwer, M.; Rabbani, S.; Herold, J.; Jiang, X.; Kleeb, S.; Lüthi, C.; Scharenberg, M.; Bezençon, J.; et al. FimH antagonists for the oral treatment of urinary tract infections: From design and synthesis to in vitro and in vivo evaluation. *J. Med. Chem.* **2010**, *53*, 8627–8641. [CrossRef] [PubMed]
61. Scharenberg, M.; Schwardt, O.; Rabbani, S.; Ernst, B. Target selectivity of FimH antagonists. *J. Med. Chem.* **2012**, *55*, 9810–9816. [CrossRef] [PubMed]
62. Jiang, X.; Abgottspon, D.; Kleeb, S.; Rabbani, S.; Scharenberg, M.; Wittwer, M.; Haug, M.; Schwardt, O.; Ernst, B. Antiadhesion therapy for urinary tract infections—A balanced PK/PD profile proved to be key for success. *J. Med. Chem.* **2012**, *55*, 4700–4713. [CrossRef]
63. Mena-Barragán, T.; García-Moreno, M.I.; Sevšek, A.; Okazaki, T.; Nanba, E.; Higaki, K.; Martin, N.I.; Pieters, R.J.; García-Fernandez, J.M.; Ortiz Mellet, C. Probing the inhibitor versus chaperone properties of SP2-iminosugars towards human β-glucocerebrosidase: A picomolar chaperone for Gaucher disease. *Molecules* **2018**, *23*, 927. [CrossRef]
64. Markham, A. Migalastat: First global approval. *Drugs* **2016**, *76*, 1147–1152. [CrossRef]
65. Dugger, S.A.; Platt, A.; Goldstein, D.B. Drug development in the era of precision medicine. *Nat. Rev. Drug Discov.* **2018**, *17*, 183–196. [CrossRef]
66. García-Moreno, M.I.; de la Mata, M.; Sánchez-Fernández, E.M.; Benito, J.M.; Díaz-Quintana, A.; Fustero, S.; Nanba, E.; Higaki, K.; Sánchez-Alcázar, J.A.; García Fernández, J.M.; et al. Fluorinated chaperone-β-cyclodextrin formulations for β-glucocerebrosidase activity enhancement in neuronopathic Gaucher disease. *J. Med. Chem.* **2017**, *60*, 1829–1842. [CrossRef]
67. Prescher, H.; Frank, M.; Gütgemann, S.; Kuhfeldt, E.; Schweizer, A.; Nitschke, L.; Watzl, C.; Brossmer, R. Design, synthesis, and biological evaluation of small, high-affinity Siglec-7 ligands: Toward novel inhibitors of cancer immune evasion. *J. Med. Chem.* **2017**, *60*, 941–956. [CrossRef]
68. Prescher, H.; Gütgemann, S.; Frank, M.; Kuhfeldt, E.; Watzl, C.; Brossmer, R. Synthesis and biological evaluation of 9-N-oxamyl sialosides as Siglec-7 ligands. *Bioorg. Med. Chem.* **2015**, *23*, 5915–5921. [CrossRef]
69. Prescher, H.; Schweizer, A.; Kuhfeldt, E.; Nitschke, L.; Brossmer, R. New human CD22/Siglec-2 ligands with a triazole glycoside. *ChemBioChem* **2017**, *18*, 1216–1225. [CrossRef]
70. Prescher, H.; Schweizer, A.; Kuhfeldt, E.; Nitschke, L.; Brossmer, R. Discovery of multifold modified sialosides as *human* CD22/Siglec-2 ligands with nanomolar activity on B-cells. *ACS Chem. Biol.* **2014**, *9*, 1444–1450. [CrossRef]
71. Collins, B.E.; Blixt, O.; Han, S.; Duong, B.; Li, H.; Nathan, J.K.; Bovin, N.; Paulson, J.C. High-affinity ligand probes of CD22 overcome the threshold set by *cis* ligands to allow for binding, endocytosis, and killing of B cells. *J. Immunol.* **2006**, *177*, 2994–3003. [CrossRef]
72. Sommer, R.; Wagner, S.; Rox, K.; Varrot, A.; Hauck, D.; Wamhoff, E.-C.; Schreiber, J.; Ryckmans, T.; Brunner, T.; Rademacher, C.; et al. Glycomimetic, orally bioavailable LecB inhibitors block biofilm formation of *Pseudomonas aeruginosa*. *J. Am. Chem. Soc.* **2018**, *140*, 2537–2545. [CrossRef]

73. Tomašić, T.; Hajšek, D.; Švajger, U.; Luzar, J.; Obermajer, N.; Petit-Haertlein, I.; Fieschi, F.; Anderluh, M. Monovalent mannose-based DC-SIGN antagonists: Targeting the hydrophobic groove of the receptor. *Eur. J. Med. Chem.* **2014**, *75*, 308–326. [CrossRef]
74. Wagner, S.; Hauck, D.; Hoffmann, M.; Sommer, R.; Joachim, I.; Müller, R.; Imberty, A.; Varrot, A.; Titz, A. Covalent lectin inhibition and application in bacterial biofilm imaging. *Angew. Chem. Int. Ed.* **2017**, *56*, 16559–16564. [CrossRef]
75. Chang, J.; Patton, J.T.; Sarkar, A.; Ernst, B.; Magnani, J.L.; Frenette, P.S. GMI-1070, a novel pan-selectin antagonist, reverses acute vascular occlusions in sickle cell mice. *Blood* **2010**, *116*, 1779–1786. [CrossRef]
76. Telen, M.J.; Wun, T.; McCavit, T.L.; De Castro, L.M.; Krishnamurti, L.; Lanzkron, S.; Hsu, L.L.; Smith, W.R.; Rhee, S.; Magnani, J.L.; et al. Randomized phase 2 study of GMI-1070 in SCD: Reduction in time to resolution of vaso-occlusive events and decreased opioid use. *Blood* **2015**, *125*, 2656–2664. [CrossRef]
77. Gabius, H.-J.; Siebert, H.-C.; André, S.; Jiménez-Barbero, J.; Rüdiger, H. Chemical biology of the sugar code. *ChemBioChem* **2004**, *5*, 740–764. [CrossRef]
78. Searle, M.S.; Williams, D.H. The cost of conformational order: Entropy changes in molecular associations. *J. Am. Chem. Soc.* **1992**, *114*, 10690–10697. [CrossRef]
79. Perret, S.; Sabin, C.; Dumon, C.; Pokorná, M.; Gautier, C.; Galanina, O.; Ilia, S.; Bovin, N.; Nicaise, M.; Desmadril, M.; et al. Structural basis for the interaction between human milk oligosaccharides and the bacterial lectin PA-IIL of *Pseudomonas aeruginosa*. *Biochem. J.* **2005**, *389*, 325–332. [CrossRef]
80. Marotte, K.; Sabin, C.; Préville, C.; Moumé-Pymbock, M.; Wimmerová, M.; Mitchell, E.P.; Imberty, A.; Roy, R. X-ray structures and thermodynamics of the interaction of PA-IIL from *Pseudomonas aeruginosa* with disaccharide derivatives. *ChemMedChem* **2007**, *2*, 1328–1338. [CrossRef]
81. Imberty, A.; Chabre, Y.M.; Roy, R. Glycomimetics and glycodendrimers as high affinity microbial anti-adhesins. *Chem. Eur. J.* **2008**, *14*, 7490–7499. [CrossRef]
82. Rinnbauer, M.; Ernst, B.; Wagner, B.; Magnani, J.; Benie, A.J.; Peters, T. Epitope mapping of sialyl LewisX bound to E-selectin using saturation transfer difference NMR experiments. *Glycobiology* **2003**, *13*, 435–443. [CrossRef]
83. Somers, W.S.; Tang, J.; Shaw, G.D.; Camphausen, R.T. Insights into the molecular basis of leukocyte tethering and rolling revealed by structures of P- and E-selectin bound to SLeX and PSGL-1. *Cell* **2000**, *103*, 467–479. [CrossRef]
84. Kolb, H.C.; Ernst, B. Development of tools for the design of selectin antagonists. *Chem. Eur. J.* **1997**, *3*, 1571–1578. [CrossRef]
85. Thoma, G.; Magnani, J.L.; Patton, J.T.; Ernst, B.; Jahnke, W. Preorganization of the bioactive conformation of sialyl LewisX analogues correlates with their affinity to E-selectin. *Angew. Chem.* **2001**, *113*, 1995–1999. [CrossRef]
86. Sager, C.P.; Fiege, B.; Zihlmann, P.; Vannam, R.; Rabbani, S.; Jakob, R.P.; Preston, R.C.; Zalewski, A.; Maier, T.; Peczuh, M.W.; et al. The price of flexibility—A case study on septanoses as pyranose mimetics. *Chem. Sci.* **2018**, *9*, 646–654. [CrossRef]
87. Moog, K.E.; Barz, M.; Bartneck, M.; Beceren-Braun, F.; Mohr, N.; Wu, Z.; Braun, L.; Dernedde, J.; Liehn, E.A.; Tacke, F.; et al. Polymeric selectin ligands mimicking complex carbohydrates: From selectin binders to modifiers of macrophage migration. *Angew. Chem. Int. Ed.* **2017**, *56*, 1416–1421. [CrossRef]
88. Zhang, X.; Yao, W.; Xu, X.; Sun, H.; Zhao, J.; Meng, X.; Wu, M.; Li, Z. Synthesis of fucosylated chondroitin sulfate glycoclusters: A robust route to new anticoagulant agents. *Chem. Eur. J.* **2018**, *24*, 1694–1700. [CrossRef]
89. Bücher, K.S.; Konietzny, P.B.; Snyder, N.L.; Hartmann, L. Heteromultivalent glycooligomers as mimetics of blood group antigens. *Chem. Eur. J.* **2019**, *25*, 3301–3309. [CrossRef]
90. Cecioni, S.; Imberty, A.; Vidal, S. Glycomimetics versus multivalent glycoconjugates for the design of high affinity lectin ligands. *Chem. Rev.* **2015**, *115*, 525–561. [CrossRef]
91. Bertolotti, B.; Sutkeviciute, I.; Ambrosini, M.; Ribeiro-Viana, R.; Rojo, J.; Fieschi, F.; Dvořáková, H.; Kašáková, M.; Parkan, K.; Hlaváčková, M.; et al. Polyvalent C-glycomimetics based on L-fucose or D-mannose as potent DC-SIGN antagonists. *Org. Biomol. Chem.* **2017**, *15*, 3995–4004. [CrossRef]
92. García-Moreno, M.I.; Ortega-Caballero, F.; Rísquez-Cuadro, R.; Ortiz Mellet, C.; García Fernandez, J.M. The impact of heteromultivalency in lectin recognition and glycosidase inhibition: An integrated mechanistic study. *Chem. Eur. J.* **2017**, *23*, 6295–6304. [CrossRef]

93. Ordanini, S.; Varga, N.; Porkolab, V.; Thépaut, M.; Belvisi, L.; Bertaglia, A.; Palmioli, A.; Berzi, A.; Trabattoni, D.; Clerici, M.; et al. Designing nanomolar antagonists of DC-SIGN-mediated HIV infection: Ligand presentation using molecular rods. *Chem. Commun.* **2015**, *51*, 3816–3819. [CrossRef]
94. Boden, S.; Reise, F.; Kania, J.; Lindhorst, T.K.; Hartmann, L. Sequence-defined introduction of hydrophobic motifs and effects in lectin binding of precision glycomacromolecules. *Macromol. Biosci.* **2019**, e1800425. [CrossRef]
95. Berzi, A.; Ordanini, S.; Joosten, B.; Trabattoni, D.; Cambi, A.; Bernardi, A.; Clerici, M. Pseudo-mannosylated DC-SIGN ligands as immunomodulants. *Sci. Rep.* **2016**, *6*, 35373. [CrossRef]
96. Pérez-Castells, J.; Hernández-Gay, J.J.; Denton, R.W.; Tony, K.A.; Mootoo, D.R.; Jiménez-Barbero, J. The conformational behaviour and P-selectin inhibition of fluorine-containing sialyl LeX glycomimetics. *Org. Biomol. Chem.* **2007**, *5*, 1087–1092. [CrossRef]
97. Asensio, J.L.; Espinosa, J.F.; Dietrich, H.; Cañada, F.J.; Schmidt, R.R.; Martín-Lomas, M.; André, S.; Gabius, H.-J.; Jiménez-Barbero, J. Bovine heart galectin-1 selects a unique (syn) conformation of C-lactose, a flexible lactose analogue. *J. Am. Chem. Soc.* **1999**, *121*, 8995–9000. [CrossRef]
98. Asensio, J.L.; Cañada, F.J.; Cheng, X.; Khan, N.; Mootoo, D.R.; Jiménez-Barbero, J. Conformational differences between O- and C-glycosides: The α-O-Man-(1→1)-β-Gal/α-C-Man-(1→1)-β-Gal case—A decisive demonstration of the importance of the *exo*-anomeric effect on the conformation of glycosides. *Chem. Eur. J.* **2000**, *6*, 1035–1041. [CrossRef]
99. Espinosa, J.-F.; Bruix, M.; Jarreton, O.; Skrydstrup, T.; Beau, J.-M.; Jiménez-Barbero, J. Conformational differences between C- and O-glycosides: The α-C-mannobiose/α-O-mannobiose case. *Chem. Eur. J.* **1999**, *5*, 442–448. [CrossRef]
100. O'Hagan, D.; Rzepa, H.S. Some influences of fluorine in bioorganic chemistry. *Chem. Commun.* **1997**, *0*, 645–652. [CrossRef]
101. Berber, H.; Brigaud, T.; Lefebvre, O.; Plantier-Royon, R.; Portella, C. Reactions of difluoroenoxysilanes with glycosyl donors: Synthesis of difluoro-C-glycosides and difluoro-C-disaccharides. *Chem. Eur. J.* **2001**, *7*, 903–909. [CrossRef]
102. Moreno, B.; Quehen, C.; Rose-Hélène, M.; Leclerc, E.; Quirion, J.-C. Addition of difluoromethyl radicals to glycals: A new route to alpha-CF2-D-glycosides. *Org. Lett.* **2007**, *9*, 2477–2480. [CrossRef]
103. Hirai, G.; Watanabe, T.; Yamaguchi, K.; Miyagi, T.; Sodeoka, M. Stereocontrolled and convergent entry to CF2-sialosides: Synthesis of CF2-linked ganglioside GM4. *J. Am. Chem. Soc.* **2007**, *129*, 15420–15421. [CrossRef]
104. Tony, K.A.; Denton, R.W.; Dilhas, A.; Jiménez-Barbero, J.; Mootoo, D.R. Synthesis of β-C-*galacto*-pyranosides with fluorine on the pseudoanomeric substituent. *Org. Lett.* **2007**, *9*, 1441–1444. [CrossRef]
105. Dondoni, A.; Catozzi, N.; Marra, A. Concise and practical synthesis of C-glycosyl ketones from sugar benzothiazoles and their transformation into chiral tertiary alcohols. *J. Org. Chem.* **2005**, *70*, 9257–9268. [CrossRef]
106. Poulain, F.; Serre, A.-L.; Lalot, J.; Leclerc, E.; Quirion, J.-C. Synthesis of α-CF2-mannosides and their conversion to fluorinated pseudoglycopeptides. *J. Org. Chem.* **2008**, *73*, 2435–2438. [CrossRef]
107. Johnson, C.R.; Johns, B.A. Suzuki cross-coupling of carbohydrates: Synthesis of β-arylmethyl-C-glycosides and aryl-scaffolded trisaccharide mimics. *Synlett* **1997**, *12*, 1406–1408. [CrossRef]
108. Dondoni, A.; Catozzi, N.; Marra, A. Stereoselective synthesis of α- and β-L-C-fucosyl aldehydes and their utility in the assembly of C-fucosides of biological relevance. *J. Org. Chem.* **2004**, *69*, 5023–5036. [CrossRef]
109. Dondoni, A.; Scherrmann, M.-C. Thiazole-based synthesis of formyl C-glycosides. *J. Org. Chem.* **1994**, *59*, 6404–6412. [CrossRef]
110. Redjdal, W.; Ibrahim, N.; Benmerad, B.; Alami, M.; Messaoudi, S. Convergent synthesis of N,S-bis glycosylquinolin-2-ones via a Pd-G3-XantPhos precatalyst catalysis. *Molecules* **2018**, *23*, 519. [CrossRef]
111. Céspedes Dávila, M.F.; Schneider, J.P.; Godard, A.; Hazelard, D.; Compain, P. One-pot, highly stereoselective synthesis of dithioacetal-α,α-diglycosides. *Molecules* **2018**, *23*, 914. [CrossRef]
112. Illyés, T.-Z.; Balla, S.; Bényei, A.; Kumar, A.A.; Timári, I.; Kövér, K.E.; Szilágyi, L. Exploring the syntheses of novel glycomimetics. Carbohydrate derivatives with Se-S- or Se-Se-glycosidic linkages. *ChemistrySelect* **2016**, *1*, 2383–2388. [CrossRef]
113. Zhu, F.; O'Neill, S.; Rodriguez, J.; Walczak, M.A. Stereoretentive reactions at the anomeric position: Synthesis of selenoglycosides. *Angew. Chem. Int. Ed.* **2018**, *57*, 7091–7095. [CrossRef]

114. Marcaurelle, L.A.; Bertozzi, C.R. New directions in the synthesis of glycopeptide mimetics. *Chem. Eur. J.* **1999**, *5*, 1384–1390. [CrossRef]
115. Mydock-McGrane, L.; Cusumano, Z.; Han, Z.; Binkley, J.; Kostakioti, M.; Hannan, T.; Pinkner, J.S.; Klein, R.; Kalas, V.; Crowley, J.; et al. Antivirulence C-mannosides as antibiotic-sparing, oral therapeutics for urinary tract infections. *J. Med. Chem.* **2016**, *59*, 9390–9408. [CrossRef]
116. Brument, S.; Sivignon, A.; Dumych, T.I.; Moreau, N.; Roos, G.; Guérardel, Y.; Chalopin, T.; Deniaud, D.; Bilyy, R.O.; Darfeuille-Michaud, A.; et al. Thiazolylaminomannosides as potent antiadhesives of type 1 piliated *Escherichia coli* isolated from Crohn's disease patients. *J. Med. Chem.* **2013**, *56*, 5395–5406. [CrossRef]
117. Chalopin, T.; Alvarez Dorta, D.; Sivignon, A.; Caudan, M.; Dumych, T.I.; Bilyy, R.O.; Deniaud, D.; Barnich, N.; Bouckaert, J.; Gouin, S.G. Second generation of thiazolylmannosides, FimH antagonists for *E. coli*-induced Crohn's disease. *Org. Biomol. Chem.* **2016**, *14*, 3913–3925. [CrossRef]
118. Sivignon, A.; Bouckaert, J.; Bernard, J.; Gouin, S.G.; Barnich, N. The potential of FimH as a novel therapeutic target for the treatment of Crohn's disease. *Expert. Opin. Ther. Targets* **2017**, *21*, 837–847. [CrossRef]
119. Alvarez Dorta, D.; Chalopin, T.; Sivignon, A.; de Ruyck, J.; Dumych, T.I.; Bilyy, R.O.; Deniaud, D.; Barnich, N.; Bouckaert, J.; Gouin, S.G. Physiochemical tuning of potent *Escherichia coli* anti-adhesives by microencapsulation and methylene homologation. *ChemMedChem* **2017**, *12*, 986–998. [CrossRef]
120. Böhm, H.-J.; Banner, D.; Bendels, S.; Kansy, M.; Kuhn, B.; Müller, K.; Obst-Sander, U.; Stahl, M. Fluorine in medicinal chemistry. *ChemBioChem* **2004**, *5*, 637–643. [CrossRef] [PubMed]
121. Ganapathy, M.E.; Huang, W.; Wang, H.; Ganapathy, V.; Leibach, F.H. Valacyclovir: A substrate for the intestinal and renal peptide transporters PEPT1 and PEPT2. *Biochem. Biophys. Res. Commun.* **1998**, *246*, 470–475. [CrossRef]
122. Inui, K.; Terada, T.; Masuda, S.; Saito, H. Physiological and pharmacological implications of peptide transporters, PEPT1 and PEPT2. *Nephrol. Dial. Transpl.* **2000**, *15*, 11–13. [CrossRef]
123. Nielsen, D.S.; Lohman, R.-J.; Hoang, H.N.; Hill, T.A.; Jones, A.; Lucke, A.J.; Fairlie, D.P. Flexibility versus rigidity for orally bioavailable cyclic hexapeptides. *ChemBioChem* **2015**, *16*, 2289–2293. [CrossRef]
124. Jornada, D.H.; dos Santos Fernandes, G.F.; Chiba, D.E.; de Melo, T.R.F.; dos Santos, J.L.; Chung, M.C. The prodrug approach: A successful tool for improving drug solubility. *Molecules* **2015**, *21*, 42. [CrossRef]
125. He, G.; Massarella, J.; Ward, P. Clinical pharmacokinetics of the prodrug oseltamivir and its active metabolite Ro 64-0802. *Clin. Pharmacokinet.* **1999**, *37*, 471–484. [CrossRef]
126. Kleeb, S.; Jiang, X.; Frei, P.; Sigl, A.; Bezençon, J.; Bamberger, K.; Schwardt, O.; Ernst, B. FimH antagonists: Phosphate prodrugs improve oral bioavailability. *J. Med. Chem.* **2016**, *59*, 3163–3182. [CrossRef]
127. Copeland, R.A.; Pompliano, D.L.; Meek, T.D. Drug-target residence time and its implications for lead optimization. *Nat. Rev. Drug Discov.* **2006**, *5*, 730–739. [CrossRef]
128. Kleeb, S.; Pang, L.; Mayer, K.; Eris, D.; Sigl, A.; Preston, R.C.; Zihlmann, P.; Sharpe, T.; Jakob, R.P.; Abgottspon, D.; et al. FimH antagonists: Bioisosteres to improve the in vitro and in vivo PK/PD profile. *J. Med. Chem.* **2015**, *58*, 2221–2239. [CrossRef]
129. Mizuno, N.; Niwa, T.; Yotsumoto, Y.; Sugiyama, Y. Impact of drug transporter studies on drug discovery and development. *Pharmacol. Rev.* **2003**, *55*, 425–461. [CrossRef]
130. Holodniy, M.; Penzak, S.R.; Straight, T.M.; Davey, R.T.; Lee, K.K.; Goetz, M.B.; Raisch, D.W.; Cunningham, F.; Lin, E.T.; Olivo, N.; et al. Pharmacokinetics and tolerability of oseltamivir combined with probenecid. *Antimicrob. Agents Chemother.* **2008**, *52*, 3013–3021. [CrossRef]
131. Chan, A.K.C.; Paredes, N.; Thong, B.; Chindemi, P.; Paes, B.; Berry, L.R.; Monagle, P. Binding of heparin to plasma proteins and endothelial surfaces is inhibited by covalent linkage to antithrombin. *Thromb. Haemost.* **2004**, *91*, 1009–1118. [CrossRef]
132. Young, E.; Prins, M.; Levine, M.N.; Hirst, J. Heparin binding to plasma proteins, an important mechanism for heparin resistance. *Thromb. Haemost.* **1992**, *67*, 639–643. [CrossRef]
133. Hazelard, D.; Compain, P. Square sugars: Challenges and synthetic strategies. *Org. Biomol. Chem.* **2017**, *15*, 3806–3827. [CrossRef]
134. Eggink, L.L.; Spyroulias, G.A.; Jones, N.G.; Hanson, C.V.; Hoober, J.K. A peptide mimetic of 5-acetylneuraminic acid-galactose binds with high avidity to siglecs and NKG2D. *PLoS ONE* **2015**, *10*, e0130532. [CrossRef]
135. Garber, K.C.A.; Wangkanont, K.; Carlson, E.E.; Kiessling, L.L. A general glycomimetic strategy yields non-carbohydrate inhibitors of DC-SIGN. *Chem. Commun.* **2010**, *46*, 6747–6749. [CrossRef] [PubMed]

136. Mahmoud, A.M.; Wilkinson, F.L.; Jones, A.M.; Wilkinson, J.A.; Romero, M.; Duarte, J.; Alexander, M.Y. A novel role for small molecule glycomimetics in the protection against lipid-induced endothelial dysfunction: Involvement of Akt/eNOS and Nrf2/ARE signaling. *Biochim. Biophys. Acta* **2017**, *1861*, 3311–3322. [CrossRef]
137. Dayde, B.; Pierra, C.; Gosselin, G.; Surleraux, D.; Ilagouma, A.T.; Laborde, C.; Volle, J.-N.; Virieux, D.; Pirat, J.-L. Synthesis of unnatural phosphonosugar analogues. *Eur. J. Org. Chem.* **2014**, *2014*, 1333–1337. [CrossRef]
138. Eggink, L.L.; Roby, K.F.; Cote, R.; Hoober, J.K. An innovative immunotherapeutic strategy for ovarian cancer: CLEC10A and glycomimetic peptides. *J. Immunother. Cancer* **2018**, *6*, 28. [CrossRef]
139. Theis, T.; Johal, A.S.; Kabat, M.; Basak, S.; Schachner, M. Enhanced neuronal survival and neurite outgrowth triggered by novel small organic compounds mimicking the LewisX glycan. *Mol. Neurobiol.* **2018**, *55*, 8203–8215. [CrossRef] [PubMed]
140. Langford-Smith, A.W.W.; Hasan, A.; Weston, R.; Edwards, N.; Jones, A.M.; Boulton, A.J.M.; Bowling, F.L.; Rashid, S.T.; Wilkinson, F.L.; Alexander, M.Y. Diabetic endothelial colony forming cells have the potential for restoration with glycomimetics. *Sci. Rep.* **2019**, *9*, 2309. [CrossRef]
141. Kieber-Emmons, T.; Luo, P.; Qiu, J.; Agadjanyan, M.; Carey, L.; Hutchins, W.; Westerink, M.A.; Steplewski, Z. Peptide mimicry of adenocarcinoma-associated carbohydrate antigens. *Hybridoma* **1997**, *16*, 3–10. [CrossRef]
142. Westerink, M.A.J.; Giardina, P.C.; Apicella, M.A.; Kieber-Emmons, T. Peptide mimicry of the meningococcal group C capsular polysaccharide. *Proc. Natl. Acad. Sci. USA* **1995**, *92*, 4021–4025. [CrossRef]
143. Basak, S.; Birebent, B.; Purev, E.; Somasundaram, R.; Maruyama, H.; Zaloudik, J.; Swoboda, R.; Strittmatter, W.; Li, W.; Luckenbach, A.; et al. Induction of cellular immunity by anti-idiotypic antibodies mimicking GD2 ganglioside. *Cancer Immunol. Immunother.* **2003**, *52*, 145–154. [CrossRef]

© 2019 by the author. Licensee MDPI, Basel, Switzerland. This article is an open access article distributed under the terms and conditions of the Creative Commons Attribution (CC BY) license (http://creativecommons.org/licenses/by/4.0/).

MDPI
St. Alban-Anlage 66
4052 Basel
Switzerland
Tel. +41 61 683 77 34
Fax +41 61 302 89 18
www.mdpi.com

Pharmaceuticals Editorial Office
E-mail: pharmaceuticals@mdpi.com
www.mdpi.com/journal/pharmaceuticals

www.ingramcontent.com/pod-product-compliance
Lightning Source LLC
LaVergne TN
LVHW071952080526
838202LV00064B/6729